**Acupuncture in Modern Medicine**
http://dx.doi.org/10.5772/46017
Edited by Lucy L. Chen and Tsung O. Cheng

**Contributors**

Takashi Seki, Hsieh, Ping-Chung Leung, Wen-Long Hu, Yu-Chiang Hung, I-Ling Hung, Yutaka Takaoka, Yoichiroh Hosokawa, Aki Sugano, Akihiko Ito, Mika Ohta, Zhonghua Fu, Ryan Shepherd, Stephen Meyer, Yoshimasa Koyama, Ting Bao, Lizhen Wang, Peter Chin Wan Fung, Sungchul Kim, Sandra Silvério Lopes, Irmgard Simma, Masahiko Tsuchiya, Lucy L Chen, Raheleh Khorsan, Tsung O. Cheng, Alexandra York

**Published by InTech**

Janeza Trdine 9, 51000 Rijeka, Croatia





**Publishing Process Manager** Ana Pantar
**Technical Editor** InTech DTP team
**Cover** InTech Design team

Additional hard copies can be obtained from orders@intechopen.com

Acupuncture in Modern Medicine, Edited by Lucy L. Chen and Tsung O. Cheng
p. cm.
ISBN 978-953-51-1020-0

For EU product safety concerns:
IN TECH d.o.o., Prolaz Marije Krucifikse Kozulić 3, 51000 Rijeka, Croatia,
info@intechopen.com or visit our website at intechopen.com.

# Meet the editors

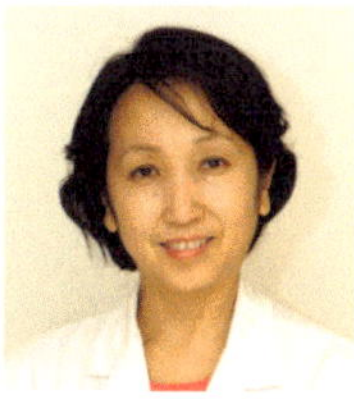

Dr. Lucy L. Chen is an Assistant Professor at Harvard Medical School and a board-certified anesthesiologist and pain medicine specialist by the American Board of Anesthesiology. She has been an attending physician at the Massachusetts General Hospital (MGH) for over a decade. Dr. Chen is a Principle Investigator and Co-investigator on several NIH RO1 grants to study the role of alternative medicine in pain management, opioid analgesia and opioid induced hyperalgesia. She led Acupuncture Clinic at the MGH Center for Pain Medicine and served as the credentialing director for acupuncture privilege at MGH. She is the director of Complementary and Alternative Medicine Research Unit at the MGH Center for Translational Pain Research. She has served as grant reviewer for NIH study section and as a reviewer for many medical journals and published a number of original papers, reviews and book chapters. She has been invited to speak at many local, regional and national conferences on the topic of acupuncture and complementary alternative medicine.

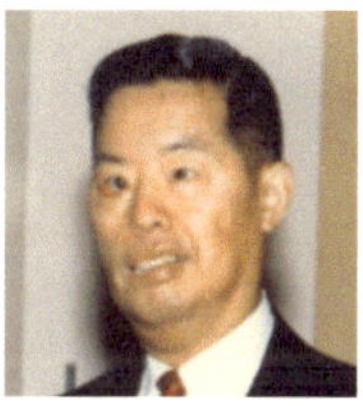

Dr. Tsung O. Cheng is a Professor of Medicine at the George Washington University, Washington, D.C. and board-certified in both Internal Medicine and Cardiovascular Disease. He is the author of over 1556 articles and 24 books or book chapters. He has lectured extensively around the world.

Dr. Cheng delivered the Second Paul White Lecture of the American College of Cardiology in 1973, entitled "Cardiology in People's Republic of China". He was the first Chinese-American physician to visit People's Republic of China in 1972, and then in 1973 introduced to China selective cine coronary arteriography which laid the foundation for percutaneous coronary interventions in modern China. Dr. Cheng has served as visiting professor in Oxford, Hamburg, Hannover, Düsseldorf, Paris, Geneva, Bern, Zurich, McMaster, Cairo, Madrid, Córdoba, Las Palmas, Rome, Milan, Pisa, Athens, Istanbul, Melbourne, Sydney, Johannesburg, Cape Town, Peking Union Medical College, Capital University, Beijing and as honorary professor in Sun-Yatsen University of Medical Science, Tongji Medical University, Shanghai Second Medical University, Tsingtao Medical College, University of Natal, Durban, S. Africa, University of Cape Town, Morón University in Buenos Aires, Argentina, and Beijing Hospital in China. He was awarded the first Lifetime Achievement Distinguished Researcher Award by The George Washington University, Washington, DC in 2007. He is well known both inside and outside China. He has recently been appointed the Roving Ambassador for Chinese Cardiovascular Science and International Consulting Editor for China by the

International Journal of Cardiology. He is listed in Who's Who in America, Who's Who in the World, and Who's Who in Shanghai, China from Overseas among such notables as the world renowned architect I.M. Pei and former Secretary of Labor Elaine L. Chao.

# Contents

# Preface

Acupuncture has been one of the most significant components of the healthcare system in East Asia for thousands of years. It has rapidly evolved as a therapeutic modality in the modern west medicine system over the last few decades. In the United States, acupuncture has gained much interest since President Nixon's trip to China in 1972. A nationwide survey in 1998 showed that office visits seeking alternative therapies are twice as many as those for primary care and there are estimated five million visits to acupuncture practices alone. Acupuncture needles have been classified as medical equipment, subject to the same standards for medical needles, syringes, surgical scalpels since 1996. The National Institutes of Health (NIH) organized a Consensus Development Conference on Acupuncture in 1997. The Conference recognized that acupuncture has been extensively practiced by many healthcare providers to treat a wide variety of medical problems including pain conditions. A major benefit of acupuncture therapy is that adverse events are substantially lower than that of many medications and commonly accepted medical procedures. In the meantime, scientific research has lead to the increasing understanding of acupuncture's mechanisms, physiologic impacts, and therapeutic effects. These promising developments in research and clinical application of acupuncture therapy have established a new field of integrative medicine that combines complementary and alternative medicine including acupuncture with western-style medical practice.

Despite the progress in acupuncture therapy as an alternative treatment modality, current clinical research on acupuncture still faces a number of challenges. For example, although many studies on acupuncture treatment have been published, their scientific merits may be limited by the study design and non-standardized acupuncture practices. It remains difficult to maintain true blindness to patients and, in some cases to investigators, in clinical trials. Non-specific needling (i.e. placing an acupuncture needle at an unintended acupoint) or sham needling may elicit some response similar to that of active acupuncture treatment, making it difficult to interpret trial outcomes because it is difficult to separate the placebo effect from the actual acupuncture effect.

With regard to the practice of acupuncture, a plan for acupuncture treatment is often highly individualized for a given condition and varies from one practitioner to another. As such, it is rather difficult to compare treatment outcomes if a given clinical condition is treated with different settings including acupoints, needling techniques (e.g., electrical versus manual), duration of treatment for each session, and between-session intervals. Therefore, concerted efforts should be made to standardize acupuncture clinical trials in order to improve scientific merits of such trials. Nonetheless, it can be anticipated that complementary medicine, including acupuncture, will play a growing and positive role in pain management.

This book offers comprehensive updates of current knowledge in acupuncture practice and research. 18 chapters are divided into four categories: 1) Acupuncture Research; 2) New Developments in Acupuncture; 3) Acupuncture Therapy for Clinical Conditions and 4) Assessment and Accessibility of Acupuncture Therapy. The book is intended for physicians, acupuncturists, medical students and other healthcare providers who are interested in acupuncture therapy and research. These chapters are written by experienced and well-recognized acupuncture practitioners, clinicians and researchers from both private and academic settings. The topics discussed in this book provide 1) a unique look at the current status and new trends of acupuncture research, 2) comprehensive and analytic reviews of acupuncture therapy for clinical disorders and conditions, and 3) up-to-date developments reviewed by both scientists and clinicians.

Finally we sincerely thank the authors for their dedication and enormous contributions to this project. We are also grateful to InTech Publisher for their support which made it possible to publish this important book. As physicians and researchers, we hope the renewed interest in acupuncture therapy and research will take a deep root in the minds and practices of many physicians and healthcare providers in order to accelerate the integration of acupuncture into modern medicine.

**Dr. Lucy L. Chen, M.D.**
Massachusetts General Hospital,
Harvard Medical School,
Boston, MA, USA

**Dr. Tsung O. Cheng, M.D.**
George Washington University
Medical Center,
Washington, D.C., USA

## Dedication

*I dedicate this book to my family for their love and support. I also dedicate this book to my patients for allowing me to do the most rewarding job in the world as a physician: to care for those who are suffering.*

**Lucy L. Chen**

Section 1

# Acupuncture Research

Chapter 1

# Current Trends in Acupuncture Research: From Analgesia to Physiological Function of Brain

Chen Wei-Liang and Hsieh Ching-Liang

Additional information is available at the end of the chapter

http://dx.doi.org/10.5772/55184

## 1. Introduction

Acupuncture has been used for different kinds of disorders for a long period of time in Asian [1] and currently been accepted by western countries by virtue of its obvious efficacy and scientific evidences on basic and clinical studies. As a part of Traditional Chinese Medicine (TCM), acupuncture may be the most evident therapy among all other complementary and alternative medicines (CAMs). This chapter is going to discuss current trends in basic acupuncture research and clinical trials.

Early findings of acupuncture analgesia inspired following studies with the opioid- and serotonin-mediated descending inhibitory pathways [2]. In central nervous system (CNS), acupuncture, especially electroacupuncture (EA), activates many cortical and subcortical regions involved in these pathways. Noteworthy, the EA effects are frequency-dependent. For example, lower frequency EA (1-5Hz) possesses prominent anti-hyperalgesic and anti-inflammatory effects whereas higher (100Hz) one has more effect on cortical serotoninergic system. Accordingly, different frequency EA initiates different pathways. At more peripheral level, the analgesic effects of acupuncture are partly explained by modulation of synaptic plasticity and cholinergic reflex. The relationship between cholinergic reflex and acupuncture has been postulated for decades. Currently, more and more evidences support this assumption [3]. Electrophysiology is a promising tool to investigate neurophysiology. Compelling evidences have clarified the acupuncture effect on electrophysiological profiles. One of the important contributions of electrophysiology is to consolidate the idea that acupuncture act through high cortical conditioning. In addition to traditional histological and electrophysiological studies, advent of neural functional imaging provides more impetus for CNS functioning during acupuncture [4]. Since CNS is the major modulator of homeostasis, acupuncture also effectively to regulate metabolic penal, such as blood glucose and lipid.

In the eras of randomized control trial (RCT), acupuncture need to be verified by more rigid method. In addition to methodological and sham designs, we found that acupoint selection and assessment tool are equally important. Especially in trials for pain syndromes, inadequacy of acupoint or outcome measurement often elicits biased conclusion. The idea is that there are three distinct physiological effects of acupuncture, namely, point-specific effect, placebo and non-specific physiologic effects to needle insertion; some of them overlap with sham and placebo controls which are the methods widely used in current acupuncture RCTs. Several cases in point will be discussed in this chapter.

Among many acupuncture RCTs that have been published in the past decades, pain syndromes are explored most extensively. The present chapter is going to take chronic headache, low back pain, osteoarthritis and postoperative pain as examples. Although most of the data suggested better outcomes after acupuncture treatment, we can still find the fact that not every pain syndrome is suitable for standardized and inflexible acupuncture trials. Another encouraging issue currently is using acupuncture to treat neurological disorder, such as stroke and peripheral neuropathy. Acupuncture now is a rising star for the treatment of stroke. Many pioneer trials have demonstrated the beneficial effect of acupuncture treatment on stroke rehabilitation. Others will also be mentioned here are disorders such as metabolic syndrome and atopic disorders. The nature of uncontrollable inflammation of these lingering disorders makes them the next in the spotlight, since postulated role of acupuncture may regulate inflammation.

From analgesic effect of acupuncture to physiological function of brain, acupuncture researches have made their own mark on scientific world.

## 2. Mechanism of acupuncture analgesia

### 2.1. Inspiring findings from the studies of mechanisms of Acupuncture Analgesia (AA)

Analgesic effect is the most studied one among the variety clinical applications of acupuncture. As the scientists all over the world have devoted themselves into this field, several evidences are brought forward [1, 2]. The starting place is gate control theory [5]. It is believed that acupuncture stimulation activates larger Aβ nerve fiber which then "gates" the nociceptive signals from Aδ and C nerve fibers in substantia gelatinosa (SG) in spinal dorsal horn. However, gate control theory can only explain transient and local AA within the same and adjacent dermatomes where painful areas are. Gating control cannot produce distal and prolonged AA. Therefore, widespread regulation elicited by acupuncture at spinal and supraspinal levels has been the central question to be addressed for decades.

http://dx.doi.org/10.5772/55184

To view the whole picture of AA, quick review of central endogenous opioid system and descending inhibitory pathways is necessary. Purification of β-endorphin, enkephalin and dynorphin in late 1970s [6] gave rise to the accelerated progress on the understanding of central endogenous opioid systems, as well as mechanism of AA. The arcuate nucleus in hypothalamus and periaqueduct gray (PAG) in midbrain are the major locations releasing beta-endorphin and enkephalin [7]. Arcuate nucleus projects endorphinergic axons to PAG, and then PAG sends endorphinergic axons to nucleus raphes magnus (NRM). This arcuate-PAG-NRM axis is the center of "descending inhibitory pathway". For example, stimulating PAG with electrical or opioids produces analgesia [7]. NRM has widespread serotoninergic projection to spinal cord, and mainly has synapse with enkephalinergic inhibitory interneurons in SG of spinal dorsal horn. Another counterpart descending inhibitory pathway of arcuate-PAG-NRM axis involves parabranchial nucleus (PBN). Unlike arcuate nucleus, PBN releases dynorphin instead of beta-endorphin or enkephalin to PAG. In both descending pathways, spinal endogenous opioid presynaptically knocks out/down nociceptive signals [8]. The relationship between the abovementioned endogenous opioid system and AA date back to 1970s, illustrated by the finding that Naloxone, an nonselective antagonist to opioid receptors, attenuates analgesic effect of acupuncture in human [9] and mice [10].

Based on progress of the knowledge of different endogenous opioids, compelling evidences have more directly revealed the relationship between AA and endogenous opioids [11-13]. Furthermore, researches also demonstrated the characterized frequency-dependent effect of EA on the release of different endogenous [14]. This early observation inspired later researches on EA. The most well-known ones are conducted by Han's group. The frequency-dependent characteristic of EA hasn't been elucidated until the experiments of his group. They reported that in EA, frequency of electrical stimulation determines the pathway it could activate [15]. For example, by using a cross-tolerance technique, lower frequency (2 Hz) EA produces analgesia through μ- and δ-opioid receptors and that higher frequency (100 Hz) EA through the κ-opioid receptor. They concluded that 2 Hz EA stimulates the release of β-endophin, enkephalin and endomorphin [16, 17] within the network of the CNS and that 100 Hz EA releases dynorphin [18]. Taken together with descending inhibitory pathways, lower frequency (2Hz) EA is postulated to active arcuate-PAG-NRM pathway and higher (100Hz) one to activate PBN-PAG-NRM.

Although we have already known that AA is speculated emanated form endogenous opioids and related descending inhibitory pathways [11, 19], hypothalamus-pituitary axis is still a possible source of endogenous opioids mediated AA [10]. These two mechanisms (hormone and neurotransmitter) are not mutually exclusive because different stimulating protocol, not only frequency but pulse width of EA, can yield different effects [20]. We assume that hormonal mechanism produces its analgesic effect via anti-inflammation in a gradual mode whereas endogenous opioids are transmitted faster in descending inhibitory pathway.

Another salient part of descending inhibitory pathway is serotoninergic NRM-spinal neuron. Serotonin was suggested as an analgesic transmitter in an early study [14], and EA can activate these serotoninergic NRM neurons [21]. This analgesic effect of EA diminishes after p-chlorophenylalanine (serotonin synthesis inhibitor) injection [22]. Therefore, serotonin is pointed to a role of AA. Evidence suggests that serotonin level increases in spinal cord after EA [23] and that its precursor (5-hydroxytryptophan) responds to enhanced analgesia at 2 Hz EA [24].

As to a neurotransmitter, it is always important to understand its receptor subtypes. There are several serotonin (5-HT) receptor subtypes in CNS. The 5-HT1 and 5-HT3 subtypes locate in the spinal dorsal horn and their agonists have been found to reduce pain [25, 26]. The 5-HT1a subtype is also an autoreceptor within the NRM. Antagonists for different subtypes of serotonin receptors, namely 5-HT1a, 5-HT2 and 5-HT3, have been used to elucidate their roles in AA. It has been found that EA analgesia is blocked by 5-HT1a and 5-HT3 antagonists at both lower and higher frequencies; whereas, EA analgesia is enhanced by 5-HT2 antagonist at high frequency (100 Hz) [24]. The results form these serotonin studies demonstrated another frequency-dependent characteristic of AA and are supported by later studies [27, 28].

The exact effect of serotonin in spinal cord is to activate inhibitory interneurons postsynaptically via the serotoninergic NRM-spinal terminals. The enkephalin-containing inhibitory interneurons knock out/down nociceptive signals through μ/δ-opioid receptors on presynaptic Aδ and C-fibers (heterosynaptic plasticity)[29]. EA, both lower and higher frequencies, can activate this mechanism mentioned above through 5-HT1a and 5-HT3 receptors. In contrast, the 5-HT2 receptor subtype increases the transmission of nociceptive signal [26]. It is also an excitatory receptor in the cortex and the hippocampus [30]. Higher frequency EA might decrease the serotonin concentration within the cortex; therefore it acts as a sedative. As a result, higher frequency EA elicits analgesic effect via both the descending pain inhibitory pathway and the cortical modulation.

In conclusion AA is mediated by the arcuate nucleus-PAG-NRM-spinal cord [19, 31] and PBN-PAG-NRM-spinal cord axes [18, 32]. These axes are activated frequency-dependently by lower or higher frequency EA. By injecting dynorphin antiserum to PAG decreases the analgesic effect of higher frequency; in contrast, the β-endorphin antiserum decreases the analgesic effect of lower frequency EA [18]. In addition, higher frequency EA can further involve in cortical serotonergic transmission, along with the NRM-spinal pathway.

### 2.2. Current researches in hyperalagesia models

Synaptic plasticity is the central mechanism of several neurological physiology and pathology, such as memory formation, epilepsy and hyperalgesia. One pattern of synaptic plasticity is homosynaptic, which means the change is only within synaptic cleft. If the change involved a second synapse, it is a heterosynaptic pattern. Interneurons usually play important roles in a heterosynaptic synaptic plasticity. Since acupuncture has capability to modulate nociception through spinal cord inhibitory interneurons in SG, synaptic plasticity becomes an appealing subject to address AA. Chemical-induced local inflammation or inflammation came from nerve injury lead to a series of changes of peripheral and central sensitization (hyperalgesia), including undertrophed and overtrophed changes (e.g. change of nerve growth factors; NGF) of nerve ending, of upregulating specific kinds of dorsal root ganglion (DRG) receptors, of long-term potentiation (LTP) and long-term depression (LTD) on spinal dorsal horn neurons [33]. Hence, more recently researches focus on the acupuncture-mediated synaptic plasticity and anti-hyperalgeic effect in neuropathic pain animal models [20, 34-37].

Nerve injury and following local inflammatory response induce cytokines (IL1, IL6 and TNF-alpha) and NGF, which are related to hyperalgesia [38]. NGF is the central mediator of peripheral sensitization. Binding with tyrosine kinase receptor A (trkA), NGF induces catastrophic cascade in DRG neuron. For example, NGF-induced over-expression of ASIC3 [39] and transient receptor potential valloid type 1 (TRPV1) [40] result in increased cation permeability on DRG cell membrane and spontaneous activation. Current research showed that lower frequency EA prevents NGF-induced trafficking of TRPV1 and Substance P (SP) from DRG to peripheral skin [41].

Interestingly, NGF also induces expression of peripheral opioid receptors on inflammatory nerve endings at late stage [42]. This seems to be a compensatory reaction which responses to hyperalgesia. In peripheral inflammatory tissue, immune cells express endogenous opioid and bind to opioid receptors on peripheral nerve endings [43]. Research showed that analgesia of EA is mediated by this inhibitory binding on nerve endings [36]. From Sekido's research, local blockade of opioid receptors decreased the analgesic effect of EA rather than systemic blockade. Therefore, in early stage of hyperalgesia, EA regulates NGF-mediated changes in peripheral tissues, whereas in late stage EA enhances opioid-mediated leukocyte-neuron interaction.

DRGs play an important role in peripheral sensitization. Up-regulating receptors such as purinergic receptor P2X3, Acid-Sensing Ion Channel 3 (ASIC3) and TRPV1 increase response of nociceptor to noxious stimulation [33]. Our study showed that acupuncture reverses the mechanical hyperalgesia in both carrageenan- and complete Freund's adjuvant (CFA)-induced mice model by attenuating expression of ASIC3 on DRG [37]. Other evidences have suggested anti-hyperalgesic effect of acupuncture through P2X3 [44], TRPV1 [45] and P35/P25 [46]receptors attenuation. These studies implied that acupuncture affects neuron sensitization at level of receptor proteins.

Within spinal cord, there are various inhibitory interneurons modulating the synaptic plasticity. For example, inhibitory enkephalinergic neurons increase after nociceptive stimulation [47]. This inhibition blocks the ascending nociceptive signal from peripheral Aδ and C-fibers, as well as regulates synaptic plasticity and LTP contributing to the development of hyperalgesia [33]. Evidences have shown that acupuncture reduces hyperalgesia through spinal dorsal horn interneuron. For example, in CFA- and paclitaxel-evoked hyperalgesia models, intrathecal injection of opioid receptors antagonist reverse the anti-hyperalgesia effect induced by acupuncture [36, 48, 49]. These evidences suggested that acupuncture elicits anti-hyperalgesic effect via opioid receptors. However, the roles of different opioid receptors (μ, δ and κ) are not identical in different animal models. In paclitaxel model, clear evidence has shown that 10Hz EA acts through all three opioid receptors but in CFA model EA, only through μ- and δ-opioid receptors [35, 48, 50]; This conflict implies that animal models, different treatment protocols (timing of needling and selection of acupoints) and tools of assessment can influence the result even when the stimulating frequency is similar.

Ionotropic glutamate receptors (NMDA, AMPA and KA receptors) are involved in LTP in DRG. Prseynaptically tetanus burst opens the postsynapse NMDA receptors and influx of calcium through NMDA up-regulates expression of AMPA receptor. Spontaneous discharge of DRG neurons in hyperalgesia animal facilitates LTP [51]. Therefore, the dorsal horn neuron is more sensitive to glutamate after LTP. EA has been found to prevent LPT by down-regulating AMPA and NMDA receptors in SG [29]. Indirect evidences that excitatory amino acid antagonists can enhance the anti-hyperalgesic effect of EA also support glutamate receptor-mediated anti-hyperalgsia of acupuncture [52, 53].

In conclusion, acupuncture reverses hyperalgesia at both peripheral and spinal levels. The effect is multifactorial but mainly through regulation of synaptic plasticity.

### 2.3. The role of Central Nervous System (CNS) on acupuncture treatments

We have known from the previous two sections that AA is mediated by descending inhibitory pathway and synaptic plasticity, but how acupuncture activates them is still blurred. It is believed that the sensation of "De Qi" during acupuncture treatments is the major determinant of therapeutic effectiveness. "De Qi" is, not a pain sensation, characterized with numbness, dullness, soreness or heaviness, therefore the sensory cortex and related structures has been postulated contributing to activation of abovementioned mechanisms. According to our studies, acupuncture can alter the sensory processing in CNS. For instance, electrophysiological studies have revealed that needling at specific acupoints suppresses the sympathetic skin response [54], cutaneous reflex [55] and blink reflex [56] supraspinally. These results suggested that acupuncture doesn't change the monosynaptic reflex at the brainstem and spinal level. Indeed, utilizing auditory endogenous potentials (P300), we elucidated that cerebral cortex is the major location where acupuncture interferes sensory processing [57].

In consistence with our early electrophysiology studies, current functional magnetic resonance imaging (fMRI) studies have demonstrated the importance of cerebral cortex. Given the intricate theory of TCM and the complicated networks of the CNS, the complexness of physiological response of acupuncture is not surprising. Functional magnetic resonance image (fMRI) was once regarded as a novel tool to elucidate the CNS effect of acupuncture. Indeed, Ho's group suggested that certain brain regions were activated in experimental animals with point-specific property [58, 59]. In human subjects, needling at traditional analgesic points (ST36 and LI4) can enhance the signals of analgesic matrix (hypothalamus and nucleus accumbens) and reduce the signals of pain perception area (limbic system) [60]. However, some results cannot be duplicated due to the sophisticated data process and analysis for the blood oxygenation-level dependent (BOLD) signals. For example, conflict results arise from two studies that tried to elucidate acupoint specificity by analyzing BLOD responses to vision-related acupoints [61, 62].

Most of the early fMRI studies have analyzed neural activities in an acute and spatial pattern. Lin's group noticed that carryover effects of block design (on- and off-treatment) would complicate the interpretation of acupuncture fMRI study [63]. Therefore, currently a group focuses on effects of acupuncture on functional connectivity on resting-state. They have found that acupuncture can exert sustained and specific effects on resting brain networks [4, 61, 64-66]. Among all the brain regions, anterior cingulated cortex (ACC) has been studied most extensively [65, 67, 68]. ACC has wide connection with other cortical region and hippocampus, amygdala and hypothalamus. Therefore it is correlated with memorial (hippocampus), affective (amygdala) and physiological (hypothalamus) components of pain [69]. Indeed, in a hyperalgesic animal model, destruction of rostral ACC eliminates the anti-hyperalgesic effect of acupuncture [67]. However, the role of whole cerebral cortex plays in AA is still inconclusive, more delicate electrophysiology and functional imaging studies are needed.

In conclusion, functional studies (electrophysiology and fMRI) have revealed extensive effect of acupuncture on cerebral cortex. However, it is still controversial whether this effect is specific to acupuncture or not.

### 2.4. The role of Autonomic Nervous System (ANS) on acupuncture treatments

Autonomic anti-inflammatory reflex elicited by acupuncture has been postulated by virtue of acupuncture's anti-inflammation effect and ability to poise autonomic nervous system (ANS). It has been showed that long term EA can regulate immune cells such as T and B cell in lymph nodes [70] and splenic natural killer (NK) cells [71] in mouse. Elimination of immune regulation by naloxone [71] implied EA as an opioid-mediated immune modulator. In hyperalgesic animal models, inflammatory responses (edema and hyperalgesia) reduced by EA [72-74] is also mediated by opioids [75]. However, the fact that local injection of naloxane isn't able to eliminate the immediate anti-inflammation effect of EA [73, 75] may imply a faster neuronal pathway way other than opioid-mediated one. Indeed, EA is capable to adjust inflammatory profiles in the CNS. In the hypothalamus, commonly regarded as homeostasis center, the expression of mRNA of proinflammatory cytokines by lipopolysaccharide stimulation is reduced after EA [76]. Proteomic analysis has revealed that inflammatory protein levels are normalized in the hypothalamus after EA stimulation [77]. Taken together, a CNS-mediated non-opioid anti-inflammatory effect of acupuncture is implicated.

Although hypothalamus-pituitary-adrenal axis has been implicated to mediate the anti-inflammatory effect of acupuncture [59, 76-79], current focus is more on ANS [3, 80] by virtue of its more immediate response to acupuncture. Many researchers have found that acupuncture can regulate the function of the ANS in different kinds of physiology parameters [81-84]. But our question here is whether ANS also mediates the anti-inflammation effect of acupuncture. In enodtoxin-induced sepsis model, survival benefits of EA are mediated by central muscurinic and peripheral nicotinic receptors [3]. This result demonstrated the involvement of cholinergic systems in EA-mediated anti-inflammation, congruent with previous study [27]. Among various cortical areas, ACC receives lots of cholinergic terminals. Thanks to the advent of fMRI, it is more feasible to assess the neural connection within CNS. Current study suggested that acupuncture, via prefrontal cortex (PFC)-perigenual ACC (pgACC)-arcuate-PAG axis, could regulate ANS in spatial pattern [68]. This axis has strong interconnection to descending inhibitory pathways and may be the common pathway of analgesic and anti-inflammatory effect of acupuncture.

In conclusion, the anti-inflammation effect of acupuncture is evident. In terms of the overlapping between cholinergic reflex and descending inhibitory pathways, acupuncture is speculated to be able to activate cortical ANS centers such as PFC and ACC.

### 2.5. Effect of acupuncture on metabolism

Acupuncture effect on hypothalamus nucleus (i.e. arcuate) implies its homeostatic characteristic. In contrast to reductionism of early modern medicine, TCM views living organism in systemic way. Emphasis is placed on holistic treatment in TCM theory. Therefore, acupuncture effect on metabolism has been the central of attention in scientific world. Current studies have shown that acupuncture on spleen and stomach meridians can regulate appetite and body weight through central mechanism[85, 86]. Therefore, acupuncture has been regarded as a novel alternative for controlling metabolic syndrome.

Insulin resistance is the major alteration of non-insulin dependent diabetes mellitus (NIDDM, type II DM) and metabolic syndrome. A series of studies on diabetic animal model has proven anti-diabetes effect of acupuncture. CV12 (Zhongwan) is a common acupoint used to regulate digestive function. Fifteen Hz EA at CV12 had hypoglycemic effect in normal and model rats of non-insulin-dependent diabetes mellitus (Type II DM)[87]. Likewise in analgesia studies, this hypoglycemic effect is also mediated by opioid [88, 89] and serotonin [90]. Fifteen Hz EA at bilateral ST36 (Zusanli) can further improve insulin sensitivity [91] by lowering free fatty acid in model rats of insulin-resistance [92]. Our study has also revealed that EA at ST36 can modulate the blood glucose and increase metabolic rate in the cellular level [93]. These results imply the clinical feasibility of acupuncture treatment for metabolic syndrome.

## 3. Clinical trials in acupuncture treatment

### 3.1. Important precautions for acupuncture trials

Study design is very crucial for acupuncture trials. Randomized control trial (RCT) is the minimal requirement for any modern clinical trial. However, for acupuncture trials, other precautions should be considered. Current acupuncture trials have to follow the standards of reporting interventions in controlled trials of acupuncture (STRICTA) [94]. To evaluate the validity of any acupuncture trial, additional emphasis should be placed along with STRICTA. The first one is "blinding method". Double-blinded RCT means neither practitioner nor patient is aware of the content of treatment. However, it is virtually impossible for acupuncture trial since the practitioner have to delivery acupuncture or sham treatment according to the protocol and group assignment correctly. Therefore, blind to assessor and patient is relatively more important in acupuncture trials to avoid bias.

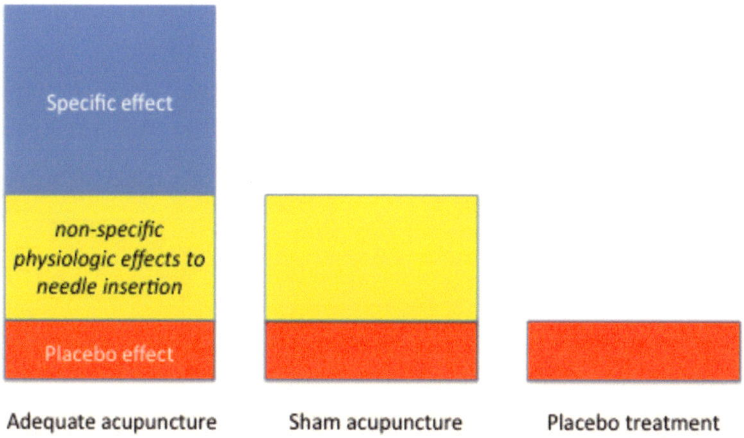


**Figure 1.** Three effects of acupuncture treatment. Left column is the three compositions of acupuncture treatment, namely, specific effect, non-specific physiology effect to needle insertion and placebo effect. Sham acupuncture such as minimal acupuncture (middle column) doesn't consist of specific effect. The right is placebo like mock TENS or Streitberger's placebo needles.

The second one is the design of sham treatment. It is commonly accepted that acupuncture has three major therapeutic characteristics (figure 1.), *point-specific effect, placebo and non-specific physiologic effects to needle insertion* [95]. Before going further into these three effects, two terms should be clarified ahead. Although often being used alternatively in many articles, the terms, sham acupuncture and placebo procedure, are not entirely equal in their meanings [96]. Pragmatically, sham acupuncture is defined as an ineffective and improper form of real acupuncture treatment. Sham acupuncture can elicit both the placebo and the non-specific physiologic effect to needle insertion. However, a placebo procedure should be really inert (namely, this procedure is not allowed to induce any physiological response, including the non-specific physiologic effect to needle insertion). Therefore, if a trial is to compare real acupuncture and blank negative control (no treatment control), the efficacy of acupuncture seemly cannot obtain conclusion (figure 2A). The therapeutic effect can either arise from *point-specific effect, placebo or non-specific physiologic effects to needle insertion* in acupuncture group. It is the usually case in early clinical trial. If a trial compared acupuncture with placebo treatment such as mock transcutaneous electrical nerve stimulation (TENS), then conclusion will be, at best, acupuncture elicits non-specific physiologic effects because, without needling, mock TENS cannot rule out the possibility of non-specific effect in acupuncture treatment. Only when a trial used minimal penetrating acupuncture at non-acupoints as sham treatment, then the therapeutic effect of real acupuncture can be deduced (figure 2B).

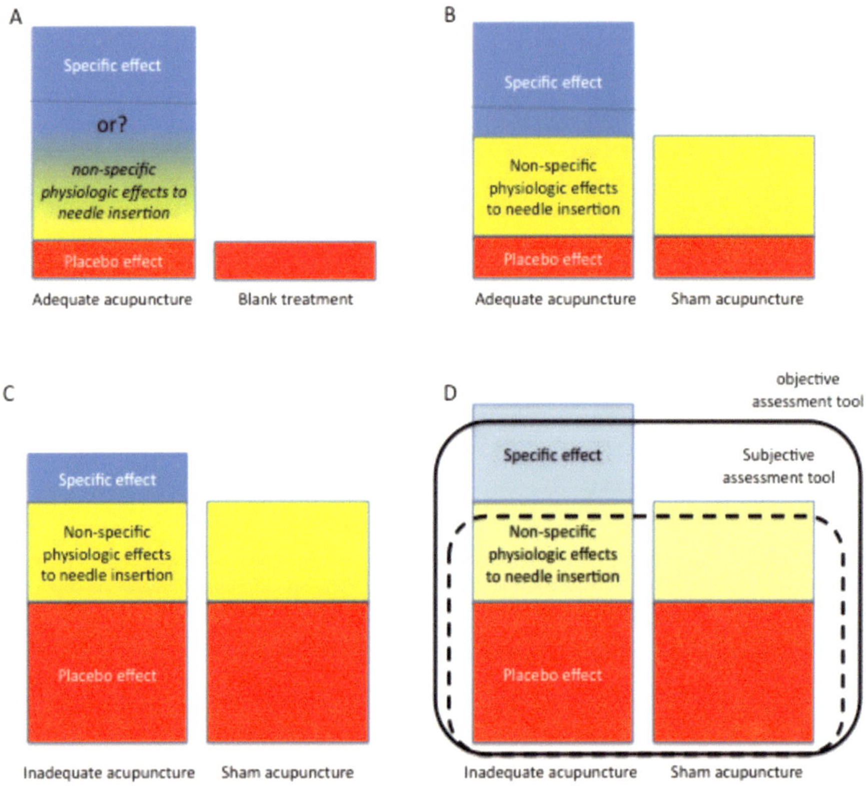


**Figure 2.** Different inadequacies jeopardize the RCT results. A, the lack of sham acupuncture makes assessment of real effect of acupuncture difficult. It is impossible to distinguish specific effect and non-specific effect of acupuncture without sham control. B, with sham acupuncture, the specific effect is more detectable. C, if the acupuncture treatment wasn't designed adequately, the specific effect of real acupuncture will be less significant along with the stronger placebo effects (the condition occurs often in migraine treatment). D, dashed line box is the area that subjective assessment tool (such as pain severity) can measure. Solid line represents the objective assessment condition. Without objective tool, specific effect could be ignored and significance between real and sham acupuncture vanish.

During early times, placebo effect of acupuncture is always a problem when it comes to clinical trials. As the advent of sham procedures and devices, how to diminish the non-specific effect of acupuncture dominates in modern acupuncture trials. One way is to maximally enhance the specific effect of acupuncture. Adequate point selection thus becomes important. For example, it happened in clinical trials to use identical acupoints for every patient in treatment group. Although it seems reasonable to do that, better choice is individualized acupoint selection according to meridian and TCM diagnosis. Otherwise, it will just like using penicillin for any pathogens in pneumonia cases. Inadequate point selection in real acupuncture treatment will obtain only non-specific and placebo effect, like minimal acupuncture (figure 2C). Above is the third precaution.

The final precaution is the outcome assessment, is especially important in analgesia trials. Because pain is a very subjective symptom and acupuncture is a time-consuming treatment, placebo effect is usually amplified in both sham control and real acupuncture groups. If a trial only assessed the outcome by subjective method such as visual analog scale (VAS) and then the chance of overestimating placebo effect will increase and the chance to detect specific effect will decrease. This is especially true when an inadequate point selection occurs in a trial using minimal acupuncture as sham treatment (figure 2D). Therefore it is always important to assess outcome with objective parameters (such as range of motion or dosage of medication) along with objective ones (such as VAS or quality of life).

### 3.2. Pain syndromes

Pain syndromes are the most commonly conducted clinical trials using acupuncture all over the world because of the strong evidence of AA in experimental models. This section will only discuss some most-studied disorders, chronic headache, low back pain (LBP), osteoarthritis of the knee (OAK) and postoperative pain.

#### *3.2.1. Chronic headache*

Before the era of RCT, early non-randomized or non-controlled studies [97] have already found that acupuncture treatment can mitigate the severity and the times of migraine attack in a short- and long-lasting pattern. RCT further confirmed the efficacy of real acupuncture on an short- and long-term patterns [98] as well as its effect compared with conventional medication (metoprolol) [99]. However, like other early clinical trials, there are several inadequacies within these trials. For example, these trials are flawed by absence of concealment of allocation to groups and blurred explanation of dropout and withdrawal. These inadequacies make the result less convincing [100]. Another bias of early acupuncture trial is the lack of placebo or sham group, so that it had been assumed that acupuncture placebo effect dominates. Indeed, some researchers supported this assumption by their finding that acupuncture isn't superior to placebo [101-103].

In the introduction, we emphasize the importance of point selection. Originated from TCM, it would be better to choose acupoints according to TCM diagnosis and meridian theory. Therefore it is not surprising that some trials [101-103] concluded acupuncture as a placebo because of their point selection. For example, none of abovementioned studies used the TCM diagnosis (individualized assessment of patient's constitution regardless of their disorder) to choose acupoints. But if with individualized treatment, current trial conducted in Brazil was able to reveal better pain relieve during real acupuncture than minimal acupuncture [104].

Although it would be better to go according to TCM and meridian theory, it is very difficult to reproduce this kind of research conducted under the thinking process of TCM for its high experimental requirements and complicity [103]. Treatments delivered by different practitioners or strategies always result in different outcomes. Sometimes, it depends on how experienced the practitioners are; therefore current guideline (STRITCA) asks trialists to report the qualification of their acupuncture practitioners. Indeed, a previous trial found that acupuncture is a better preventive treatment for full blown migraine even in those patients who had previous received ineffective acupuncture therapy [105]. By treating those patients within 48 hours after migraine attack, acupuncture can prevent mild migraine from exacerbating to full blown one. Interestingly, in this trial (n=179), most of the participants (80%) had previously received acupuncture for migraine without good success. This phenomenon confirms the idea that adequate trial design influences the trial result.

In conclusion, acupuncture is an effective tool to eliminate headache pain during attack and has short-term analgesic effect [106]. However, for lingering disorders like migraine, prevention is way more important than treatment for acute flare up. Acupuncture has been found to be more effective than Flunarize [107] and topiramate [108] for migraine prophylaxis. Although these studies revealed a positive result for acupuncture therapy, without an adequate sham or placebo design, it is still hard to elucidate acupuncture's real prophylactic effect from these studies. Indeed, one month after ending treatments, the difference between real and sham acupuncture on pain reduction and numbers of attack became insignificant [104]. Further well-designed trials are needed to elucidate the prophylactic effect of acupuncture on chronic migraine

There is no consensus as to whether acupuncture is superior to sham acupuncture for treating tension-type headache (TTH)[109]. Very few good quality trials have been conducted and their conclusions are conflicting. Different researchers can conclude even the same data differently. For instance, the result of one trial that implied no difference between real acupuncture and superficial acupuncture (at non-acupoit without De Qi) was conducted in 1992 [110]. However, later reviews reevaluated the data from the Tavola's study and found positive results favoring real acupuncture group [100, 111]. These reviews concluded that acupuncture was an effective strategy for treating TTH but they also pointed out the most difficult issue of acupuncture research is the placebo effect. Like migraine studies, some researches have concluded that acupuncture is a placebo [112, 113].

Since the placebo effect of acupuncture analgesia is difficult to retort in headache trials, researchers have tried to evade this effect by investigating the existence of any additional phenomenon of acupuncture. For instance, in Karsta's trial [114], they found that although acupuncture did not significantly decrease the severity of TTH attack in comparison to sham, it can objectively increase the pressure pain threshold. In other words, both groups felt the same degree of pain but acupuncture group had higher pain threshold. The explanation for this discrepancy between perception of pain and pain threshold is based on the strong placebo effect of real acupuncture. During the treatments, real acupuncture and sham acupuncture can reduce the perception of pain, in part mediated by placebo effect. It is especially the case because TTH is related to emotional stressor and both treatments can offer participants a relieved experience. But if this placebo effect is stronger enough in both treatments, then the specific effect (decreased pain threshold) of real acupuncture will be masked by placebo due to sampling and statistic limitation. This again reinforces our precaution that subjective parameters (pain severity) should be assessed along with objective ones (pain threshold).

Applying this conclusion to the migraine research, it is easily to speculate that there are certain specific therapeutic effects of real acupuncture causing objective changes in the patients with migraine, as the change of the pressure pain threshold in patients with TTH treated by real acupuncture. Indeed current trial suggested real acupuncture changes heart rate variability

(HRV) despite there are no significant difference in pain severity between placebo and real acupuncture [115]. Although this HRV change isn't easily correlated to migraine, ANS alteration may reflect hormonal, hemodynamic, electrophysiological or neural changes that can influence migraine.

In conclusion, acupuncture is effective in treating chronic headache. Because chronic headache may have psychogenic symptom component, the benefit of acupuncture might be partly contributed to the placebo effect of acupuncture; however, acupuncture dose elicit specific therapeutic effects that sham acupuncture dose not produce. Future trials should focus on develop objective assessment tools.

### 3.2.2. *Lower back pain*

Low back pain (LBP) may be the most popular pain condition for acupuncture trials. Although LBP is a self-limiting disease [116], it is a major cause of medical expenses, absenteeism and disablement [117]. Acupuncture is one of the most common complementary therapies for LBP. Early RCTs showed that acupuncture is superior to no treatment [118-120] in the pain scores, the dosages of pain pills, the limitation of activity and total hours of pain per. However, these early trials possess many serious flaws, such as poor description of statistical analysis and study protocol (including point selection, duration, interval, stimulation type and so on), small patient numbers, and unclear outcome measurements. As in chronic headache, these kinds of problems perplex most early clinical trials [121]. In these early clinical trials, we can also notice that the validity of a trial is correlated with the results. More valid the trials are, more likely the negative results are shown [122]. Therefore, again, it had been speculated that acupuncture is placebo effect [123]. However, current meta-analysis showed encouraging result of acupuncture treatment for patient with chronic LBP. Immediately after treatments, patients received acupuncture significantly had better reduction in pain intensity than placebo group [124]. However, long-term benefit cannot be observed in this meta-analysis. More RCTs may be needed to clarify the long-term effect, but more rigid design is equal important, especially for "point selection" and "outcome assessment".

Interestingly, compared with minimal acupuncture, individualized point selection in acupuncture treatment elicited better result in pain reduction [125]; whereas fixed point brought out non-superior pain reduction [123]. In both studies, acupuncture was used as a supplement to standard treatments. The phenomenon that acupuncture at individualized acupoints was more effective than minimal acupuncture but equal result of acupuncture at fixed point and minimal acupuncture implies the importance of strong non-specific and placebo effect of minimal acupuncture and fixed point strategy. Chronic LBP is not a specific diagnosis; it may consist of different disorders in different trials. If adequate acupuncture treatment cannot be given, non-specific and placebo effect then head up.

Outcome assessment by VAS and functional disability is still prevalent in acupuncture RCTs. However, the following example will ascertain again the importance of objective assessment tool. Being conducted in Germany [126] with considerable large numbers of volunteers and a firm methodological design, this research had been a strong cons of beneficial effect of acupuncture. The researchers aimed to determine whether acupuncture has a better therapeutic effect for chronic LBP than the minimal acupuncture (sham) and no treatment. After a long period of follow-up (8, 26 and 52 weeks) and with multiple measurements of outcomes (VAS; SF-36, 36-Item Short-Form Quality of Life Questionnaire; SES, Schmerzempfindungs-skala (questionnaire for assessing the emotional aspects of pain); ADS, Allgemeine Depres-sionsskala (depression scale)), they concluded that acupuncture is better than no treatment but not better than sham acupuncture in pain relief. Only slightly improvement (compared with sham acupuncture) in functional outcome (SF-36 and times of limited function) in the acu-puncture group was observed between baseline and follow-up periods. However, read it details, a significant pain relief of acupuncture treatment will be found if according to the need of medication in their discussion portion. Acupuncture group need less medication and has better functional outcomes than sham one. Dose that turn out to be strong pros of beneficial acupuncture effect?

Another interesting question is how long the acupuncture analgesia can last. According to a 2-years follow-up study, acupuncture can induce an analgesic effect in chronic LPB patients for at least 2 years [127]. Furthermore, an observational study [128] investigated the patients' out-comes after acupuncture. This observation included a total of 2564 patients treated by 1607 practitioners. It was shown that both functional outcomes and pain severity improved. In addition, the study also suggested that acupuncture could prevent LBP change to a chronic state.

In conclusion, acupuncture is a valid strategy for chronic LBP treatment. It can reduce the severity of and improve the functional outcomes in patients. Acupuncture seems to be a specific treatment rather than a placebo, although some authors do not agree. Combination of acupuncture and conventional interventions is a better choice for patient with chronic LBP.

### 3.2.3. Osteoarthritis of the Knees (OAK)

In TCM, OAK has long been treated by acupuncture. The major discomforts associated with OAK are pain and dysfunction of movement. Early pilot study revealed that acupuncture relieved pain and improved function in patients with OAK [129]. A later small RCT (n=73) confirmed that acupuncture group is superior in pain and functional outcomes to standard care group, even 4 weeks after treatment had been terminated [130]. However, take the non-specific and placebo effects into account, these results aren't convincing.

It is worth mentioning an interesting sham treatment used in Berman's trial [131]. First, they used plastic guidance tubes to mask their procedure. With the plastic tubes covering the true acupoints on the skin, the participants, who had never undergo prior acupuncture therapy, were not able to tell whether or not the needles were being inserted. In the acupuncture group, the needles were inserted (with De Qi sensation); in the sham group, the needles were not inserted. In addition to acupuncture at the acupoints that are commonly used for relieving knee pain, the researchers also needled at distal sham points on the abdomen that did not correspond to knee pain. The sham points were also covered by plastic guidance tubes. In the acupuncture group, the needles were not inserted into the sham points, whereas in the sham group, the needles were inserted into. Therefore, in the acupuncture group, the patients received real needling at the true acupoints and sham needling at the sham points; in the sham group, the patients received sham needling at the true acupoints and real needling at the sham points. In this crossover way, they can investigate effects of both placebo (true acupoints without needling) and non-specific physiologic effects to needle insertion (sham acupoints with needling) at the same time. The study comprised a total of 570 patients randomized into 3 groups, true acupuncture, sham acupuncture and education. Treatment was tapered over 26 months (2 treatments every week for 8 weeks; 1 treatment every week for 2 weeks; 1 treatment every 2 weeks for 4 weeks; and 1 treatment per month for 12 weeks). After a long period of follow-up (26 weeks post-baseline period), there are still 142 and 141 participants available in the acupuncture and sham groups, respectively. Most of the participants in both true and sham acupuncture groups reported that they had received true acupuncture. This suggested that this sham treatment is a credible blinding procedure and this sham acupuncture might elicit a similar degree of placebo effect as true acupuncture. Those who were received true acupuncture experienced better pain and functional outcomes; however, a significant difference in pain relief between the groups was not observed until 14 weeks. This implies that true acupuncture improves short-term and long-term functional outcomes, whereas the analgesia effect takes longer time to be elicited.

Other studies also suggested similar results that acupuncture is a benefit to the patients with OAK; however these studies showed that acupuncture can also elicited a short-term analgesia effect [132, 133]. These conflicting results might be due to the different placebo procedures or different treatment protocols.

In conclusion, although few reported discouraging results [134, 135], most of the trials published so far have shown preferable result of real acupuncture, especially in short-term pain and functional outcomes [136]. It is worth noting that, unlike acupuncture for chronic LBP, there is a general consensus among most studies that acupuncture is an effective treatment for OAK. Furthermore, its effectiveness (both in pain relief and functional improvement) seems not caused by the placebo or non-specific effects. This difference in effectiveness between these two diseases (LBP and OAK) might be due to the characteristics of the diseases. LBP is a heterogeneous syndrome comprising various disorders; it is an ambiguous and indistinct term. In contrast, OAK is a relatively clear and precise term to LBP. The diagnosis of OAK needs to meet many clinical criteria including imaging findings. Accordingly, there is less heterogeneity in OKA population than LBP.

#### 3.2.4. Post-operative Pain

The prototype of modern acupuncture analgesia research is the minor surgeries such as thyroidectomy under acupuncture anesthesia performed in Mainland China [137]. Although in some recent reports it did not achieve excellent result [138, 139], this issue still fascinates researcher to assess the difference of anesthesia dose between acupuncture and control group [140, 141]. It has been shown that the fentanyl dose for anesthesia maintenance is significant lower in patient group who also receive auricular acupuncture than sham one [140]. Instead of acupuncture anesthesia, it is more common to use acupuncture as painkiller after surgery (post-operative pain). Previous trials have shown both equivocal [142] and negative results [143] of acupuncture for post-operative pain relieving. A more rigorous trial has demonstrated that acupuncture elicited a short-term analgesia effect in patients after oral surgery [144]. In that study, acupuncture group received real needle treatment with De Qi needling sensation. Those in the placebo group were not needled, but instead received treatment with discernible tapped sensation by plastic tube on the area next to the acupoints chosen in the acupuncture group. In this way, the feeling that they have been treated in the placebo group can produce a placebo effect on them. Significantly longer post-operative pain-free period; delayed for sensing moderate pain and the need for the first dose of rescue pain medication was observed in the acupuncture group. However, these effects did not last longer than one week. This phenomenon suggests that acupuncture can elicit a short-term analgesic effect, in consistent with other pain syndromes. The acupuncture treatment timing for postoperative pain control is another interesting issue that has been studied in two different trials. In detail, these two trials were conducted by needling at similar acupoints (local ST6 and ST7 and distant LI4 among others) and a similar stimulation (manual acupuncture to achieve the De Qi sensation) but their results are opposite. Ekblom's trial has shown that there is no different of pain severity between the acupuncture and placebo group. The most obvious difference in study design between these two trials is the timing of intervention. The optimal timing of acupuncture are shown to be immediately after an operation [144] rather than before or 2-4 hours after an operation. A pretreatment of acupuncture attempted to prevent post-operative pain of oral surgery is in vain and as well as delayed acupuncture [143]. Based on the above study, we can assume that the timing of acupuncture intervention determined its analgesic effect on post-operative pain.

Acupuncture analgesia has also been studied in patients after the major abdominal surgery and it has been suggested that preoperative EA elicited no preventive analgesia after hysterectomy [142]. In this study, EA (100 Hz) was begun 20 minutes before skin incision and maintain until the end of the operation; the patients in the control group did not receive EA. The authors found no significant differences between two groups in pain severity, analgesics requirement and patients' stress states. However, this result is not consistent with a latter findings that shown the total amount of morphine [145] or fentanyl [146] required for pain control was significantly less in patients who received preoperative acupuncture than in patients in the control group. In Lin's trial, there were four groups included (control group without needling, sham EA group with needling but no electric stimulation, low-EA group with 2 Hz electric stimulation and high-EA with 100 Hz) and acupuncture treatment was performed 20 minutes before the induction of anesthesia. The analgesic effect is significant in patients who received higher frequency EA.

The conflict between these three trials can be contributed to the timing of intervention again. According to section 1 in this chapter, acupuncture analgesia is mediated by the regulation of CNS; however, under anesthesia, the CNS might not be able to activate neuronal and hormonal systems, which are correspond to acupuncture analgesia. In Christensen's study EA started after induction of anesthesia; therefore the analgesia effect of acupuncture may be reduced or eliminated by anesthesia. However, In Lin's and Coura's studies, acupuncture was performed before induction of anesthesia in order to elicit reliable CNS reactions.

Transcutaneous nerve electric stimulation (TENS) is a procedure that the electrodes are directly stuck on the skins. Although, the possible mechanism of TENS was found to be different from that of traditional acupuncture or EA [147], we still can compared a study using TENS with Lin's [145] study to clarify the role of electric stimulation plays in analgesic effect. TENS at specific acupoints (ST36) has been shown to be more effective at inducing analgesia than TENS at non-acupoints after lower abdominal surgeries [148]. This phenomenon suggested that the analgesic effect is determined by the location the stimulation is given instead by electric stimulation that we apply. Therefore, we can speculate that both sham EA and real EA at non-acupoints cannot induce an effective analgesic effect as that in Lin's study [145].

Taken together, acupuncture and TENS at specific acupoints may provided a valid strategy for post-operative analgesia. The best timing to introduce acupuncture is 20-30 minutes before induction of anesthesia in major abdominal surgery and immediately after oral surgery.

### 3.3. Metabolic syndrome

Using acupuncture and herbal medicine to control weight is very popular in oriental countries. The beneficial effect of acupuncture on metabolism drives clinicians to conduct clinical trial on weight reduction and hypertension. There are two different methods of acupuncture for weight reduction, somatic (body) and auricular (ear) acupuncture. Both of them have their advantages. For example, somatic acupuncture is claimed to be able to enhance local fat metabolism [149], and auricular acupuncture is more convenient in clinical practicing. Indeed, crossover and pilot trials have documented benefit effect of EA on body weight (BW), BMI and waist circumference (WC) in obese women [150, 151]. Bimodal somatic acupoints, including CV6, CV9, ST28, K14 locally on abdomen and ST36, ST40, SP6 distally on legs, were chosen according to TCM theory in these trials. The effectiveness of this kind of bimodal point selection strongly implied the involvement of the CNS and related homeostatic nuclei (activated by diatal acupoints) in additional to focal metabolic effect (activated by local abdomen acupoints). As to auricular acupuncture, assumed mechanisms for weight reduction are involved the ANS (sympathomimetic effect) [152], leptin and ghrelin[153]. However, there is no RCT to verify the acupuncture effect on weight loss and we are suggesting future RCTs to compare the effect of either local (abdomen) or distal (leg, arm, aricular) acupoints roles.

### 3.4. Neurological disorders

Since major effective site of acupuncture stimulation is the brain, it has been used for treating neurological diseases other than pain. One of the popular topics is the effect of acupuncture treatment on stroke rehabilitation. For example, early trials have suggested that electric stimulation at some acupoints enhanced the neurological function in patients with hemiplegic stroke [154] and spinal cord injury[155]. Further RCT implied more balance improvement in stroke patients treated by true manual acupuncture [156]. Compared with control group who received acupuncture treatment without the sensation of "De Qi", true manual acupuncture at GV20 (Baihui) and 4 Spirit acupoints elicited an immediate effect on several balance parameters. It is important to understand the effect of stimulation modalities. In animal study, optimal scalp EA (5-20Hz) can increase blood flow during acute infraction, reduce infraction area and restore blood flow after acute infraction [157]. Our previous animal studies have revealed that EA at ST36 (Zusanli) increased the cerebral blood flow (CBF) in cerebral ischemia rats [158].

Acupuncture at GV20 (Baihui) enhanced the dopamine level and protected the neurons from apoptosis in the ischemia-reperfusion injured brains of rats [159]. Consistently, RCT also suggests scalp EA (2Hz) but not sham EA, improve functional outcomes after acupuncture [160]. It seems that adequate stimulation protocol is the major determinant of acupuncture treatment effect for ischemic brain injury. For example, RCT using 100Hz scalp EA cannot produce superior functional recovery in stroke patients compared with mock TENS [161].

In addition to scalp acupuncture, EA (1Hz) at cognition-related acupoints enhanced the cognitive function in patients with stroke [162]. Lin's group concluded that EA at PC6 (Neiquan) and HT7 (Shenmen) shown a promising effect for rehabilitation in stroke patients. Taken together, acupuncture treatments have benefit effects on the ischemic brain.

Another common acupuncture indication is peripheral neuropathy. As mentioned in previous section (see Current researches in hyperalgesia models), EA can attenuate hyperalgesia at peripheral and central level. Current research showed acupuncture can reduce severity of neuropathic pain in different neuropathies [163-165], but another sham control trial didn't support acupuncture [166]. More RCTs are needed to elucidate the real effect of acupuncture on peripheral neuropathies.

### 3.5. Asthma and atopic diseases

Anti-inflammation effect of acupuncture through ANS and immune systems make it a possible treatment for atopic diseases such as asthma, allergic rhinitis and eczema, but only few trials have been published in asthma [167, 168], allergic rhinitis [169] and eczema [170], therefore no conclusion can be made so far. However, in Scheewe's trial, acupuncture can improve rehabilitation response and the peak expiratory flow variability differs significantly, which means that acupuncture seems able to stabilize asthmatic airway. Further RCTs are needed to elucidate acupuncture effect on asthma.

## 4. Conclusion

From basic studies on AA to RCTs, current acupuncture researches illustrate us the diversities and possibilities of this traditional medicine playing an role in modern medicine. Commonly accepted by western countries, acupuncture studies first began at analgesia. The analgesic effect may be originated from cerebral cortex, brainstem, spinal dorsal horn, DRG to peripheral tissues. The study of the acupuncture mechanism and exact pathway are still in process. However, involvement of AAC, hypothalamus, PAG, NRM is more evident to date. Inhibitory interneuron and ANS are current focuses on acupuncture research. Results form these studies to date have shown effects of acupuncture on synaptic plasticity and cholinergic reflex. The clinical trials of pain syndromes have offered different level of evidences to support basic studies on AA. Short-term pain relief can be observed in migraine, chronic low back pain, post-operative pain and osteoarthritis of the knee. The effect of acupuncture seems longer in osteoarthritis and low back pain.

Since CNS has been long believed to initiate acupuncture effect, functional studies such as fMRI and electrophysiology have been utilized to test it. The results confirmed the crucial role of CNS on acupuncture-mediated therapeutic effects. But it is also suggested some limitations of these tools. For example, spatial analysis of brain activity by fMRI is not as adequate as analysis of brain network connectivity. As to clinical trials, stroke is a current concern. Many trials suggested better functional outcomes in stroke patients treated with acupuncture. The effect is frequency-dependent, lower frequency (1-5 Hz) EA is more effective.

Diabetes and obesity are two major modern healthy issues all over the world. In animal models, the acupuncture effect on blood glucose is mediated by serotonin and endogenous opioids. The influence of acupuncture on metabolism also occurs at cellular level. Therefore, it is believed acupuncture can enhance metabolism in general and it has been used as a tool for weight reduction. Currently, no rigid RCTs available to verify the real effect of acupuncture on body weight. So is true for Asthma. Preliminary report suggested acupuncture can stabilize airway, but, like weight reduction, the effect is still unclear in the lack of rigid RCTs.

## 5. Summary

Being one of the major categories of complementary and alternative medicines (CAMs), acupuncture might be the most explored one. Despite current acupuncture researches have explored more diverse phenomenon such as anti-inflammation and regulation of homeostasis, neural system is still the main target. Early studies suggested that the central opioids and serotonin mediate analgesic effect of acupuncture. Current studies further illustrated the roles of synaptic plasticity and cholinergic reflex in acupuncture treatment. It is believed that acupuncture is able to modulate hyperalgesia and inflammation at levels of receptor proteins. Although the central nervous system (CNS) has been studied extensively, acupuncture effect on cerebral cortex is still in the scientific spotlight. Function imaging and electrophysiology studies have shown complicated networks that acupuncture involves in. Take the whole CNS into account; axes composing certain CNS regions are activated by acupuncture. For example, the anterior cingulated cortex (ACC)-arcuate-periagueductal gray (PAG)-nucleus raphes magnus (NRM) axis participates in analgesic effect of lower frequency electroacupuncture (EA).

Series of studies consolidated the beneficial effect of acupuncture on animal model of diabetes that blood glucose and insulin statuses are influenced by EA. These effects are also partly mediated by opioid and serotonin. In real clinical setting, acupuncture is used for weight reduction rather than for diabetes. Some current trials have validated its effectiveness as to weight reduction. Clinical trials on pain syndromes, stroke, neuropathy and asthma also have revealed different degrees of benefit of acupuncture treatment. Clinical research work on acupuncture has been carry on for many decades, most dominant in pain syndromes, namely chronic headache, low back pain, osteoarthritis and post-operative pain. However, some study result may possess inadequacies, such as fixed acupoint selection and the lack of objective assessment.

## Author details

Chen Wei-Liang[1,4,5] and Hsieh Ching-Liang[1,2,3*]

*Address all correspondence to: clhsieh@mail.cmuh.org.tw

1 Graduate Institute of Acupuncture Science, China Medical University, Taichung, Taiwan

2 Acupuncture Research Center, China Medical University, Taichung, Taiwan

3 Graduate Institute of Integrated Medicine, China Medical University, Taichung, Taiwan

4 Division of Neurology, Department of Pediatrics, University of Colorado School of Medicine, Aurora, CO 80045, USA

5 Children's Hospital Colorado, Aurora, CO 80045, USA

## References

[1] Chen WL, Hsieh CL. Acupuncture research in Taiwan. *Taiwan J Obstet Gynecol* 2012;51(2)179-185.

[2] Lin JG, Chen WL. Acupuncture analgesia: a review of its mechanisms of actions. *Am J Chin Med* 2008;36(4)635-645.

[3] Song JG, Li HH, Cao YF, *et al.* Electroacupuncture improves survival in rats with lethal endotoxemia via the autonomic nervous system. *Anesthesiology* 2012;116(2)406-414.

[4] Liu P, Zhou G, Yang X, *et al.* Power estimation predicts specific function action of acupuncture: an fMRI study. *Magn Reson Imaging* 2011;29(8)1059-1064.

[5] Melzack R, Wall PD. Pain mechanisms: a new theory. *Science* 1965;150(3699)971-979.

[6] Simantov R, Snyder SH. Morphine-like peptides in mammalian brain: isolation, structure elucidation, and interactions with the opiate receptor. *Proc Natl Acad Sci U S A* 1976;73(7)2515-2519.

[7] Heinricher MM, Tavares I, Leith JL, *et al.* Descending control of nociception: Specificity, recruitment and plasticity. *Brain Res Rev* 2009;60(1)214-225.

[8] Budai D, Fields HL. Endogenous opioid peptides acting at mu-opioid receptors in the dorsal horn contribute to midbrain modulation of spinal nociceptive neurons. *J Neurophysiol* 1998;79(2)677-687.

[9] Mayer DJ, Price DD, Rafii A. Antagonism of acupuncture analgesia in man by the narcotic antagonist naloxone. *Brain Res* 1977;121(2)368-372.

[10] Pomeranz B, Cheng R, Law P. Acupuncture reduces electrophysiological and behavioral responses to noxious stimuli: pituitary is implicated. *Exp Neurol* 1977;54(1)172-178.

[11] Pert A, Dionne R, Ng L, *et al.* Alterations in rat central nervous system endorphins following transauricular electroacupuncture. *Brain Res* 1981;224(1)83-93.

[12] Clement-Jones V, McLoughlin L, Tomlin S, *et al.* Increased beta-endorphin but not met-enkephalin levels in human cerebrospinal fluid after acupuncture for recurrent pain. *Lancet* 1980;2(8201)946-949.

[13] Kiser RS, Khatami MJ, Gatchel RJ, *et al.* Acupuncture relief of chronic pain syndrome correlates with increased plasma met-enkephalin concentrations. *Lancet* 1983;2(8364)1394-1396.

[14] Cheng RS, Pomeranz B. Electroacupuncture analgesia could be mediated by at least two pain-relieving mechanisms; endorphin and non-endorphin systems. *Life Sci* 1979;25(23)1957-1962.

[15] Chen XH, Han JS. Analgesia induced by electroacupuncture of different frequencies is mediated by different types of opioid receptors: another cross-tolerance study. *Behav Brain Res* 1992;47(2)143-149.

[16] Han Z, Jiang YH, Wan Y, *et al.* Endomorphin-1 mediates 2 Hz but not 100 Hz electroacupuncture analgesia in the rat. *Neurosci Lett* 1999;274(2)75-78.

[17] Huang C, Wang Y, Chang JK, *et al.* Endomorphin and mu-opioid receptors in mouse brain mediate the analgesic effect induced by 2 Hz but not 100 Hz electroacupuncture stimulation. *Neurosci Lett* 2000;294(3)159-162.

[18] Han JS. Acupuncture: neuropeptide release produced by electrical stimulation of different frequencies. *Trends Neurosci* 2003;26(1)17-22.

[19] He LF. Involvement of endogenous opioid peptides in acupuncture analgesia. *Pain* 1987;31(1)99-121.

[20] Lao L, Zhang RX, Zhang G, *et al.* A parametric study of electroacupuncture on persistent hyperalgesia and Fos protein expression in rats. *Brain Res* 2004;1020(1-2)18-29.

[21] Liu X, Zhu B, Zhang SX. Relationship between electroacupuncture analgesia and descending pain inhibitory mechanism of nucleus raphe magnus. *Pain* 1986;24(3)383-396.

[22] Tsai H, Chen Y, Lin J. Effect of electroacupuncture analgesia on serotoninergic neurons in rat central nervous system. *Chinese Pharmacology Journal* 1989;41(2)123-126.

[23] Tsai HY, Lin JG, Inoki R. Further evidence for possible analgesic mechanism of electroacupuncture: effects on neuropeptides and serotonergic neurons in rat spinal cord. *Jpn J Pharmacol* 1989;49(2)181-185.

[24] Chang FC, Tsai HY, Yu MC, *et al.* The central serotonergic system mediates the analgesic effect of electroacupuncture on ZUSANLI (ST36) acupoints. *J Biomed Sci* 2004;11(2)179-185.

[25] Danzebrink RM, Gebhart GF. Evidence that spinal 5-HT1, 5-HT2 and 5-HT3 receptor subtypes modulate responses to noxious colorectal distension in the rat. *Brain Res* 1991;538(1)64-75.

[26] Eide PK, Hole K. The role of 5-hydroxytryptamine (5-HT) receptor subtypes and plasticity in the 5-HT systems in the regulation of nociceptive sensitivity. *Cephalalgia* 1993;13(2)75-85.

[27] Baek YH, Choi DY, Yang HI, *et al.* Analgesic effect of electroacupuncture on inflammatory pain in the rat model of collagen-induced arthritis: mediation by cholinergic and serotonergic receptors. *Brain Res* 2005;1057(1-2)181-185.

[28] Kim SK, Park JH, Bae SJ, *et al.* Effects of electroacupuncture on cold allodynia in a rat model of neuropathic pain: mediation by spinal adrenergic and serotonergic receptors. *Exp Neurol* 2005;195(2)430-436.

[29] Choi BT, Kang J, Jo UB. Effects of electroacupuncture with different frequencies on spinal ionotropic glutamate receptor expression in complete Freund's adjuvant-injected rat. *Acta Histochem* 2005;107(1)67-76.

[30] Wada Y, Shiraishi J, Nakamura M, *et al.* Role of serotonin receptor subtypes in the development of amygdaloid kindling in rats. *Brain Res* 1997;747(2)338-342.

[31] Lee JH, Beitz AJ. The distribution of brain-stem and spinal cord nuclei associated with different frequencies of electroacupuncture analgesia. *Pain* 1993;52(1)11-28.

[32] Guo HF, Tian J, Wang X, *et al.* Brain substrates activated by electroacupuncture of different frequencies (I): Comparative study on the expression of oncogene c-fos and genes coding for three opioid peptides. *Brain Res Mol Brain Res* 1996;43(1-2)157-166.

[33] Campbell JN, Meyer RA. Mechanisms of neuropathic pain. *Neuron* 2006;52(1)77-92.

[34] Koo ST, Park YI, Lim KS, *et al.* Acupuncture analgesia in a new rat model of ankle sprain pain. *Pain* 2002;99(3)423-431.

[35] Huang C, Hu ZP, Long H, *et al.* Attenuation of mechanical but not thermal hyperalgesia by electroacupuncture with the involvement of opioids in rat model of chronic inflammatory pain. *Brain Res Bull* 2004;63(2)99-103.

[36] Sekido R, Ishimaru K, Sakita M. Differences of electroacupuncture-induced analgesic effect in normal and inflammatory conditions in rats. *Am J Chin Med* 2003;31(6)955-965.

[37] Chen WH, Hsieh CL, Huang CP, *et al.* Acid-sensing ion channel 3 mediates peripheral anti-hyperalgesia effects of acupuncture in mice inflammatory pain. *J Biomed Sci* 2011;1882.

[38] Groth R, Aanonsen L. Spinal brain-derived neurotrophic factor (BDNF) produces hyperalgesia in normal mice while antisense directed against either BDNF or trkB, prevent inflammation-induced hyperalgesia. *Pain* 2002;100(1-2)171-181.

[39] Mamet J, Lazdunski M, Voilley N. How nerve growth factor drives physiological and inflammatory expressions of acid-sensing ion channel 3 in sensory neurons. *J Biol Chem* 2003;278(49)48907-48913.

[40] Simonetti M, Fabbro A, D'Arco M, *et al.* Comparison of P2X and TRPV1 receptors in ganglia or primary culture of trigeminal neurons and their modulation by NGF or serotonin. *Mol Pain* 2006;211.

[41] Aloe L, Manni L. Low-frequency electro-acupuncture reduces the nociceptive response and the pain mediator enhancement induced by nerve growth factor. *Neurosci Lett* 2009;449(3)173-177.

[42] Sehgal N, Smith HS, Manchikanti L. Peripherally acting opioids and clinical implications for pain control. *Pain Physician* 2011;14(3)249-258.

[43] Stein C. The control of pain in peripheral tissue by opioids. *The New England journal of medicine* 1995;3321685-1690.

[44] Tu WZ, Cheng RD, Cheng B, *et al.* Analgesic effect of electroacupuncture on chronic neuropathic pain mediated by P2X3 receptors in rat dorsal root ganglion neurons. *Neurochem Int* 2012;60(4)379-386.

[45] Zhang Z, Wang C, Gu G, *et al.* The Effects of Electroacupuncture at the ST36 (Zusanli) Acupoint on Cancer Pain and Transient Receptor Potential Vanilloid Subfamily 1 Expression in Walker 256 Tumor-Bearing Rats. *Anesth Analg* 2012;114(4)879-885.

[46] Hwang HS, Yang EJ, Lee SM, *et al.* Antiallodynic Effects of Electroacupuncture Combined with MK-801 Treatment through the Regulation of p35/p25 in Experimental Diabetic Neuropathy. *Exp Neurobiol* 2011;20(3)144-152.

[47] Hossaini M, Jongen JL, Biesheuvel K, *et al.* Nociceptive stimulation induces expression of Arc/Arg3.1 in the spinal cord with a preference for neurons containing enkephalin. *Mol Pain* 2010;643.

[48] Meng X, Zhang Y, Li A, *et al.* The effects of opioid receptor antagonists on electroacupuncture-produced anti-allodynia/hyperalgesia in rats with paclitaxel-evoked peripheral neuropathy. *Brain Res* 2011;141458-65.

[49] Zhang RX, Wang L, Liu B, *et al.* Mu opioid receptor-containing neurons mediate electroacupuncture-produced anti-hyperalgesia in rats with hind paw inflammation. *Brain Res* 2005;1048(1-2)235-240.

[50] Zhang RX, Lao L, Wang L, *et al.* Involvement of opioid receptors in electroacupuncture-produced anti-hyperalgesia in rats with peripheral inflammation. *Brain Res* 2004;1020(1-2)12-17.

[51] Ji RR, Kohno T, Moore KA, *et al.* Central sensitization and LTP: do pain and memory share similar mechanisms? *Trends Neurosci* 2003;26(12)696-705.

[52] Zhang YQ, Ji GC, Wu GC, *et al.* Excitatory amino acid receptor antagonists and electroacupuncture synergetically inhibit carrageenan-induced behavioral hyperalgesia and spinal fos expression in rats. *Pain* 2002;99525-535.

[53] Zhang YQ, Ji GC, Wu GC, *et al.* Kynurenic acid enhances electroacupuncture analgesia in normal andcarrageenan-injected rats. *Brain research* 2003;966300-307.

[54] Hsieh CL, Lin JG, Li TC, *et al.* Changes of pulse rate and skin temperature evoked by electroacupuncture stimulation with different frequency on both Zusanli acupoints in humans. *Am J Chin Med* 1999;27(1)11-18.

[55] Chang QY, Lin JG, Hsieh CL. Effect of electroacupuncture and transcutaneous electrical nerve stimulation at Hegu (LI.4) acupuncture point on the cutaneous reflex. *Acupunct Electrother Res* 2002;27(3-4)191-202.

[56] Hsieh CL. The physiological mechanisms of 2 Hz electroacupuncture: a study using blink and H reflex. *Am J Chin Med* 2002;30(2-3)369-378.

[57] Hsieh CL, Li TC, Lin CY, *et al.* Cerebral cortex participation in the physiological mechanisms of acupuncture stimulation: a study by auditory endogenous potentials (P300). *Am J Chin Med* 1998;26(3-4)265-274.

[58] Chiu JH, Cheng HC, Tai CH, *et al.* Electroacupuncture-induced neural activation detected by use of manganese-enhanced functional magnetic resonance imaging in rabbits. *Am J Vet Res* 2001;62(2)178-182.

[59] Chiu JH, Chung MS, Cheng HC, *et al.* Different central manifestations in response to electroacupuncture at analgesic and nonanalgesic acupoints in rats: a manganese-enhanced functional magnetic resonance imaging study. *Canadian journal of veterinary research* 2003;6794-101.

[60] Wu MT, Hsieh JC, Xiong J, *et al.* Central nervous pathway for acupuncture stimulation: localization of processing with functional MR imaging of the brain--preliminary experience. *Radiology* 1999;212(1)133-141.

[61] Kong J, Kaptchuk TJ, Webb JM, *et al.* Functional neuroanatomical investigation of vision-related acupuncture point specificity--a multisession fMRI study. *Hum Brain Mapp* 2009;30(1)38-46.

[62] Li G, Cheung RT, Ma QY, *et al.* Visual cortical activations on fMRI upon stimulation of the vision-implicated acupoints. *Neuroreport* 2003;14(5)669-673.

[63] Ho T, Duann J, Chen C, *et al.* Carryover effects alter FMRI statistical analysis in an acupuncture study. *American journal of Chinese medicine* 2008;36(1)55-70.

[64] Feng Y, Bai L, Ren Y, *et al.* FMRI connectivity analysis of acupuncture effects on the whole brain network in mild cognitive impairment patients. *Magn Reson Imaging* 2012;30(5)672-682.

[65] Feng Y, Bai L, Zhang W, *et al.* Investigation of acupoint specificity by whole brain functional connectivity analysis from fMRI data. *Conf Proc IEEE Eng Med Biol Soc* 2011;20112784-2787.

[66] Zhong C, Bai L, Dai R, *et al.* Modulatory effects of acupuncture on resting-state networks: a functional MRI study combining independent component analysis and multivariate Granger causality analysis. *J Magn Reson Imaging* 2011;35(3)572-581.

[67] Yi M, Zhang H, Lao L, *et al.* Anterior cingulate cortex is crucial for contra- but not ipsi-lateral electro-acupuncture in the formalin-induced inflammatory pain model of rats. *Mol Pain* 2011;761.

[68] Beissner F, Deichmann R, Henke C, *et al.* Acupuncture--deep pain with an autonomic dimension? *Neuroimage* 2012;60(1)653-660.

[69] LeDoux J. The emotional brain, fear, and the amygdala. *Cell Mol Neurobiol* 2003;23(4-5)727-738.

[70] Yim YK, Lee H, Hong KE, *et al.* Electro-acupuncture at acupoint ST36 reduces inflammation and regulates immune activity in Collagen-Induced. *Evidence-based complementary and alternative medicine : eCAM* 2007;451-57.

[71] Yu Y, Kasahara T, Sato T, *et al.* Role of endogenous interferon-$\gamma$ on the enhancement of splenic NK cell activity by electroacupuncture stimulation in mice. *Journal of neuroimmunology* 1998;90176-186.

[72] Zhang RX, Lao L, Wang L, *et al.* Involvement of opioid receptors in electroacupuncture-produced anti-hyperalgesia in rats with peripheral inflammation. *Brain research* 2004;102012-17.

[73] Zhang SP, Zhang JS, Yung KKL, *et al.* Non-opioid-dependent anti-inflammatory effects of low frequency electroacupuncture. *Brain research bulletin* 2004;62327-334.

[74] Choi BT, Kang J, Jo UB. Effects of electroacupuncture with different frequencies on spinal ionotropic glutamate receptor expression in complete Freund's adjuvant-injected rat. *Acta histochemica* 2005;10767-76.

[75] Sekido R, Ishimaru K, Sakita M. Differences of electroacupuncture-induced analgeis effect in normal and inflammatory condition in rats. *The American journal of Chinese medicine* 2003;31(6)955-965.

[76] Son YS, Park HJ, Kwon OB, *et al.* Antipyretic effects of acupuncture on the lipopolysaccharideinduced fever and expression of interleukin-6 and interleukin-1b mRNAs in the hypothalamus of rats. *Neuroscience letters* 2002;31945-48.

[77] Sung HJ, Kim YS, Kim IS, *et al.* Proteomic analysis of differential protein expression in neuropathic pain and electroacupuncture treatment models. *Proteomics* 2004;42805-2813.

[78] Lee HJ, Lee B, Choi SH, *et al.* Electroacupuncture Reduces Stress-Induced Expression of c-Fos in the Brain of the Rat. *The American journal of Chinese medicine* 2004;32597-806.

[79] Lao L, Zhang RX, Zhang G, *et al.* A parametric study of electroacupuncture on persistent hyperalgesia and Fos protein expression in rats. *Brain research* 2004;102018-29.

[80] Tracey KJ. The inflammatory reflex. *Nature* 2002;420853-859.

[81] Ernst M, Lee MHM. Sympathetic vasomotor changes induced by manaul and electrical acupuncture of the hoku point visualized by thermography. *Pain* 1985;2125-33.

[82] Hsieh CL, Lin JG, Li TC, *et al.* Changes of pulse rate and skin temperature evoked by electroacupuncture stimulation with different frequency on both Zusanli Acupoint in human. *The American journal of Chinese medicine* 1999;2711-18.

[83] Hsu CC, Weng CS, Liu TS, *et al.* Effects of Electrical Acupuncture on Acupoint BL15 Evaluated in Terms of Heart Rate Variability, Pulse Rate Variability and Skin Conductance Response. *The American journal of Chinese medicine* 2006;3423-26.

[84] Anderson B, Nielsen A, McKee D, *et al.* Acupuncture and heart rate variability: a systems level approach to understanding mechanism. *Explore (NY)* 2012;8(2)99-106.

[85] Fei W, Tian de R, Tso P, *et al.* Arcuate nucleus of hypothalamus is involved in mediating the satiety effect of electroacupuncture in obese rats. *Peptides* 2011;32(12)2394-2399.

[86] Tian DR, Li XD, Wang F, *et al.* Up-regulation of the expression of cocaine and amphetamine-regulated transcript peptide by electroacupuncture in the arcuate nucleus of diet-induced obese rats. *Neurosci Lett* 2005;383(1-2)17-21.

[87] Chang SL, Lin JG, Chi TC, *et al.* An insulin-dependent hypoglycaemia induced by electroacupuncture at the Zhongwan (CV12) acupoint in diabetic rats. *Diabetologia* 1999;42(2)250-255.

[88] Lin JG, Chen WC, Hsieh CL, *et al.* Multiple sources of endogenous opioid peptide involved in the hypoglycemic response to 15 Hz electroacupuncture at the Zhongwan acupoint in rats. *Neurosci Lett* 2004;366(1)39-42.

[89] Lin JG, Chang SL, Cheng JT. Release of beta-endorphin from adrenal gland to lower plasma glucose by the electroacupuncture at Zhongwan acupoint in rats. *Neurosci Lett* 2002;326(1)17-20.

[90] Chang SL, Tsai CC, Lin JG, *et al.* Involvement of serotonin in the hypoglycemic response to 2 Hz electroacupuncture of zusanli acupoint (ST36) in rats. *Neurosci Lett* 2005;379(1)69-73.

[91] Chang SL, Lin KJ, Lin RT, *et al.* Enhanced insulin sensitivity using electroacupuncture on bilateral Zusanli acupoints (ST 36) in rats. *Life Sci* 2006;79(10)967-971.

[92] Lin RT, Tzeng CY, Lee YC, *et al.* Acute effect of electroacupuncture at the Zusanli acupoints on decreasing insulin resistance as shown by lowering plasma free fatty acid levels in steroid-background male rats. *BMC Complement Altern Med* 2009;926.

[93] Tseng CS, Shen WC, Cheng FC, *et al.* Dynamic change in energy metabolism by electroacupuncture stimulation in rats. *Am J Chin Med* 2005;33(5)767-778.

[94] MacPherson H, Altman DG, Hammerschlag R, *et al.* Revised STandards for Reporting Interventions in Clinical Trials of Acupuncture (STRICTA): extending the CONSORT statement. *PLoS Med* 2010;7(6)e1000261.

[95] Lin JG, Chen WL. Review: acupuncture analgesia in clinical trials. *Am J Chin Med* 2009;37(1)1-18.

[96] Lewith GT, Machin D. On the evaluation of clinical effects of acupuncture. *Pain* 1983;16111-127.

[97] Boivie J, Brarrberg G. Are the long lasting effect on migraine headache after one series of acupuncture treatment? *The American journal of Chinese medicine* 1987;1569-75.

[98] Vincent CA. A controlled trial of the treatment of migraine by acupuncture. *Clinical Journal of Pain* 1989;5305-312.

[99] Hesse J, Mogelcang B, Simosen H. Acupuncture versus metoprolol in migraine prophylaxis: a randomized trial of trigger point inactivation. *Journal of Internal Medicine* 1994;235451-456.

[100] Melchar D, Linde K, Fischer P, *et al.* Acupuncture for recurrent headaches: a systematic review of randomized controlled trials. *Cephalalgia* 1999;19779-786.

[101] Linde M, Fjell A, Carlsson J, *et al.* Role of the needling per se in acupuncture as prophylaxis for menstrually related migraine: a randomized placebo-controlled study. *Cephalalgia* 2004;2541-47.

[102] Linde K, Streng A, Jürgens S, *et al.* Acupuncture for patients with migraine: A randomized controlled trial. *JAMA* 2005;293(17)2118-2125.

[103] Alecrim-Andrade J, Maciel-Júnior J, Cladellas X, *et al.* Acupuncture in migraine prophylaxis: a randomized sham-controlled trial. *Cephalalgia* 2006;26520-529.

[104] Alecrim-Andrade J, Maciel-Junior JA, Carne X, *et al.* Acupuncture in migraine prevention: a randomized sham controlled study with 6-months posttreatment follow-up. *Clin J Pain* 2008;24(2)98-105.

[105] Melchart D, Thormaehlen J, Hager S, *et al.* Acupuncture versus placebo versus sumatriptan for early treatment of migraine attacks: a randomized controlled trial. *Journal of Internal Medicine* 2003;253181-188.

[106] Li Y, Liang F, Yang X, *et al.* Acupuncture for treating acute attacks of migraine: a randomized controlled trial. *Headache* 2009;49(6)805-816.

[107] Allais G, Lorenzo CD, Quirico PE, *et al.* Acupuncture in the prophylactic treatment of migraine without aura: A comparison with Flunarizine. *headache* 2002;42855-861.

[108] Yang CP, Chang MH, Liu PE, *et al.* Acupuncture versus topiramate in chronic migraine prophylaxis: a randomized clinical trial. *Cephalalgia* 2011;31(15)1510-1521.

[109] Vernon H, McDermaid CS, Hagino C. Systematic review of randomized clinical trials of complementary/alternative therapies in the treatment of tension-type and cervicogenic headache. *Complementary Therapies in Medicine* 1999;7142-155.

[110] Tavola T, Gala C, Conte G, *et al.* Traditional Chinese acupuncture in tension-type headache: a controlled study. *Pain* 1992;48325-329.

[111] Manias P, Tagaris G, Karageorgiou K. Acupuncture in headache: A critical review. *Clinical Journal of Pain* 2000;16334-339.

[112] White A, Resch K, Chan J, *et al.* Acupuncture for episodic tension-type headache: a multicentre randomized controlled trial. *Cephalalgia* 2000;20632-637.

[113] Karst M, Reinhard M, Thum P, *et al.* Needle acupuncture in tension-type headache: a randomized, placebo-controlled study. *Cephalalgia* 2001;21637-642.

[114] Karst M, Rollnik JD, Fink M, *et al.* Pressure pain threshold and needle acupuncture in chronic tension-type headache: a double-blind placebo-controlled study. *Pain* 2000;88199-203.

[115] Backer M, Grossman P, Schneider J, *et al.* Acupuncture in migraine: investigation of autonomic effects. *Clin J Pain* 2008;24(2)106-115.

[116] Andersson GB. Epidemiological feature of chronic low-back pain. *Lancet* 1999;354581-585.

[117] Tulder MWv, Koes BW, Bouter LM. A cost-of-illness study of back pain in the Netherlands. *Pain* 1995;62233-240.

[118] Coan RM, Wang G, Ku SL, *et al.* The acupuncture treatment of low back pain: a randomized controlled study. *The American journal of Chinese medicine* 1980;8(2)181-189.

[119] Gunn CC, Milbrandt WE, Little AS, *et al.* Dry needling of muscle motor points for chronic low-back pain. *Spine* 1980;5279-291.

[120] Garvey TA, Marks MR, Wiesel SW. A prospective, randomized, double-blind evaluation of trigger-point injection therapy for low -back pain. *Spine* 1989;14962-964.

[121] Ernst E, White AR. Acupuncture for Back Pain: A Meta-Analysis of Randomized Controlled Trials. *Archives of internal medicine* 1998;1582235-2241.

[122] Smith LA, Oldman AD, McQuay HJ, *et al.* Teasing apart quality and validity in systematic reviews: an example from acupuncture trials in chronic neck and back pain. *Pain* 2000;86119-132.

[123] Leibing E, Leonhardt U, Koester G, *et al.* Acupuncture treatment of chronic low-back pain – a randomized, blinded,placebo-controlled trial with 9-month follow-up. *Pain* 2002;96189-196.

[124] Furlan AD, Yazdi F, Tsertsvadze A, *et al.* A systematic review and meta-analysis of efficacy, cost-effectiveness, and safety of selected complementary and alternative medicine for neck and low-back pain. *Evid Based Complement Alternat Med* 2012;2012953139.

[125] Molsberger AF, Mau J, Pawelec DB, *et al.* Does acupuncture improve the orthopedic management of chronic low back pain – a randomized, blinded, controlled trial with 3 months follow up. *Pain* 2002;99579-587.

[126] Brinkhaus B, Witt CM, Jena S, *et al.* Acupuncture in patients with chronic low back pain. *Archives of internal medicine* 2006;166450-457.

[127] Thomas KJ, MacPherson H, Thorpe L, *et al.* Randomised controlled trial of a short course of traditional acupuncture compared with usual care for persistent non-specific low back pain. *BMJ* 2006;333(7569)623.

[128] Weidenhammer W, Linde K, Streng A, *et al.* Acupuncture for chronic low back pain in routine care: A multicenter observational study. *Clinical Journal of Pain* 2007;23128-135.

[129] Berman BM, Lao L, Greene M, *et al.* Efficacy of tranditional chinese acupuncture in the treatment of symptomatic knee osteoarthritis: a pilot study. *Osteoarthritis Cartilage* 1995;3139-142.

[130] Berman BM, Singh BB, Lao L, *et al.* A randomized trial of acupuncture as an adjunctive therapy in osteoarthritis of the knee. *rheumatology* 1999;38346-354.

[131] Berman BM, Lao L, Langenberg P, *et al.* Effectiveness of acupuncture as adjunctive therapy in osteoarthritis of the Knee. *Annals of internal medicine* 2004;141901-910.

[132] Vas J, Méndez C, Perea-Milla E, *et al.* Acupuncture as a complementary therapy to the pharmacological treatment of osteoarthritis of the knee: randomised controlled trial. *BMJ* 2004;329.

[133] Witt C, Brinkhaus B, Jena S, *et al.* Acupuncture in patients with osteoarthritis of the knee: a randomised trial. *Lancet* 2005;366136-143.

[134] Scharf H-P, Mansmann U, Streitberger K, *et al.* Acupuncture and knee osteoarthritis: A three-armed randomized trial. *Annals of internal medicine* 2006;14512-20.

[135] White P, Bishop FL, Prescott P, *et al.* Practice, practitioner, or placebo? A multifactorial, mixed-methods randomized controlled trial of acupuncture. *Pain* 2012;153(2)455-462.

[136] White A, Foster NE, Cummings M, *et al.* Acupuncture treatment for chronic knee pain: a systematic review. *rheumatology* 2007;46384-390.

[137] Kho HG, Egmong JV, Zhuang CF, *et al.* The patterns of stress response in patients undergoing thyoid surgery under acupuncture anaesthesia in China *Acta Anaesthesiologica Scandinavica* 1990;34563-571.

[138] Kvorning N, Christiansson C, Akeson J. Acupuncture facilitates neuromuscular and oculomotor responses to skin incision with no influence on auditory evoked potentials under sevoflurane anaesthesia. *Acta Anaesthesiologica Scandinavica* 2003;471073-1078.

[139] Kvorning N, Christiansson C, Beskow A, *et al.* Acupuncture fails to reduce but increases anaesthetic gas required to prevent movement in response to surgical incision. *Acta Anaesthesiologica Scandinavica* 2003;47818-822.

[140] Wetzel B, Pavlovic D, Kuse R, *et al.* The effect of auricular acupuncture on fentanyl requirement during hip arthroplasty: a randomized controlled trial. *Clin J Pain* 2011;27(3)262-267.

[141] Chu DW, Lee DTT, Chan TTF, *et al.* Acupuncture Anaesthesia in inguinal hernia repair. *ANZ journal of surgery* 2003;73125-127.

[142] Christensen PA, Rotne M, Vedelsdal R, *et al.* Electroacupuncture an anaesthesia for hysterectomy. *British journal of anaesthesia* 1993;71835-838.

[143] Ekblom A, Hansson P, Thomsson M, *et al.* Increased postoperative pain and consumption of analgesia following acupuncture. *Pain* 1991;44241-247.

[144] Lao L, Bergman S, Hamilton GR, *et al.* Evaluation of acupuncture for pain control after oral surgery. *Archives of otolaryngology--head & neck surgery* 1999;1999567-572.

[145] Lin J-G, Lo M-W, Wen Y-R, *et al.* The effect of high and low frequency electroacupuncture in pain after lower abdominal surgery. *Pain* 2002;99509-514.

[146] Coura LE, Manoel CH, Poffo R, *et al.* Randomised, controlled study of preoperative electroacupuncture for postoperative pain control after cardiac surgery. *Acupunct Med* 2011;29(1)16-20.

[147] Pertovaara A, Kemppainen P, Johansson G, *et al.* Dental analgesia produced by non-painful, low-frequency stimulation is not influenced by stress or reversed by naloxone. *Pain* 1982;13379-384.

[148] Chen L, Tang J, White PF, *et al.* The effect of location of transcutaneous electrical nerve stimulation on postoperative opioid analgesic requirement: Acupoint versus nonacupoint stimulation. *Anesthesia and analgesia* 1998;871129-1135.

[149] Zhang H, Peng Y, Liu Z, *et al.* Effects of acupuncture therapy on abdominal fat and hepatic fat content in obese children: a magnetic resonance imaging and proton magnetic resonance spectroscopy study. *J Altern Complement Med* 2011;17(5)413-420.

[150] Hsu CH, Hwang KC, Chao CL, *et al.* Effects of electroacupuncture in reducing weight and waist circumference in obese women: a randomized crossover trial. *Int J Obes (Lond)* 2005;29(11)1379-1384.

[151] Hsu CH, Hwang KC, Chao CL, *et al.* Electroacupuncture in obese women: a randomized, controlled pilot study. *J Womens Health (Larchmt)* 2005;14(5)434-440.

[152] Shen EY, Hsieh CL, Chang YH, *et al.* Observation of sympathomimetic effect of ear acupuncture stimulation for body weight reduction. *Am J Chin Med* 2009;37(6)1023-1030.

[153] Hsu CH, Wang CJ, Hwang KC, *et al.* The effect of auricular acupuncture in obese women: a randomized controlled trial. *J Womens Health (Larchmt)* 2009;18(6)813-818.

[154] Wong AM, Su TY, Tang FT, *et al.* Clinical trial of electrical acupuncture on hemiplegic stroke patients. *Am J Phys Med Rehabil* 1999;78(2)117-122.

[155] Wong AM, Leong CP, Su TY, *et al.* Clinical trial of acupuncture for patients with spinal cord injuries. *Am J Phys Med Rehabil* 2003;82(1)21-27.

[156] Liu SY, Hsieh CL, Wei TS, *et al.* Acupuncture stimulation improves balance function in stroke patients: a single-blinded controlled, randomized study. *Am J Chin Med* 2009;37(3)483-494.

[157] Zhou F, Guo J, Cheng J, *et al.* Electroacupuncture increased cerebral blood flow and reduced ischemic brain injury: dependence on stimulation intensity and frequency. *J Appl Physiol* 2011;111(6)1877-1887.

[158] Hsieh CL, Chang QY, Lin IH, *et al.* The study of electroacupuncture on cerebral blood flow in rats with and without cerebral ischemia. *Am J Chin Med* 2006;34(2)351-361.

[159] Chuang CM, Hsieh CL, Li TC, *et al.* Acupuncture stimulation at Baihui acupoint reduced cerebral infarct and increased dopamine levels in chronic cerebral hypoperfusion and ischemia-reperfusion injured sprague-dawley rats. *Am J Chin Med* 2007;35(5)779-791.

[160] Hsing WT, Imamura M, Weaver K, *et al.* Clinical Effects of Scalp Electrical Acupuncture in Stroke: A Sham-Controlled Randomized Clinical Trial. *J Altern Complement Med* 2012.

[161] Hopwood V, Lewith G, Prescott P, *et al.* Evaluating the efficacy of acupuncture in defined aspects of stroke recovery: a randomised, placebo controlled single blind study. *J Neurol* 2008;255(6)858-866.

[162] Chou P, Chu H, Lin JG. Effects of electroacupuncture treatment on impaired cognition and quality of life in Taiwanese stroke patients. *J Altern Complement Med* 2009;15(10)1067-1073.

[163] Yang CP, Wang NH, Li TC, *et al.* A randomized clinical trial of acupuncture versus oral steroids for carpal tunnel syndrome: a long-term follow-up. *J Pain* 2011;12(2)272-279.

[164] Schroder S, Liepert J, Remppis A, *et al.* Acupuncture treatment improves nerve conduction in peripheral neuropathy. *Eur J Neurol* 2007;14(3)276-281.

[165] Shiflett SC, Schwartz GE. Effects of acupuncture in reducing attrition and mortality in HIV-infected men with peripheral neuropathy. *Explore (NY)* 2011;7(3)148-154.

[166] Penza P, Bricchi M, Scola A, *et al.* Electroacupuncture is not effective in chronic painful neuropathies. *Pain Med* 2011;12(12)1819-1823.

[167] Scheewe S, Vogt L, Minakawa S, *et al.* Acupuncture in children and adolescents with bronchial asthma: a randomised controlled study. *Complement Ther Med* 2011;19(5)239-246.

[168] Choi JY, Jung HJ, Kim JI, *et al.* A randomized pilot study of acupuncture as an adjunct therapy in adult asthmatic patients. *J Asthma* 2010;47(7)774-780.

[169] Brinkhaus B, Witt CM, Jena S, *et al.* Acupuncture in patients with allergic rhinitis: a pragmatic randomized trial. *Ann Allergy Asthma Immunol* 2008;101(5)535-543.

[170] Pfab F, Huss-Marp J, Gatti A, *et al.* Influence of acupuncture on type I hypersensitivity itch and the wheal and flare response in adults with atopic eczema - a blinded, randomized, placebo-controlled, crossover trial. *Allergy* 2010;65(7)903-910.

Chapter 2

# Nitric Oxide in Acupuncture Mechanism

Masahiko Tsuchiya

Additional information is available at the end of the chapter

http://dx.doi.org/10.5772/54165

## 1. Introduction

In Japan and other parts of East Asia, acupuncture is an important component of traditional medicine, where it is widely used for pain relief and other healing effects for a variety of disorders [1]. However, studies in the United States and European countries that investigated the effectiveness of acupuncture have been inconclusive or equivocal [2], and the mechanism of acupuncture is not fully elucidated [3]. Recent findings suggest specific neural pathways that transmit acupuncture stimulation to distant body areas via the central nervous system, which may support traditional meridian theory [4]. In addition to such a possible central mechanism, a peripheral mechanism has also been suggested to be active in acupuncture treatment, as several studies have noted increases in skin temperature and muscular blood perfusion at acupuncture sites [5-8].

Nitric oxide (NO) is a key regulator of vascular tone and blood flow in local circulation, the importance of which has been well documented in various *in vitro* and *in vivo* studies [9, 10]. There have been several findings indicating that the level of NO can vary according to pathophysiological events and metabolic alteration. Considering the effects of acupuncture on local perfusion, an involvement of NO in the acupuncture mechanism can be speculated.

NO typically functions in a very limited area, while its half-life is short and the amount produced is small. In addition, food or water intake, daily activity or time of measurement, and the activities of various resident bacteria can greatly affect the amount of NO-related metabolites such as nitrite and nitrate, thus interfering with determination of actual NO level [11-13]. Therefore, it is quite difficult to demonstrate true changes in local NO concentration coupled with physiological or pathological effects in individuals or at the organ level. Furthermore, it is highly controversial whether acupuncture used in animals and humans is exactly the same in regard to physiological and anatomical considerations, and findings obtained only in animal studies may be of limited significance [3]. Thus, to demonstrate the involvement of NO in the acupuncture mechanism, evidence obtained with human subjects is absolutely necessary.

Our laboratory has been investigating traditional medicine from the standpoint of Western medicine and basic science, and has also extensively studied reactive oxygen species (ROS) and NO metabolism in various physiological and pathological conditions [9, 10]. Through these studies, we have found strong evidence that changes in NO level are coupled with biological functions in human subjects [12,13]. In this chapter, such results demonstrating the functions NO in the human body will be briefly shown, followed by findings showing that acupuncture has a significant impact on the level of NO at the same magnitude as shown in those results [14], which may validate the notion that NO has an important function in the mechanism of acupuncture.

## 2. NO in human respiratory system

### 2.1. Study design

To clarify the effect of NO on pulmonary gas exchange, the relationship between exhaled NO and arterial blood gases was studied in healthy human subjects.

### 2.2. Methods

Exhaled NO and arterial blood gases were analyzed in 23 healthy non-smokers without airway inflammation (20 males, 3 females; 41±4 [mean ± SD] years old) in a special clean room, in which the concentration of NO was less than 4 parts per billion (ppb). In order to minimize environmental external NO, the subjects remained in the room for at least 1 hour before measurement were performed. Previous studies have reported that exhaled NO was increased in asthmatic patients and others with airway inflammation, and may possibly reflect the inflammatory status of the airway [15, 16]. Therefore, subjects with upper or lower respiratory inflammation were strictly excluded from the present study. In addition, measurements were performed at the same time each day after more than 10 hours of fasting to eliminate the effects of external NO metabolites from diet. These careful procedures were considered important to determine the exact concentration of exhaled NO.

After 1 hour in the special clean room, blood samples were anaerobically obtained from the radial artery of each subject, then analyzed for arterial blood gases (pH, $PaO_2$, $PaCO_2$) with a blood gas analyzer (Model 288; Chiron, MA). Next, exhaled NO was measured using a chemiluminescence NO analyzer CML-500 (Shimizu, Kyoto, Japan). Each subject was instructed to perform a slow vital capacity maneuver over 30-40 seconds into unobstructed tubing while wearing nose clips. Air samples were continuously collected through a side arm as the plateau concentration at the end of expiration.

### 2.3. Results

Analysis of the exhaled air samples revealed that the concentrations of exhaled NO ranged from 13 to 53 ppb. Values for $PaO_2$, $PaCO_2$, and pH in the blood samples were 88.9±2.0 mmHg, 40.2±0.8 mmHg, and 7.40±0.01, respectively. Among these examined parameters, arterial $PaO_2$ was significantly correlated with the concentration of exhaled NO (Figure 1). However, no significant correlation was found between that concentration and pH or $PaCO_2$.

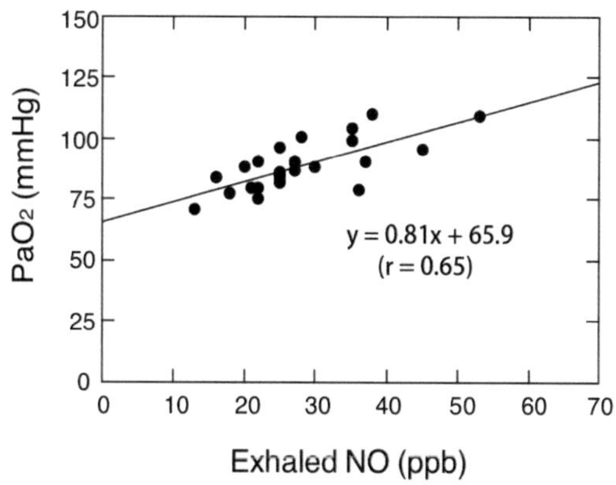


**Figure 1.** Relationship between $PaO_2$ and exhaled NO. Exhaled air samples were collected from 23 healthy subjects using a slow vital capacity maneuver. $PaO_2$ was significantly correlated with the concentration of exhaled NO (r = 0.65).

### 2.4. Interpretation

Our findings indicate that exhaled airway NO is involved in arterial oxygenation in the respiratory system. This is not surprising when considering the potent effects of NO on vascular and/or airway smooth muscular tone, which may control ventilation-to-perfusion matching in the respiratory system. Theoretically, NO concentrations in respiratory gas exchange are not equal throughout the respiratory zone, as they are dependent on the amount of inspirable NO generated in the upper airway in addition to intrinsic NO generated in the lower respiratory zone. Thus, a well-ventilated zone, which requires much perfusion, could receive much more NO than a poorly ventilated one. In this manner, airway NO actively controls gas exchange in the respiratory system, even though its concentration is very low.

## 3. NO in human circulatory system; adverse effects of cigarette smoking

### 3.1. Study design

Cigarette smoke contains superoxide and other reactive oxygen species (ROS) [17-19], thus it has been speculated that some of the adverse effects of smoking may be caused by oxidative damage to endothelial cells, resulting in NO shortage. To investigate this possibility, changes in plasma level of NO and other antioxidants in healthy subjects with a cigarette smoking habit after smoking a single cigarette were compared between those divided into real smoking and sham smoking groups.

### 3.2. Methods

Changes in plasma concentrations of nitrate plus nitrite, used as an index of NO formation in the circulation, as well as changes in plasma concentrations of major antioxidants (ascorbic acid, cysteine, methionine, uric acid) in healthy young smokers after smoking a single cigarette were measured. Subject number, age, height, weight, and smoking history in the smoking group were 20, 28±4 (mean ± SD) years old, 169±8 cm, 61±7 kg, and 6±3 pack-years (number of cigarettes in packs smoked daily times number of years), respectively, while those in the sham smoking group were 15, 27±3 years old, 170±8 cm, 61±8 kg, and 6±2 pack-years, respectively, which were not significantly different.

Both food and water contain substantial amounts of nitrate, thus it is especially important to control those factors before attempting to determine endogenous plasma NO formation in humans [11, 20]. We limited and standardized the food and water intake by the subjects prior to the experiment, in which all were asked to not eat for 10 hours, and not drink or smoke for 6 hours prior to the experiment. Measurements were performed at the same time each day while the subjects were at rest. Blood was sampled at the following intervals: just prior to smoking a cigarette, 5 minutes after smoking that cigarette, and again 60 minutes later.

### 3.3. Results

The plasma concentration of nitrate plus nitrite was significantly decreased by 3.4±1.1 μM in the smoking group after smoking a single cigarette as compared with the sham smoking group (23.9±1.1 μM in the smoking group vs. 27.3±1.2 μM in the sham smoking group) (Figure 2). The concentrations of antioxidants (ascorbic acid, cysteine, methionine, uric acid) were also significantly decreased. After 60 minutes, all parameters returned to pre-experimental levels. In the sham smoking group subjects, no significant changes were noted.

### 3.4. Interpretation

These results show that smoking a single cigarette decreases the plasma concentration of nitrate plus nitrite, as well as ascorbic acid and other antioxidants. We previously demonstrated that cigarette smoke contains superoxide and a large number of other ROS [17-19]. Inhalation of these ROS by smoking increases oxidative stress in smokers, and induces a reduction in NO and antioxidant levels. Since an adequate level of NO is essential for sufficient coronary circulation, such transient changes contribute to coronary vasoconstriction, which is routinely observed after smoking [21,22].

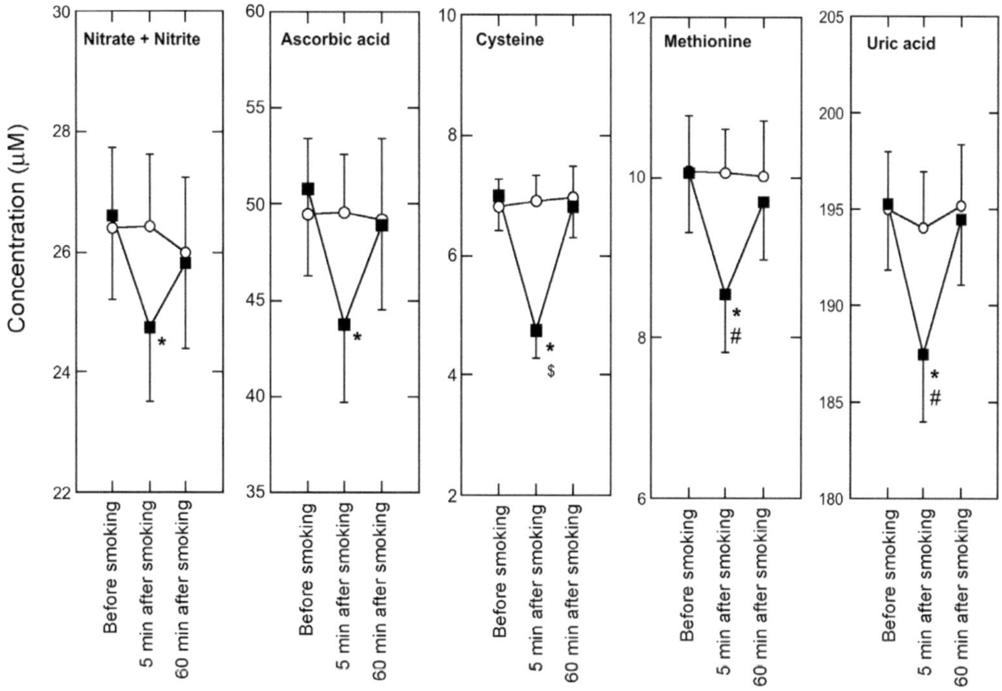


**Figure 2.** Changes in plasma concentrations (mean ± SD) of nitrate and nitrite, ascorbic acid, cysteine, methionine, and uric acid in smokers at 5 and 60 minutes after smoking a single (closed square) or sham (open circle) cigarette. * *P*< 0.01 *vs.* values before smoking, $ *P*< 0.01 *vs.* corresponding values in control group, # *P*< 0.05 *vs.* corresponding values in control group.

# 4. Change in concentration of NO required for physiological effects

It is difficult to compare NO concentrations in the respiratory system by measuring exhaled breath (13-53 ppb range) with those in the circulatory system by measuring plasma (23.9-27.3 μM range). However, it is important to note that units of ppb are considered to present a more precise scale than units of μM. Thus, based on our results, it seems certain that NO functions in the human body in a range less than μM depending on the environmental condition.

# 5. NO in acupuncture treatment in humans; effects on local circulation

## 5.1. Study design

NO is a key regulator of local circulation, and the development and persistence of pain can be affected by changes in circulation. Thus, we speculated that acupuncture can regulate NO levels. We studied the effects of acupuncture on local NO levels and circulation in a randomized, double blind, crossover study with healthy human subjects.

### 5.2. Methods

#### Procedures for acupuncture

Twenty subjects (28±5 years old [mean±SD], height 169±6 cm, weight 65±7 kg) with no knowledge of or experience with acupuncture therapy were randomly assigned to initially undergo either real or sham acupuncture treatment using computer-generated random numbers. All acupuncture treatments were performed at the same time of day, and none of the subjects ate for 10 or drank for 6 hours prior to treatment, the same as in the study of cigarette smoking. For the real acupuncture group, the subjects were blindfolded and received acupuncture at the Li4, P6, L6, and H5 acupoints in a forearm by a well-trained acupuncturist (Figure 3). In Japan, these acupoints are considered to be effective for relieving muscle and joint pain in the forearm and hand. Each acupoint was manually stimulated twice for 1 minute each by finely twisting the needle, according to standard acupuncture technique, then the needle was left *in situ* for 10 minutes. Sham acupuncture subjects were similarly blindfolded, and the same true acupoints were tapped with an empty plastic needle tube. Palpation of the surface of the skin was induced with a blunt adherent instrument for the same period as with the true acupuncture. One week after the first treatment (real or sham), the same subjects underwent the opposite treatment (real or sham acupuncture) performed in the same manner as described above.

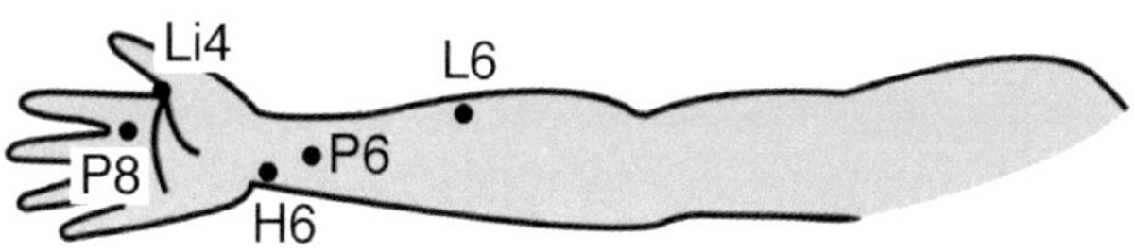


**Figure 3.** Acupoints used in the study.

#### Measurements of change in palmar circulation in acupunctured forearm

Before, and 5 and 60 minutes after acupuncture, subcutaneous circulation in the palm on the side of the treated forearm was investigated using a laser tissue blood flow meter (FLO-N1, Omegawave, Tokyo, Japan) by an investigator who did not know whether the subjects had undergone real or sham acupuncture [23]. The laser tissue blood flow meter allows measurement of microvascular blood flow in tissue at approximately 1-4 mm deep below the probe. The flow probe was placed at the center of the palm and allowed to stabilize, then the average reading over a period of 5 minutes was obtained.

#### Measurements of NO formation in acupunctured forearm

Following the measurement of microcirculation, 2 ml of whole blood from an axillary vein was drawn from the subject and collected into heparinized tubes. NO generation in blood was determined using an HPLC (high performance liquid chromatography) method by measuring the plasma concentrations of nitrate and nitrite [12], and confirmed by an ESR (electron spin resonance) method that directly measured NO signals [24], as described below.

**a.** HPLC method

Plasma was isolated by centrifugation of the collected blood samples (5 minutes at 750 x *g*, 4°C) and deproteinized by addition of an equal volume of methanol. The samples were then applied to an HPLC system (ENO-20, EICOM, Kyoto, Japan) to determine nitrate and nitrite concentrations. Nitrate and nitrite were separated using a reverse-phase column (NO-PAK), after which nitrate was reduced to nitrite in a reduction column packed with copperized cadmium (NO-RED) at 35°C. The nitrite was then mixed with Griess reagent in a reaction coil and change in absorbance was monitored at 540 nm. The flow rate of the mobile phase, which consisted of 10% methanol containing 0.15 M $BaCl_2$-$NH_4Cl$ and 0.5 g/l EDTA-4Na, was 0.33 ml/minute. Griess reagent was delivered at a rate of 0.1 ml/minute.

**b.** ESR method

The remainder of the blood sample (400 μl) was quickly transferred to ESR tubes (4 mm inner diameter) and frozen with liquid nitrogen, then analyzed by an ESR method at 110 K using a JES-RE1X spectrometer (JOEL, Tokyo) with 100 kHz field modulation. ESR analysis was conducted with a microwave power of 8 mW at a frequency of 9.099 GHz, 325±50 mT field, 3-minute sweep time, 0.125-mT modulation amplitude, and 0.1-second time constant. As a positive control, fresh non-treated blood was incubated for 10 minutes with NOC7 ([1-hydroxy-2-oxo-3-(N-methyl-3-aminopropyl)-3-methyl-3-aminopropyl]-3-methyl-1-triazene), which chemically generates NO with a half-life of 5 minutes.

**Chemicals**

Reagents for HPLC analysis were obtained from EICOM (Kyoto, Japan) and NOC7 was obtained from Dojin Co. (Kumamoto, Japan). Other reagents used were of analytical grade.

### 5.3. Results

**Palmar circulation in acupunctured forearm**

Prior to receiving acupuncture, microvascular blood flow in the palm of the forearm that underwent real acupuncture did not differ from that in the forearm that underwent sham acupuncture (Figure 4-A). At 5 and 60 minutes after acupuncture, microvascular blood flow in the palm of the sham acupunctured forearm was unchanged, while that in the real acupunctured side was significantly increased as compared with both the pre-acupuncture and sham values.

**NO formation in acupunctured forearm: HPCL study**

Prior to receiving acupuncture, there were no differences in regard to plasma concentrations of nitrate plus nitrite between the real and sham acupuncture groups (Figure 4-B). After acupuncture as well, no significant changes in plasma concentrations of nitrate plus nitrite were noted in either the non-treated forearm in subjects who underwent real acupuncture or those that underwent sham treatment. However, that concentration in the acupunctured forearm was significantly increased as compared with both the pre-acupuncture value and values obtained for the opposite non-treated and sham-acupunctured forearms at 5 and 60 minutes after real acupuncture treatment. Plasma concentration of nitrate plus nitrite was 24.6±6.1 μM in the acupunctured forearm before acupuncture, 27.5±6.5 (mean±SD) μM at 5 minutes after acupuncture, and 27.1±6.6 μM at 60 minutes. Thus, the amount of increase above the pre-acupuncture value was 2.8±1.5 μM after 5 and 2.5±1.4 μM after 60 minutes.

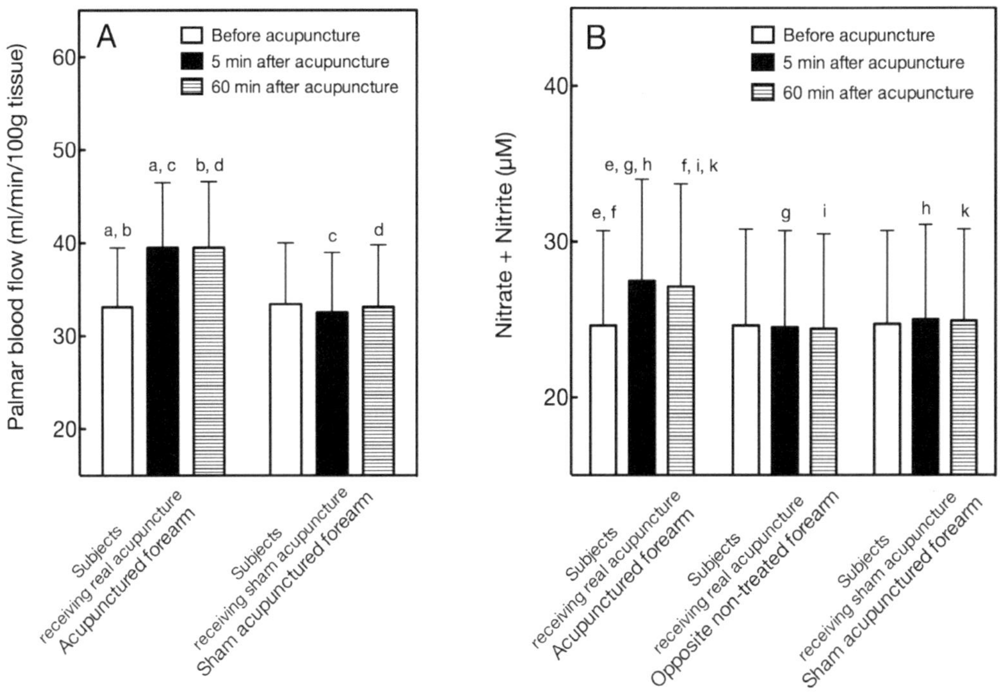


**Figure 4.** Changes in blood flow (mean±SD) in palmer subcutaneous tissue (A), and plasma concentrations of nitrate and nitrite in samples from an axillary vein (B) in subjects who received real or sham acupuncture in a forearm. Alphabetic characters of a, b, c, d, e, f, g, h, i, and k indicate a significant difference ($p < 0.05$) between values.

## NO formation: ESR study

The ESR spectrum attributed to $Cu^{2+}$ of ceruloplasmin was observed in blood samples obtained before acupuncture (Figure 5-A). At 5 minutes after acupuncture, a small peak with a *g* value of 2.0 developed and was superimposed on the $Cu^{2+}$-ceruloplasmin adduct spectrum [24] in blood samples obtained from the acupunctured forearm (arrows in Figure 5-B), but not in blood samples from the non-treated and sham forearms (data not shown). Although the ESR signal observed was small, it was assigned to the NO-hemoglobin adduct spectrum with reference to the typical ESR spectrum of NO-hemoglobin generated by incubation of NOC7, a short-lived potent NO releaser, with a fresh non-treated blood sample, as shown in Figure 5-C and D.

http://dx.doi.org/10.5772/54165

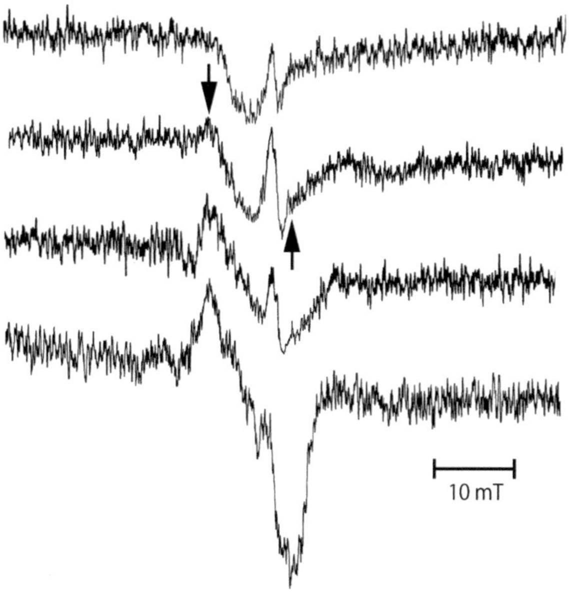


**Figure 5.** ESR spectra of blood samples from acupunctured forearm. Prior to acupuncture (A), 5 minutes after acupuncture (B), and 10 minutes after incubation of fresh non-treated blood with 15 μM (C) and 60 μM (D) of NOC7 as a positive control. Arrows in B indicate the NO-hemoglobin adduct with a *g* value of 2.0 superimposed on the originally generated $Cu^{2+}$-ceruloplasmin adduct. Detailed ESR settings are described in the text.

### Correlation between NO formation and palmar circulation

In the real acupunctured forearm, the amount of increase in microvascular blood flow in the palm above the pre-acupuncture value was significantly correlated with that in plasma concentration of nitrate plus nitrite, with a regression line of y = 2.3x and correlation coefficient (r) of 0.79 (Figure 6). In the sham forearm, no correlation was found between the amount of increase in microvascular blood flow in the palm and that in plasma concentration of nitrate plus nitrite.

## 5.4. Discussion and interpretation

We found that acupuncture increased the plasma concentration of nitrate plus nitrite in treated regions, coupled with an increase in blood flow. Although measurements of NO itself were not performed, previous studies have shown that concentrations of nitrate and nitrite, end-products of NO metabolism, are reliable indicators of NO formation *in vivo* [25].

It should be noted that blood in the axillary vein of the acupunctured forearm contained nitrate plus nitrite derived from locally generated NO in the forearm itself, in addition to that basally generated throughout the body. Thus, to confirm that basal NO generation did not affect the change in concentration of nitrate plus nitrite in blood from the acupunctured forearm, that in blood from the opposite non-treated forearm was also measured, which showed no significant change. This finding indicates that background basal NO level did not change in the present subjects. Thus, the increased NO level in the acupunctured forearm was primarily from changes that occurred in the forearm itself.

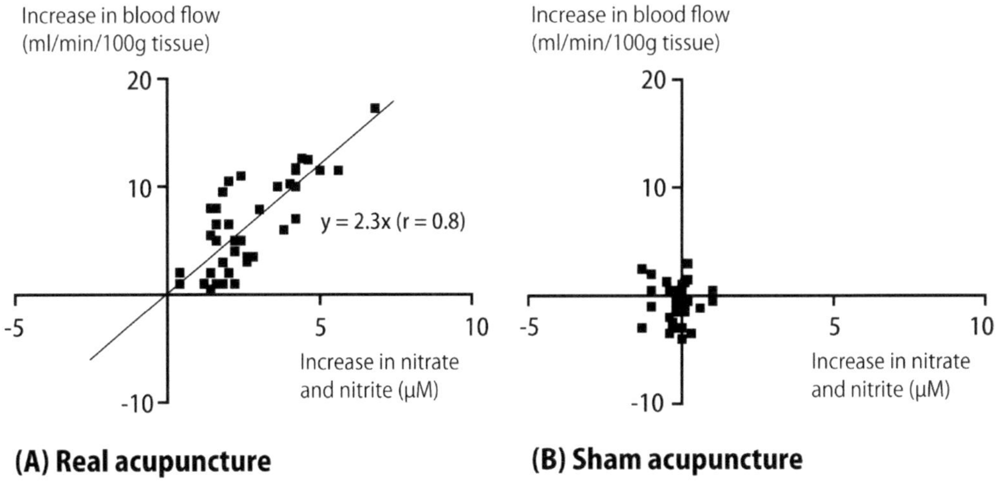


**Figure 6.** Relationship between amount of increase in palmar blood flow above the pre-acupuncture value, and that in plasma concentration of nitrate plus nitrite in real acupunctured (A) and sham-acupunctured (B) forearms. There was a significant correlation after real acupuncture, with a regression line of y = 2.3x and correlation coefficient (r) of 0.79, but not after sham acupuncture.

An ESR method was used to detect and confirm NO generation in the forearm treated with acupuncture. An advantage of ESR is that it can directly and specifically detect NO even in biological samples, whereas it is not highly sensitive and does not provide quantitative findings [26]. Because the affinity of hemoglobin for NO is very high, 300,000 times greater than that for oxygen molecules, NO generated in blood rapidly reacts with hemoglobin to form an NO-hemoglobin adduct, which is detected as a characteristic ESR spectrum and interpreted as evidence of NO generation [24]. Thus, even a small ESR peak for NO-hemoglobin, as seen in the present study, is strong and reliable evidence for NO generation in the forearm from which blood samples were collected. To the best of our knowledge, this is the first study to demonstrate that manual acupuncture treatment increases plasma NO in acupunctured regions in human subjects.

The increase in palmar microvascular blood flow seen in the acupunctured forearm side indicates that acupuncture controls regional circulation, and agrees well with previous studies that reported increases in skin temperature and muscular blood flow in regions subjected to acupuncture [5-8]. The significant correlation between the amounts of increase in blood flow and NO level in the acupunctured forearm indicates that NO-dependent mechanisms are involved in regulation of circulation by acupuncture. Regional ischemia is an important factor in development and prolongation of certain types of pain, and improvement in blood flow washes out pain-generating metabolic products [27, 28]. Thus, the regulatory effect on regional circulation through control of NO level partly accounts for the biological mechanism of the effects of acupuncture on pain.

## 6. NO a key molecule in acupuncture

The findings of NO dynamics in human subjects described in the previous sections 2 and 3 indicate that changes in NO concentration in μM amounts have a strong influence on vital body functions. Therefore, the magnitude of NO generated by acupuncture shown in the present study is of great biological significance. Furthermore, coupled physiological effects were also observed, as expected. We consider it reasonable to conclude that NO plays a key role in the effects of acupuncture. A recent animal study showed that acupuncture increased muscle blood flow to some degree, even in denervated hindlimb muscles, indicating that a local regulation mechanism may have a dominant role in acupuncture [29]. When considering the importance of NO as a biological molecule for basic vital functions [9, 10], its local regulation is a compelling candidate for an acupuncture-related molecular mechanism.

## 7. Further advancements in studies of NO metabolism related to acupuncture

Based on an understanding of the importance of NO generation in acupuncture, the question regarding which mechanism is involved becomes important. In addition to the present findings, several studies have reported higher levels of generated NO on the skin surface at meridians and acupoints in resting or acupuncture treated human subjects [30-32]. Furthermore, an increase in NO generation at certain acupoints during electrical acupuncture treatment at distant acupoints belonging to the same meridian has been shown using dermal micro-dialysis [33].

Some resident bacteria could produce NO-related metabolites, thus it is possible that the bacterial organisms in the area of the skin contribute to these NO phenomena [20, 31]. On the other hand, it should be noted that many acupoints and meridians are located close to blood vessels and peripheral neural fibers, which might express nitric oxide synthase (NOS) enzymes with various stimuli. In fact, enhancement of the expression of endothelial nitric oxide synthase (eNOS) and neuronal nitric oxide synthase (nNOS) by acupuncture was reported [34, 35], though in animal studies. Together with other studies, we suggest that the acupoint and meridian NOS system function to regulate the level of NO in acupunctured individuals with the aid of surrounding blood vessels and local neural fibers. These should be confirmed in future studies.

## 8. Conclusion

Acupuncture elevates the level of local NO in treated regions, thereby increasing local blood flow. The importance of local perfusion in patients suffering from pain suggests that these effects contribute to pain relief by acupuncture. Our findings may be useful for elucidation of the complex mechanisms underlying the clinical effects and mechanism of acupuncture.

## Author details

Masahiko Tsuchiya

Address all correspondence to: oxymasa@ea.mbn.or.jp

Department of Anesthesiology, Osaka City University Medical School, Abeno-ku, Osaka, Japan

## References

[1] Kaptchuk TJ: Acupuncture: theory, efficacy, and practice. *Ann Intern Med* 2002, 136(5):374-383.

[2] Ezzo J, Berman B, Hadhazy VA, Jadad AR, Lao L, Singh BB: Is acupuncture effective for the treatment of chronic pain? A systematic review. *Pain* 2000, 86(3):217-225.

[3] Langevin HM, Wayne PM, Macpherson H, Schnyer R, Milley RM, Napadow V, Lao L, Park J, Harris RE, Cohen M *et al*: Paradoxes in acupuncture research: strategies for moving forward. *Evid Based Complement Alternat Med* 2011, 2011:180805.

[4] Zhang ZJ, Wang XM, McAlonan GM: Neural acupuncture unit: a new concept for interpreting effects and mechanisms of acupuncture. *Evid Based Complement Alternat Med* 2012, 2012:429412.

[5] Ernst M, Lee MH: Sympathetic vasomotor changes induced by manual and electrical acupuncture of the Hoku point visualized by thermography. *Pain* 1985, 21(1):25-33.

[6] Lo SY: Meridians in acupuncture and infrared imaging. *Med Hypotheses* 2002, 58(1): 72-76.

[7] Sandberg M, Larsson B, Lindberg LG, Gerdle B: Different patterns of blood flow response in the trapezius muscle following needle stimulation (acupuncture) between healthy subjects and patients with fibromyalgia and work-related trapezius myalgia. *Eur J Pain* 2005, 9(5):497-510.

[8] Sandberg M, Lundeberg T, Lindberg LG, Gerdle B: Effects of acupuncture on skin and muscle blood flow in healthy subjects. *Eur J Appl Physiol* 2003, 90(1-2):114-119.

[9] Inoue M, Nishikawa M, Sato EF, Ah-Mee P, Kashiba M, Takehara Y, Utsumi K: Cross-talk of NO, superoxide and molecular oxygen, a majesty of aerobic life. *Free Radic Res* 1999, 31(4):251-260.

[10] Inoue M, Sato EF, Nishikawa M, Park AM, Kira Y, Imada I, Utsumi K: Cross talk of nitric oxide, oxygen radicals, and superoxide dismutase regulates the energy metabolism and cell death and determines the fates of aerobic life. *Antioxid Redox Signal* 2003, 5(4):475-484.

[11] Node K, Kitakaze M, Yoshikawa H, Kosaka H, Hori M: Reversible reduction in plasma concentration of nitric oxide induced by cigarette smoking in young adults. *Am J Cardiol* 1997, 79:1538-1541.

[12] Tsuchiya M, Asada A, Kasahara E, Sato EF, Shindo M, Inoue M: Smoking a single cigarette rapidly reduces combined concentrations of nitrate and nitrite and concentrations of antioxidants in plasma. *Circulation* 2002, 105(10):1155-1157.

[13] Tsuchiya M, Tokai H, Takehara Y, Haraguchi Y, Asada A, Utsumi K, Inoue M: Interrelation between oxygen tension and nitric oxide in the respiratory system. *Am J Respir Crit Care Med* 2000, 162(4 Pt 1):1257-1261.

[14] Tsuchiya M, Sato EF, Inoue M, Asada A: Acupuncture enhances generation of nitric oxide and increases local circulation. *Anesth Analg* 2007, 104(2):301-307.

[15] Kharitonov SA, Yates D, Robbins RA, Logan-Sinclair R, Shinebourne EA, Barnes PJ: Increased nitric oxide in exhalated air of asthmatic patients. *Lancet* 1994, 343:133-135.

[16] Persson MG, ZetterstrOm O, Agrenius V, Ihre E, Gustafsson LE: Single-breath nitric oxide measurements in asthmatic patients and smokers. *Lancet* 1994, 343:146-147.

[17] Tsuchiya M, Suzuki YJ, Cross CE, Packer L: Superoxide generated by cigarette smoke damages the respiratory burst and induces physical changes in the membrane order and water organization of inflammatory cells. *Ann N Y Acad Sci* 1993, 686:39-52.

[18] Tsuchiya M, Thompson DF, Suzuki YJ, Cross CE, Packer L: Superoxide formed from cigarette smoke impairs polymorphonuclear leukocyte active oxygen generation activity. *Arch Biochem Biophys* 1992, 299(1):30-37.

[19] Tsuchiya M, Kang M, kanbara T, Manabe M: Superoxide in cigarette smoke. *Free Radicals in Clinical Medicine* 1996, 10:34-40.

[20] Weitzberg E, Lundberg JO: Nonenzymatic nitric oxide production in humans. *Nitric Oxide* 1998, 2(1):1-7.

[21] Celermajer DS, Sorensen KE, Georgakopoulos D, Bull C, Thomas O, Robinson J, Deanfield JE: Cigarette smoking is associated with dose-related and potentially re-

versible impairment of endothelium-dependent dilation in healthy young adults. *Circulation* 1993, 88(5 Pt 1):2149-2155.

[22] Quillen JE, Rossen JD, Oskarsson HJ, Minor RL, Jr., Lopez AG, Winniford MD: Acute effect of cigarette smoking on the coronary circulation: constriction of epicardial and resistance vessels. *J Am Coll Cardiol* 1993, 22(3):642-647.

[23] Takemura S, Minamiyama Y, Inoue M, Kubo S, Hirohashi K, Kinoshita H: Nitric oxide synthase inhibitor increases hepatic injury with formation of oxidative DNA damage and microcirculatory disturbance in endotoxemic rats. *Hepatogastroenterology* 2000, 47(35):1364-1370.

[24] Minamiyama Y, Takemura S, Inoue M: Effect of thiol status on nitric oxide metabolism in the circulation. *Archives of biochemistry and biophysics* 1997, 341(1):186-192.

[25] Zeballos GA, Bernstein RD, Thompson CI, Forfia PR, Seyedi N, Shen W, Kaminiski PM, Wolin MS, Hintze TH: Pharmacodynamics of plasma nitrate/nitrite as an indication of nitric oxide formation in conscious dogs. *Circulation* 1995, 91(12):2982-2988.

[26] Tsuchiya M, Asada A, Kasahara E, Sato EF, Shindo M, Inoue M: Antioxidant protection of propofol and its recycling in erythrocyte membranes. *Am J Respir Crit Care Med* 2002, 165(1):54-60.

[27] Borg-Stein J, Simons DG: Focused review: myofascial pain. *Arch Phys Med Rehabil* 2002, 83(3 Suppl 1):S40-47, S48-49.

[28] Tullberg M, Alstergren PJ, Ernberg MM: Effects of low-power laser exposure on masseter muscle pain and microcirculation. *Pain* 2003, 105(1-2):89-96.

[29] Shinbara H, Okubo M, Sumiya E, Fukuda F, Yano T, Kitade T: Effects of manual acupuncture with sparrow pecking on muscle blood flow of normal and denervated hindlimb in rats. *Acupunct Med* 2008, 26(3):149-159.

[30] Hui B, Rong PJ, Li L, Gao XY, He W: Effects of different acupuncture stimulations on NO content in acupoint areas. *J Tradit Chin Med* 2010, 30(1):25-29.

[31] Ma SX, Li XY, Sakurai T, Pandjaitan M: Evidence of enhanced non-enzymatic generation of nitric oxide on the skin surface of acupuncture points: An innovative approach in humans. *Nitric Oxide* 2007, 17(2):60-68.

[32] Ma SX, Li XY, Smith BT, Jou NT: Changes in nitric oxide, cGMP, and nitrotyrosine concentrations over skin along the meridians in obese subjects. *Obesity (Silver Spring)* 2011, 19(8):1560-1567.

[33] Jou NT, Ma SX: Responses of nitric oxide-cGMP release in acupuncture point to electroacupuncture in human skin in vivo using dermal microdialysis. *Microcirculation* 2009, 16(5):434-443.

[34] Kim DD, Pica AM, Duran RG, Duran WN: Acupuncture reduces experimental reno-vascular hypertension through mechanisms involving nitric oxide synthases. *Micro-circulation* 2006, 13(7):577-585.

[35] Ma SX: Enhanced nitric oxide concentrations and expression of nitric oxide synthase in acupuncture points/meridians. *J Altern Complement Med* 2003, 9(2):207-215.

Chapter 3

# Acupuncture in Modulation of Immunity

Sandra Silvério-Lopes and
Maria Paula Gonçalves da Mota

Additional information is available at the end of the chapter

http://dx.doi.org/10.5772/54286

## 1. Introduction

Acupuncture is one of the Traditional Chinese Medicine (TCM) and perhaps most important, by the way the world is widely used as a treatment effective, because it is more structured in terms of legislation, education and research. Until recently it was mostly known for its analgesic effects, and has an large number of research demonstrating the benefits in this area [1,2,3].Within the thinking of acupuncture, each individual should be treated as the disturbance of energy imbalance that presents itself at the time of the session, seeking the well-known syndromic diagnosis [4]. For the same pain can have many points in common from one patient to another, but there are known as energetic characteristics that complement the individualized treatment. Some acupuncture points, but they are consecrated by its clinical efficacy, repeated year after year as part of the arsenal of the specialist training in acupuncture and traditional literature of how these professionals, translated into different languages [4,5,6]. These acupuncture points and / or their combinations and how they are applied has ensured the continuity of its increasing use by the population for this ancient technique that has survived more than 2400 years of recorded history.

Currently, the scientific world investigating acupuncture in the search, especially to understand its mechanisms of action, the "whys" of their therapeutic efficacy, as is the energy system of energy meridians of the nature of acupoints and the brain impressions stimulated by acupuncture [7,8,9]· Another line of research aims to verify the possible use of acupuncture to cure difficult diseases such as: cancer and acquired immunodeficiency syndrome (AIDS) [10,11]. Complaints such as fatigue resulting from the stress are common in acupuncture clinics, and there is research demonstrating such benefits with acupuncture in treatment of fatigue in cancer patients [12]. Many of the gains and benefits referred to as energy acupuncture are based on the classic books, such as points capable of mobilizing the qi (energy) and xue (blood) [4]. Assuming that acupuncture improves vitality, science wants to know what the neuro-endocrine mechanisms, underlying biochemical [11]. Another line investigates whether these potential benefits can be extended to groups specific so far little exploited in research as gerontes, children and athletes [13].From the perspective of public health efforts are priorities immunologically vulnerable individuals, those most likely to get sick in the face of epidemics such as: children, elderly, pregnant women, immunosuppressed and immunodeficient [14].When comparing those most vulnerable, with the demands of patients in the acupuncture clinics, as well as in the research, notes that there are large numbers of elderly (gerontes), but very little children, pregnant women, immunosuppressed and imunodeficient patients. We believe the demand is low due to cultural issues, such as children and pregnant women afraid of needles. In immunodeficient and immunosuppressed patients there is no guidance of the benefits that acupuncture could provide, and some cultural preconceptions that isolate this resource as the possibility of complementary medicine, especially in the Western.The structure of this chapter, a brief look behind the immunity from the perspective of Traditional Chinese Medicine (TCM), then moving on to a more detailed study the applicability of acupuncture in the modulation of immunity, through a literature review, whose main focus is described in the methodology.

## 2. The pathogenesis and immunity against the perspective of Traditional Chinese Medicine (TCM)

The Traditional Chinese Medicine (TCM) has its pillars to support in philosophical foundations of Taoism, in a period of human history where there was no technological capabilities of modern diagnostics and treatments to cure of diseases. A need for greater interaction with the nature in the preservation of life, caused the man to develop a greater capacity for observing the natural cycles of climate change, time for crops, for work and home, the search for food, and therefore the preservation of health. As a result of observation and interaction with nature, the man identified prime materials for the cure of diseases and health preservation. Sustained for historical reasons there arose a form of healing spread in a philosophical and symbolic language, which for many today who do not study acupuncture / TCM appears be something still considered "mystical" or alien to Western rational mind. To understand the issue of immunity from the standpoint of TCM, it is necessary to recall some concepts that we will describe.

For TCM, the concept of health is the harmony or balance between yin and yang, or a perfect movement of the energy flow inside the body. Yin and yang are in turn defined as part of complementary and contradictory phenomena of nature and relate to each other [5].

From this reference, was formulated ratings patterns as well as supporting the symptoms syndromic, for example to be classified as ***Yin***; night, cold, weak, pale, chronic pathologic processes, fatigue, and classified as ***Yang*** their opposites; days, heat, strong, hyperemic, sharp,vitality. From the perspective western modern, we can say that there is a possible equivalence of classified the Sympathetic Nervous System (SNS) as *yang* and the Parasympathetic (SNP) as *Yin*.Is independent if the language to be Taoist symbolic or modern scientific, the body this whole time looking for this balance.Its is a dynamic process, and continue to sustain life. For the TCM the relationship health *vs* disease or loss of balance between *Yin* and *Yang* is related to the factors of resistance and organic etiological factors. Every day we face the many forms of climate change exposure, emotional imbalance, microorganisms, mechanical trauma, pollution, food with big load of pesticides and / or preservatives, these factors are considered etiological factors.The resistance factors in turn, are called in TCM with defense energy (*wei qi)* and are represented by the skin, mucous membranes, hair, controlling the opening and closing the pores and the sphincters of the body. An example that can illustrate when the body is affected by climate change like the wind-chill, it makes the hair stand on end in a shiver of cold, forming a protective voluminous layer and sequentially the pores are closed. In this state of trial protection as cited in this example, the body would result in the closing of the pores to retain the internal heat, which continued for more time will become pathological. This inbalance is expressed by some physiologic indicators of syndromic diagnosis of TCM.

Another example are some cases of urinary incontinence in the elderly, where the deficiency of *Yang* energy, represented by the weakness pelvic floor muscles, predisposes to not control the sphincters.

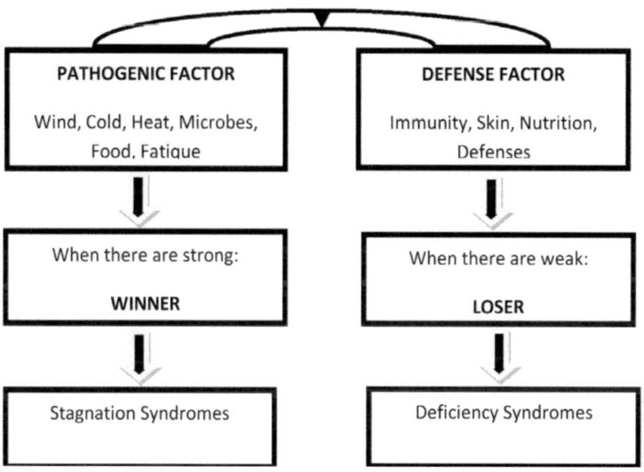


**Figure 1.** Pathogenic Factors *vs* Defense Factors

In this Figure 1 is showing two situations where the disease is established, because the defense factors are weak, or because the pathogenic factors are very strong, as occurs in viral epidemics where there is often an apparently healthy

Individual' immune profile might get sick. It is necessary to remember that when the TCM was formulated more than 2400 years ago, we had no knowledge of physiology, anatomy, biochemistry, and so little understanding of the immunology currently available for modern science. Is understandable within the context of the time theories were based on possibilities resources and understanding of man's relationship with the natural phenomena.

# 3. Applicability of acupuncture in the modulation of immunity: A literature review

## 3.1. Initial considerations and objectives

It is consistent the applicability of acupuncture in various phatological conditions.The modern science research resources to enhance health and quality of life. We understand that all possibilities to become viable are welcome. Although there are benefits of acupuncture modulation of immunity, there are gaps of knowledge,such as the best treatment techniques, which would be the best biochemical markers, which are the best acupoints.There is much information about research in this area, but they are highly dispersed, which causes difficulties in the conclusions, and thus clinical applicability.

The aim therefore of this review is to compile and discuss the scientific literature regarding the efficacy of acupuncture in modulation immunity.

## 3.2. Methodology

As from the selected article was organized some data that can help to support future work or point out gaps in knowledge,regarding the applicability of acupuncture in the modulation to immunity, choice of biochemical markers and immunomodulators acupuncture points.The use of systematic reviews as a means of research methodology, has increased,and has been shows to be of great contribuition and impacto internationally 1 [15]. To organize this chapter were considered scientific papers from journals, scientific repositories, MEDLINE, PUBMED, bibliography of articles on manual search, the Cochrane Library. The keywords "acupuncture and/or electroacupuncture in treatment of :"cancer", "immunossupressed"," immunodeficiency","allergic process","inflammation process","AIDS" and "modulation to immunity with acupuncture and/or electroacupuncture ".The reference lists of studies retrieved were examined to capture any other potentially relevant articles.

**The inclusion criteria were:**

**a.** Publication between january 2001 to december 2011.(The period was limited intentionally, because they understand that there was growing improvement in the methodology of scientific research, as well as growing interest in the field of acupuncture).

**b.** Clinical interventions and / or case studies, contain a description of immunological and biochemical markers, as well as the acupuncture points.

**c.** Experimental studies in human and / or animal,contain a description of immunological and biochemical markers, as well as the acupuncture points.

**d.** Reviews of clinical effectiveness of acupuncture, involving the key words.

**e.** Study of mechanisms of action of acupuncture modulation of immunity.

**Studies were excluded if they:**

a. Used mixed intervention whith other therapeutic techniques besides acupuncture and electroacupuncture, such as medication, surgery, physiotherapy.

b. Used mixed intervention whith other techniques of Traditional Chinese Medicine such as: moxibustion, herbal medicine,hot needles, auriculotherapy,bleeding and cupping.

**From the variables studied aimed to answer the following questions:**

a. Acupuncture is effective to strengthen the immunity?

b. What are the diseases or conditions are more studied?

c. What are the most appropriate markers to study the immunomodulatory effects of acupuncture?What are the most appropriate acupuncture points and designated for immunity?

d. What are the acupuncture techniques most frequently used in research on modulation of immunity ?

### 3.3. Results

The initial search identified 79 studies the databases. After reading these articles should were select and evaluated 67 relevant papers(Table 1 and 2). Table 1 shows the experimental and clinical studies with acupuncture,by humans and animals.In the Table 2 only the studies for style of a systematic review and / or models involving mechanisms of action of the immunity response to acupuncture. The summary of the data, were ordered by publication date, plus their respective authors, type of population, acupuncture technique, acupuncture points used and the main results or conclusions of the studies. From these structured to Figures 2 and 3 where only the most relevant results and those that are repeated in different papers, were considered. Tables 3 to 7 are summarized also derived from the contents carried compiled.

It can be seen by looking at Figure 2, the acupuncture point more tested in experimental studies in rats and humans was St 36 (Zusanli), together making a total of 39 articles (73.5%) of articles mentioning acupuncture points tested, and with animals, especially rats(14papers) and humans( 25papers).As related to the point ST36 with the population profiles found in animals, 48% with inflammation [16,18,23,26,30,39,41,46,48,54,59], 26% of post-surgical, trauma or stress induced by cold [21,31,34,38,56,57]), 13% with cancer [48,50,58], 9% with allergic processes [42,52] and only 4% of healthy individuals [35].However in humans, there were no highlights for either disease as an object of study, and found the use of St 36 in inflammation [63], cancer [47], allergic rhinitis [17,27,29], elderdy [19,65] and athletes [24], healthy [40],depression [64] In humans, the equivalence point with ST36 (Zusanli) appears LI4 (Hegu), with 14 and 12 papers respectively, and in 8 of these items, the points LI 4, and St36 are used simultaneously. In animals there was only one papers used LI 4 acupuncture point, separately, being expressed clearly in Figure 2.

| AUTHOR | YEAR | POPULATION | TECHNIQUE | POINTS | RESULTS/CONCLUSION |
|---|---|---|---|---|---|
| LI, YN.et al [16] | 2001 | rats<br>inflammation | EA | ST36 | ↓ IL2, TNFα,IL6 |
| PETTI, FB.et al [17] | 2002 | human<br>allergic rhinitis | ACP | ST36 ,LI4 | ↓IL 10<br>↑IL2<br>IL6 did not change |
| TIAN, L.et al [18] | 2002 | rats<br>ulcerative colitis | EA | ST36 | ↓ TNFα |
| KARST, M.et al [19] | 2002 | human<br>elderly | ACP | ST36,LI4,SP6 | Neutrophil and respiratory burst did not change |
| MORI, H. et al [20] | 2002 | human<br>healthy | EA | LI4, LU6 | ↓ Heart rate, stimulates SNP and suppresses SNS, modulates immunity, normalization of lymphocytes and granulocytes. |
| CHOI, GS. et al [21] | 2002 | rats<br>hypothalamic lesion | EA | ST36 | ↑NK cells |
| KARST, M.et al [22] | 2003 | human<br>healthy | ACP | LI11 | ↑ TNFα |
| TIAN, L. et al [23] | 2003 | rats<br>ulcerative colitis | EA | ST36 | ↓ IL6,IL8, TNFα |
| AKIMOTO, T.et al [24] | 2003 | human<br>athlets | ACP | ST36, LI4, ST6,<br>LU6 | ↑ IgA salivary<br>↓ salivary cortisol |
| YU, P.et al [25] | 2003 | human<br>Behcet's disease | ACP | No cites | ↓ IgM, Zn, and recurrence rate |
| PARK, MB.et al [26] | 2004 | mice<br>inflammation | EA | ST36 | ↓ IgE,IL4,IL13,inflammation<br>INFg did not change |
| NG, DK .et al [27] | 2004 | human<br>allergic rhinitis | ACP | ST36, yintang,<br>shanyingxiang | IL6, eosinophils did not change.<br>improvements in allergic symtoms |
| JOHANSEN, M.et al [28] | 2004 | human<br>healthy | ACP | LI4 | ↑ IL2, IFNg |
| MAGNUSSON,AL.et al [29] | 2004 | human<br>allergic rhinitis | ACP | LI4,LI20,ST36,L<br>R3,LU7, yintang | ↓ IgE<br>Allergic symptoms did not change |
| SCOGNAMILLO-SZABO,<br>MRV.et al [30] | 2004 | rats<br>inflammation | ACP | ST36,DU1 | ↓ Peritoneal neutrophils and bacterias. |
| HAHM, ET .et al [31] | 2004 | rats<br>hypothalamic lesion | EA | ST36 | ↑NK cells<br>EA restores the suppression of NK cells in hypothalamic lesion |
| SCOGNAMILLO-SZABO,<br>MRV.et al [32] | 2005A | Rats peritoneal<br>inflammation | ACP | DU20, yintang,<br>KI7 | ↓ IL1b<br>TNFα,IL10 did not change.<br>Antiinflammatory effects of ACP does not involve steroids. |
| SCOGNAMILLO-SZABO,<br>MRV.et al [33] | 2005<br>B | rats peritoneal<br>inflammation | ACP | K7, yintang<br>DU20 | ↓ neutrophils, inflammation |
| WANG, J.et al [34] | 2005 | rats<br>post-surgery | EA | ST36, lan wei | ↓ Lymphocyte apoptosis by inhibiting FAS protein andimmune depletion after surgery |
| KIM, CK .et al [35] | 2005 | rats healthy | EA | ST36 | ↑ NKcells |
| KOU, W.et al [36] | 2005 | human<br>healthy | ACP | ST36, LI11,<br>SP10, DU14 | ↓ CD3 CD8 CD4<br>↓ Leukocytes and lymphocytes. |

| AUTHOR | YEAR | POPULATION | TECHNIQUE | POINTS | RESULTS/CONCLUSION |
|---|---|---|---|---|---|
| | | | | | Did not change cortisol and norepinephrine |
| ZANG, RX.et al [37] | 2005 | rats inflammation | EA | GB30 | ↓ edema, inflammation↑ corticosterone |
| SHEN, GM.et al [38] | 2006 | rats cold stress | EA | ST36 | ↓ Gastric motility and nitric oxide. |
| HUANG, CL.et al [39] | 2006 | rats inflammation (lung) | ACP | ST36 | ↓ inflammatory injury<br>↓ nitric oxide and nitric oxide synthase |
| YAMAGUCHI, N.et al [40] | 2007 | human healthy | ACP | ST36, BL18, BL20, BL23 | ↑ CD2 CD4 CD8 CD11B CD16 CD19 e CD56 by exhaustion; activates macrophages |
| YIM, YK.et al [41] | 2007 | rats inflammation arthritis | EA | ST36 | ↓ IL6, TNF, INFy |
| LEE, Y.et al [42] | 2007 | allergic mice | EA | ST36 | ↓ IL4 anti CD3 and IgE block the allergic process |
| ARRANZ, L.et al [43] | 2007 | human anxious | ACP | LI4, ST36,SP6, GB34,GB43, LI11, PC6, SI3,RN3,RN4,RN6, RN15, HT5, HT3, SJ5 | Modulates the immune system to anxiety.<br>↑ phagocytosis, NK cells, lymphocytes;<br>↓ Reactive oxygen species (ROS)↓ anxiety |
| LU, W . et al [44] | 2007 | human after chemotherapy | ACP | No cites | ↑ leukocytes in leukopenic post chemotherapy (average of 1221 cells / ul) |
| LI , YM. et al [45] | 2007 | human allergic rhinitis | EA | LI20, yintang, shanyingxiang | ↓VIP, substance P |
| HUANG, CL.et al [46] | 2007 | rats inflammation (kidney/liver) | ACP | ST36 | -**ACP before treatment**:<br>↓ injury by inflammation (kidney)<br>↑ Nitric oxide renal and NO synthase,but did not occur in liver injury.<br>- **ACP post injury**: the inflammatory process is not contained in liver and kidney. |
| YE, F .et al [47] | 2007 | human after chemotherapy | EA | ST36,SP6,PC6 | ↓ Depletion of chemotherapy<br>did not change:IgG,IgM,IgA,CD3, CD4,CD8,NK cells, leukocytes |
| MAO, HJ.et al [48] | 2008 | rabbits leukopenia+ inflammation | EA | ST36, BL17 DU 14 | ↓ leukocyte inflammatory process<br>↑ leukocytes in leukopenia. |
| ZHANG, LJ.et al [49] | 2008 | human mammary hyperplasia | EA e ACP | BL23, DU4, DU16, KI24, KI22,LR14 | ↑CD4 ,CD8 |
| LAI, M. et al [50] | 2008 | rats /cancer | EA | ST36,LR4,SP6 | ↑ IgA,IgG,IgM,CD4<br>↓CD8 |
| YAN, J.et al [51] | 2009 | rats | EA | ST37 | ↑IL4 |

| AUTHOR | YEAR | POPULATION | TECHNIQUE | POINTS | RESULTS/CONCLUSION |
|---|---|---|---|---|---|
| | | ulcerative colitis | | | ↓IL1b |
| KIM, SK.et al [52] | 2009 | mice/allergy | EA | ST36 | ↓ IL4 e IgE<br>Effects independent of frequency |
| GAO, H. et al [53] | 2009 | human allergy | ACP | DU11 | ↓ IgE, did not change symptoms |
| FERREIRA, AS.et al [54] | 2009 | rats<br>inflammation<br>(lung) | ACP | ST36 | ↓ Inflammatory process (neutrophils, lymphocytes, total leukocytes, monocytes). Acupuncture was prophylactic. |
| LU, W.et al [55] | 2009 | human after chemotherapy | EA | ST36,LI4, LI11, SP6, LR3, DU20, SP10,LU6,KI3 | CSFg did not change<br>↑ leukocytes, softened effects chemotherapy |
| WANG, J .et al [56] | 2009 | rats<br>surgical injury | EA | ST36 | Inhibits inflammatory cytokines↓ inflammation |
| WANG, K.et al [57] | 2009 | rats<br>surgical injury | EA | ST36 ,*lanwei* | ↑IL2,INFα |
| LEE, HJ.et al [58] | 2009 | rats<br>cancer | EA | ST36 | ↑ 51.46% more β endorphin in blood and 12.6% in the brain compared to the untreated group.↓ Substance P |
| SENA-FERNANDES, V.et al [59] | 2010 | rats<br>inflammation | ACP | ST36,SP6 | ST36 is better than anti-inflammatory SP6 for gastrointestinal disorders. |
| MATSUBARA, Y.et al [60] | 2010 | human sedentary | EA | ST36, LI4, LU6, ST6 | Acupuncture attenuates the decrease in salivary IgA caused by physical exhaustion. |
| KARST,M.et al [61] | 2010 | human<br>healthy | ACP | LI11 | ↑ IL8<br>TNFα,IL 10 and endorphin did not alter |
| HAN, YF. et al [62] | 2010 | human<br>leukopenic | ACP | SJ6,IG4,IG11 | ↑ $CSF_g$ , ↑ maturation of neutrophils |
| OUYANG, BS.et al [63] | 2010 | human<br>rheumatoid arthritis | ACP, EA | ST36,LI11,SJ5G B20,RM4, DU20 | ↓ IL1, IL4, IL6,IL10, |
| SUN, H. et al [64] | 2010 | human<br>depressive | EA | ST36,DU20 | ↓ IL1, IL6<br>TNFα not changed |
| PAVAO, TS.et al [65] | 2010 | human<br>elderly | ACP | LI4,ST36,SP6 | ↑ lymphocytes T |
| SILVA, MD.et al [66] | 2010 | rats<br>peritoneal<br>inflammation | ACP | SP6 | ↑ IL10 and ↓ adrenal stimulation by inflammation; not changed TNF α e IL1b |
| YUAN, SY.et al [67] | 2011 | human<br>prostatites | EA | RM3,ST29, SP9,SP6,RM4,ST 28,SP10, LR3 | ↓ IL10,IL8,TNFα |

ACP= acupuncture

EA=electroacupuncture

**Table 1.** Experimental and clinical studies on acupuncture modulation of immunity

| AUTHOR | YEAR | APPROACH | TECHNIQUE | POINTS | CONCLUSION |
|---|---|---|---|---|---|
| ZIJLSTRA, FJ.et al [68] | 2003 | immunophysiological (inflammation) | ACP | No cites | ACP has pro-inflammatory effects with ↓ TNF, and anti-inflammatory with ↑ IL10 |
| CHEN, JX et al [69] | 2006 | neuroimmunological | ACP | Meridians and acupoints | In the acupuncture point and meridians is increased norepinephrine, and modulation of L-arginine-derived nitric oxide by the SNS (sympathetic nervous system) |
| CHO, ZH. et al [70] | 2006 | neurophysiological and neuroimaging | ACP/EA | No cites | Acupuncture acts in neurophysiology and molecular basis, and its effects can be evaluated mechanisms also by functional magnetic resonance (fRMI) and tomography |
| MA, XM.et al [71] | 2007 | immunohistochemical of the meridians and acupuncture points | ACP | Meridians: Pericardium and Bladder | The nitric oxide is at high levels in the skin surface in the acupoints and meridians and no nitrate is reduced by skin bacteria. |
| KAVOUSSI, B; ROSS, BE. [72] | 2007 | immunophysiological (inflammation) | ACP | E36 mechanisms of action | ↓TNFα,IL6,IL18,IL1b macrophages. |
| CABIOGLU, MT ; CETIN, BE [73] | 2008 | neurophysiological | EA e ACP | No cites | ACP EA and modulate the immune system, for local , neuronal and neurohumoral expression. |
| PENG, G [74] | 2008 | neurophysiological | ACP | No cites | ACP makes immunomodulation by complex mechanisms of the HPA axis and cholinergic anti inflammatory pathways. |
| ROBERTS, J et al [75] | 2008 | allergic rhinits/clinical efficacy | ACP | No cites | There is no sufficient evidence that the ACP is effective.. |
| BRINKHAU, SB .et al [76] | 2008 | allergic rhinits/clinical efficacy | ACP | No cites | ACP has clinical efficacy |
| LEE, MS et al [77] | 2009 | allergic rhinits/clinical efficacy | ACP | No cites | ACP has clinical efficacyFuture studies require inclusion of groups shan, controls, and larger samples |
| TAKAHASHI,T.et al [78] | 2009 | immunophysiological | EA e ACP | No cites | - ACP modulation function and number of neutrophils;<br>↓ Apoptosis after injury and FAS protein;<br>- EA ↓ norepinephrine corticosterone B endorphin and ACTH in stress |

| AUTHOR | YEAR | APPROACH | TECHNIQUE | POINTS | CONCLUSION |
|---|---|---|---|---|---|
| HE,TF et al [79] | 2011 | rheumatoid arthritis | EA | ST36,GB39,V23 | ↓ edema, ↑ VIP (vasoactive intestinal peptide) |
| JOHNSTON,MF.et al [11] | 2011 | human and rats cancer | ACP | Mecanisms of ACP in the prevention of cancer | It increases the cytotoxic activity of NK cells by cross effect between neurotransmitters and the immune system (nitric oxide, endorphins, cytokines). |
| MANNI, L.et al [80] | 2011 | neuroimmunological | EA | No cites | There is a biochemical synergism between EA and neurotrofina NGF, which explains immunologic improvement. |

ACP= acupuncture

EA=electroacupuncture

**Table 2.** Papers with mechanism of action models of acupuncture in immunomodulation and reviews.

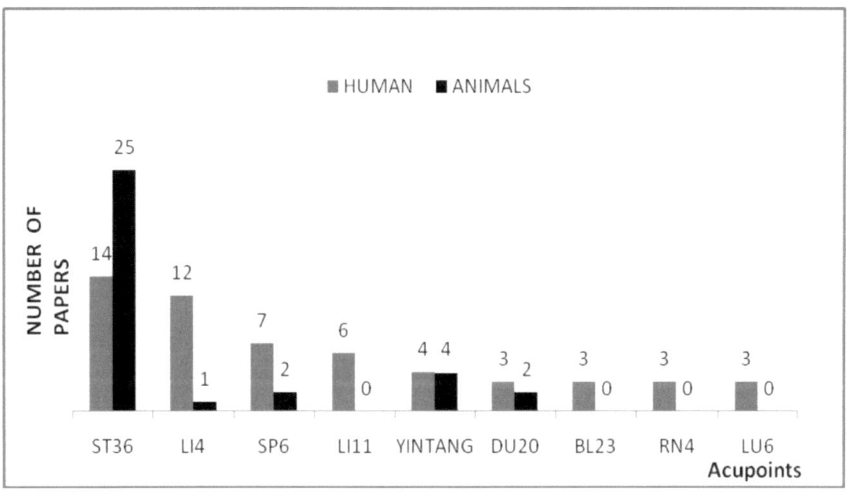


**Figure 2.** Main immunomodulators acupuncture points cited on the papers.

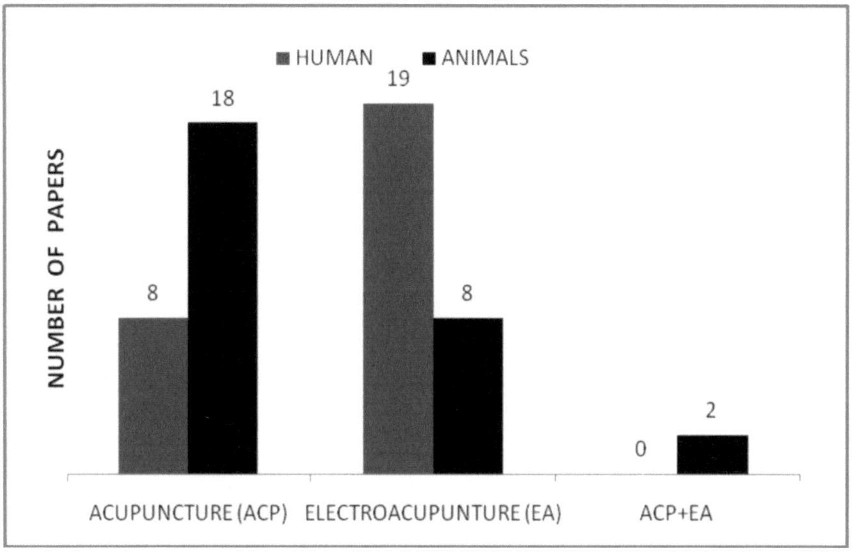


**Figure 3.** Number of papers *vs* techniques

In view of the purposes stated in the methodology of this review, prepared to Figure 3, which shows the distribution of numbers of papers regarding the use of the techniques of acupuncture (ACP) and electroacupuncture (EA) or both simultaneously (ACP + EA). Of the 56 papers that reported the technique used, 26 papers used ACP, 27 EA and 2 used both techniques (ACP + EA).

Elaborated the tables 3 to 7 on the basis of immunological and biochemical markers found in the papers of this study.

| markers | IL1β | IL2 | IL 4 | IL 6 | IL 8 | IL 10 | IL 18 | Total |
|---|---|---|---|---|---|---|---|---|
| **increase** | --- | 3 | 1 | --- | 3 | 2 | --- | 9 |
| **decrease** | 5 | 1 | 4 | 5 | 1 | 3 | 1 | 20 |
| **no change** | 1 | --- | --- | 2 | --- | 2 | --- | 5 |

**Table 3.** Number of papers that used Interleukins (IL) *vs* effects of acupuncture or electroacupuncture.

Table 3 shows the number of papers mentioning the Interleukins (IL) and immunological markers in studies with acupuncture or electroacupuncture. If we add all papers, where after acupuncture decreased the Interleukins, make up 58% versus 27%, which increased and 15% that have not changed.

| markers | CD 2 | CD 3 | CD 4 | CD 8 | CD11B | CD 16 | CD 19 | CD 56 |
|---|---|---|---|---|---|---|---|---|
| **increase** | 1 | 2 | 4 | 5 | 3 | 1 | 1 | 1 |
| **decrease** | --- | 2 | 2 | 2 | 1 | --- | --- | --- |
| **no change** | --- | --- | --- | --- | --- | --- | --- | --- |

**Table 4.** Number of papers that used markers CD vs effects of acupuncture or electroacupuncture.

Table 4 expressed a distribution of the papers mentioning the immunological markers of type CD. It is felt that there was a higher concentration in the selection of CD4 and CD8 markers. Important to note that the use of CD11b, CD16, CD19 and CD59, it is one and the same article [40]. There is a distribution of 72% of the papers where there were increases in CD, compared with 28% reduction and no article with "no change" after the intervention with acupuncture or electroacupuncture.

| markers | Leukocytes | Eosinophils | Lymphocytes | Moncytes | Neutrophils |
|---|---|---|---|---|---|
| **increase** | 3 | --- | 2 | --- | 2 |
| **decrease** | 3 | --- | 2 | 1 | 2 |
| **no change** | 1 | 1 | --- | --- | 1 |

**Table 5.** Number of papers used for Blood cells *vs* effects of acupuncture or electroacupuncture.

In the Table 5 were grouped the blood cells, relating them to their results after the intervention of acupuncture or electroacupuncture. Were the most representative use of total leukocytes, primarily found in 38% of the papers, followed by, lymphocytes and neutrophils, with 26% each, and eosinophils, monocytes with 5% each.

| markers | increase | decrease | no change |
|---|---|---|---|
| **Ig A** | 3 | --- | 1 |
| **Ig E** | --- | 4 | --- |
| **Ig M** | --- | 1 | --- |
| **IFNg/y** | 2 | 1 | 1 |
| **CSFg** | --- | 2 | --- |
| **TNFα** | 1 | 7 | 3 |
| **NK cells** | 5 | -- | --- |
| **endorphins** | --- | 13 | --- |

**Table 6.** Immune-biochemicals markers after the intervention; effects of acupuncture or electroacupuncture.

http://dx.doi.org/10.5772/54286

In the Table 6,are grouped the markers that were present in at least three or more papers. Were excluded from the markers that were cited in the minority (IgG, cortisol, CGFS, lymphocyte apoptosis, VIP (vasoactive intestinal peptide), substance P, reactive oxygen species (ROS), nitric oxide and macrophages).

| characteristics | increase | decrease | no change |
|---|---|---|---|
| **inflammation** | - | 8 | 1 |
| **symptoms** | - | 13 | 2 |

**Table 7.** Distribution of the presence of terms of service and Symptoms Inflammation X after the intervention effects with acupuncture and electroacupuncture.

To end the presentation of results was elaborated in Table 7 that grouped the papers about some terms that, although generic, were explicit in the results and / or completion of the articles studied. Since the terms chosen: **inflammation** and **clinical symptoms**. Of the articles that included in their conclusions applicability of techniques for ACP and EA the terms inflammation, in the 88% of the papers cited have demostrated decrease, and only 11,2% cited,no change in the inflamatory process.No papers cited the occurrence of increased inflamatory process.When refers to symptoms have been reported in articles 15, and these 86,6% it is stated that reduction of pathological symptoms studied, and there were no changes 13,3%. No papers mentioned that the pathological symptoms increased. Among the symptoms referred to in these papers are specific: present in respiratory allergy rhinitis, edema, depression, physical exhaustion, adverse effects of chemotherapy and anxiety.

### 3.4. Discussion

#### *3.4.1. As for immunomodulation effects and clinical efficacy*

The ACP and EA its shares in neurophysiology and molecular basis [70]·Its effects and mechanism of action can be evaluated by magnetic resonance imaging and computed tomography [70]. Ma [71] following another line of study, demonstrated the immunohistological nature of the meridians and acupoints, where he verified that there is high concentration of nitric oxide. The immunomodulatory effects of ACP and EA are confirmed by studies with diverse biochemical markers described in Table 1.

They are among the principal effects immunomodulatory:

**a.** Decrease of celular apoptopsis

**b.** Increase cytotoxic activity

**c.** Synergism biochemical between the EA and neurotrophyn(NGF)

**d.** Mobilization of corticosterone,endorphine and ACTH.

**e.** Pro-inflamatory and antinflamatory effects.

We observed that acupuncture has clinical efficacy in some situations, as in allergic processes, and in pain [1,2,3]. In other stages as inflammation can reduce or block the inflammatory process, but will depend on the stage he is and also the origin of this process. Recall for example in case of tendonitis, that acupuncture can reduce pain, edema, hyperemia, provide gain range of motion.However the origin of tendinitis is caused by repetitive strain, compression of nerve roots, weakness or muscle shortening, which in these cases need conventional physiotherapy intervention, exercise, manipulation, and / or resting muscle.Finally we have a group of pathogenic conditions where acupuncture may improve symptoms and quality of life, but the effect is still very poor immunological results and research in the area are being made, as in the case of degenerative processes, immunodeficient [10] and immunosuppressed patients [60]. In patients or cancer models, as well as elderly, where usually has low of immunity defenses, the acupuncture and electroacupuncture demonstrated in this study that increases the immunity, being a possibility of complementary therapeutic resource.In the acute or cronic inflammation and allergic processes ACP and/or EA demonstrated modulate the immune response, decreasing the hyperresponsiveness of the markers pro – inflammatory [48].

*3.4.2. As for the immunologic markers*

*3.4.2.1. Interleukins (IL)*

Interleukins (IL) constitute a class of cytokines, and soluble proteins that act as humoral regulators at nano or picomolar concentration by modulating the functional activities of cells and tissues through specific receptors of target cells [81]. In this study, we included studies of acupuncture in humans and animals, whereas several groups with different immune deficits, such as those with cancer, allergies, physical exhaustion, inflammation, and studies with healthy groups. In general there were more studies demonstrating that after acupuncture decreases interleukins, with 58% of research, compiled and summarized in Table 4. Were 27% that increased and 15% of the research there were no changes. It is understood that specificity is in the release of each group of interleukins. Some authors demonstrate that IL-6 [82] and IL10 [83] may increase after intense physical exhaustion, simulating an "inflammatory reaction" while IL8 increase but at a later continuous process of exhaustion [83]. In this review, it was shown that IL6 interleukin decreased after acupuncture in 5 of 7 of the articles has been markers, slowing a reduced immunological response. The interleukin appeared in two papers which show increase [66,68], where tree have decrease [17,63,67] and two no change [32,61], the results so far divided.Tian et al [18] in a research with EA says it is still unknown whether electroacupuncture can keep the balance between the anti-inflammatory and pro-inflamatory cytokines.He further states that the specific mechanisms of regulation of IL4, IL10 and IL13, when acupuncture have decreased these pro-inflammatory cytokines not been totally elucidated. Perhaps this explanation justifies the inconclusive results of the use of IL10 in our review.

*3.4.2.2. Blood cells*

**a.** Total leukocyte and interleukins acute stage

As for total leukocytes, as shown in Table 6, there was a decrease in 43% of research [36,48,54].Had increased by 43% [44,48,55] and in 14% of papers no change [47].Is remarkable to note that the papers that report that acupuncture increased the total leukocytes, are all with a population of leukopenic patients after chemotherapy, and in papers that report decreased after acupuncture are affected population inflammatory process. This data, demonstrate that acupuncture can both increase or decrease the inflammatory response, corroborating with Zijlstra [68], whose author claims that acupuncture has immunomodulatory effect. According to Silva [84],the leukocytes produce IL-1 and IL-6 among the main defense markers in acute inflammatory response. Looking at Table 4 the papers that were used as a marker of immune IL1, 86% after acupuncture had a decrease [32,51,63,64,72], and 14% no change [66]. The IL-1 has a similar function to the tumor necrosis factor (TNF), which is to mediate the innate immune response in especially inflammatory type.The main cellular source of IL-1 second as report by Abbas [85] are th'activated mononuclear phagocytes.

In the specific case of IL6, 75% of the papers that used this marker, decreased after acupuncture [23,41,63,64,72] against 25% no change [17,27]. It is noteworthy that all the items where IL1 and IL6 are decreased refer by population studies with inflammatory processes. This fact therefore confirms the literature and demonstrates that acupuncture can be an resource to inhibit the firing of immune responses to acute inflammatory origin. The mechanism for this increase suggests, is associated with the fact that IL-6 produced by fibroblasts and mononuclear phagocytes in response to IL-1 stimulates the hepatocytes to synthesize acute phase proteins, which act on the hypothalamus. Cooper [86] in his studies, concluded that the mechanism of action by which acupuncture makes its immunomodulatory effects are associated with stimulation of the hypothalamic-pituitary-adrenal axis, showing links between the endocrine,nervous and immune systems.

Enhancing the action of acupuncture and electroacupuncture in immunomodulation of the acute process was found 64% reduction in the articles that have been used as a marker of TNF [16,18,23,41,67,68,72],compared with 27% of the articles without change [61,64,66], and only 10% with an increase [22]. The studies in oncology are of unquestionable importance. Leukopenia is a constant in cancer patients submitted to chemotherapy.In the research compiled here, showed that the ACP and EA can modulate in a positive way by increasing leukocytes [44,48,55]. Lu, W.et al [44] came to the conclusion in a study involving humans with EA after chemotherapy there was an average increase of 1221 white cells / ul. These data are encouraging, especially if added to increase the cytotoxic activity of NK cells, as reported by other authors [11,21,31,35,43].

**b.** Lymphocyte

As for lymphocytes, no conclusive interpretation in the literature, for some authors, such as Lu et al [55] and Pavão et al [65], that acupuncture said increases lymphocytes, while others such as Kou et al [36] and Ferreira et al [54] found a decrease in their research.

This apparent contradiction of results must be interpreted in light of the the therapeutic objectives that acupuncture provides to different pathological conditions. Evaluating the articles can see that those among populations where there was an increase of lymphocytes, are patients with cancer and inflammatory processes. In these cases, therefore it is desirable that there is an increase in defenses

Furthermore, papers which show after acupuncture lymphocytes decreased were evaluated in a population with predominantly inflammatory process, therefore also a desirable result. It is concluded therefore that acupuncture has an immunomodulatory effect, can raise or lower the lymphocytes, depending on immuno-pathogenic requirements. In cellular immunity, T cells CD4+, activates macrophages to destroy phagocytosed microorganisms while CD8+ T lymphocyte,kill infected cells whiyh intracellular microbes [85]· The Complement System, consisting of serum glycoproteins and cell membrane, which along with the antibodies form the main mediators of the humoral immune response in the inflammatory process [85].The compiled studies show that acupuncture helps in stimulating this pathway of immune response, with 72% who used the results of immunochemical markers CD system, pointing to an increased presence of complement, after the intervention [40,49]. All research were performed in humans with cancer and also healthy, submitted to physical exhaustion, pointing to possibilities of acupuncture not only strengthen the immune process, but also be preventive. As for the markers of the complement system there was no consensus on what would be the most suitable. Of the five papers in the literature, the data were repeated if more CD4 + and CD8 + T cells.

The lymphocytes T, still produce CD3,IL2,IL4,IL5,IL6,IL8,IL10,IL13 and IFNy. With this comprehension is justifiable the increase demonstrated in the distribution illustrated in the Table 4. The papers, where CD3, CD4 and CD8 presented decrease after the acupuncture [36,54], were singularly at the same population profiles where there were lymphocytes decrease (stress,inflammation). Agrees, therefore desirable this decrease, like form of blocking the of the inflammatory process.

*3.4.2.3. Immunoglobulins (Ig)*

The immunoglobulins or antibodies represent a glycoproteins family related structurally, produced by the lymphocytes B, linked or secreted by cellular membrane [85].Among immunoglobulins, find IgA present in great quantity in mucosal. Akimoto [24]and Gleesen [87] show that IgA salivate decreases in exercises exhausting case, as well as the population of total lymphocytes predisposing especially athletes population the diseases of the respiratory treatment. The results expressed in the Table 6, they demonstrate that the acupuncture can increase IgA indices after exhaustion as in physical depletion cancer processes [24,50,60], signalling for acupuncture possible benefits in immunomodalation. Other immunoglobulin related in the papers was Ig E. According Abbas. [85], individuals with allergic process is found high levels of immunoglobulin IgE, in response to environment allergens, in the same way that IL4. In 100% of the papers that used IgE as markers, the results found after the acupuncture went of reduction in the serum levels [26,29,52,53].In the same way found a coherence in the citations of other authors, white respect to decrease to IL4 after the acupuncture

[26,42,52,63]. Such fact corroborates with a tendency for consensus that the acupuncture effect is immunomodulators in the allergic processes, being. Therefore IgE and IL4 are the best markers for researches and clinical support.

*3.4.2.4. Markers of adaptive immune response*

According to Abbas [85] the immunity immunity also known as it specifies is mediated by the lymphocytes and stimulated by infectious agents. It characterizes by the rare specificity of the distinct macromolecules and memory. They make her part the liberation of comprises the following cytokines: TNF$\alpha$, IFNy or gamme (g) that then it stimulates the interleukin proliferation IL2.The production of interferon IFNy (in animals) and IFNg (in humans) is produced starting from NK cells activated and lymphocytes T(effectors). Is consistent data that demostrate the correlation among the increases of NK cells and IFNy/g. The studies that were used of interferon IFNy/g with marker, there were 50% of the papers with increase [28,57], 25% with reduction [41] and 25% no change [26]after the acupuncture or eletroacupuncture. As for IL2 also followed the same line of results, with increase serum levels predominance with 75% of the papers that were used of this marker relating increase [17,28,57] and 25% decrease [15].

Although NK cells are part of the innate immune response, and not the adaptive response, this class of lymphocytes trigger the release of the adaptive response through the production of interferon (IFN). In our studies was verified in the Table 7 that in 100% of these papers,were used of the NKcells as markers, there was increase after acupuncture and electroacupuncure [11,21,31,35,43]. There were no papers that are used as a marker of NK cells expressed reduction. Therefore the result obtained in studies of NK cells are consistent to those found with IFN, demonstrating that the ACP and EA immunomodulators.

### 3.5. As for the acupuncture points

The acupuncture point is specified location along the route known as meridians. Although known by physicians for thousands of years, acupuncture points or acupoints as they are known, attracted a few decades ago the condition of being surveyed with modern resouces. Chen et al [69] showed that the acupuncture points and meridians is increased norepinephrine, and modulation of arginine,derived nitric oxide by the sympathetic nervous system (SNS). Ma et al [71] also found high concentrations of nitric oxide, and these did not suffer reduced to nitrate by bacteria in skin. The acupoint ST 36 has its original name as *Zusanli,* in chinese *ZU* means foot, and three *SAN LI* distance, translated as the point that "tones the body to walk long distances" [6]. It is a point used in clinical routine as a useful point to treat fatigue and low immunity, and analgesics, which goes against the findings in the studied articles, where the results shows that the ST36 is the most researched, both in humans and in animals.and is its present in 73.5% of the papers. We believe that this effect occurs because of the ease and stability in the anatomical containment and retention in rats when compared with other points, and because there is an established animal model in this location [52].The LI 4 was the second most cited in humans, with 12 papers. This acupoint is easily located on the back of the hand between the first and second metacarpal, within the second half of the metacarpal bone, is very suitable in the literature for improving immunity in particular inflammation, fever, and as a powerful analgesic [4,5]. However it is observed that no uniformity in relation to the use of this point in the human population under study, with respect to pathologies. It was used in work with proposed immunity in asthmatic subjects, anxious, healthy, sedentary and athletes. In animals, however there was only one article that used the LI 4.

We believe that is due to the high pain sensitivity, found in the distal portion of forepaws and little anatomical support, which would make the containment of animals and maintenance of the needles.Although escarces research, the use of aggregate LI 4 acupoint appears to others. Can not conclude therefore that the immunomodulatory effect shown is resulting from the isolated use of LI 4, as occurred with ST36.

### 3.6. The use of techniques of acupuncture (ACP) and electroacupuncture (EA)

The act of dry needling, known with acupuncture is the most technique standard of Traditional Chinese Medicine. Known millennially is widely used in clinical and research of acupuncture in humans and / or animals. In our study we noticed an homogenic distribution between the techniques, in the papers that used the ACP with 47% against 49% who used EA, and 4% with both techniques: ACP + EA. It was found as expressed in Figure 3 a greater number of papers with ACP in humans, animals and against EA was correspondingly higher. As the technique of acupuncture to more classic and old, it's understandable that it is more accepted in research with humans, both for its ease of operation, whether the receptivity of the volunteer. Recalling that there for fear of "get a shock," in EA justification is consistent with other authors [2].

Electroacupuncture compared with classical acupuncture with dry needling, is relatively more recent In approaching to research, and clinical applicability has much to be investigated, especially as regards the physical parameters that EA should follow to achieve their therapeutic effects [3], although their use is spreading might rate around the world. Cabioglu [73] dont differs in its conclusions, the ACP and EA, allocating both the fact that modulate the immune system for local, neuronal and neurohumoral expression.

The ways in which EA works in the body is well studied with regard to their analgesic effects [2], but very little about their imunomodulatory effects in order to differentiate it from ACP. In our studies we found only one papers [78] which conclude that differences in the various substances to be detected, demonstrated in Table 2. The way the immune mechanism of action of EA suggested by this author proposes that EA inhibits excessive ACTH in the processes of stress. Johnston et al [11] studying the mechanism of action of ACP on cancer prevention found that there is an increase of cytotoxic activity of NK cells by cross effect between neurotransmitters and immune system (nitric oxide, endorphins, and cytokines). Remember that EA in the case of the effect of electric current enhances the release of endorphins, a mechanism already well studied in analgesia [3].By crossing the use of EA to the research, it was not found relationship as the selection of immune-biochemical markers. However the majority of studies with EA,were carried with inflammation experimental models. It is believed that because of the ease induction of inflammation in animal models it has been a relevant factor and consequently represented by a large percentage (70%) of perpers with EA.

## 4. Final remarks

The studies compiled in this chapter, shows that the ac and EA are effective in the modulation of immunity.In these final remarks aimed to answer the questions proposed in this study.

The best markers for acute inflammatory processes are: IL1, IL6 and TNF alpha, and it is desired decrease in majority cases with ACP and EA. The best markers for allergic processes are IgE and IL4.

With respect to count of eosinophil cell, was not conclusive for the scarce number of papers in whith they where present. There were no articles describing the C-reactive protein (CRP) as a biochemical marker. We recommend its use in future research. Is relevancy the number of papers that relate in their conclusions, the reference to the generic term of "inflammation" as well as of "clinical symptoms". As described in the methodology, were excluded studies which were based on exclusively on symptomatic evaluation, but in 15 papers appear in their conclusions with immunological and / or biochemical markers, the terminology such as inflammation and symptoms. We believe it is a way to supplement the data by adding a reference to qualitative and quantitative, which has its importance and merit. The ST36(Zusanli) acupoint, was the most studied regarding immunomodulation in humans and animals and to for demonstrating satisfactory effects. We recommends your use in the clinic and research. The LI 4(*Hegu*) acupoint was so as screened for the ST36. However all the research this point appears along with others. We suggest to research the LI 4 acupoint in modulation of immunity, in an isolated manner, because can not conclude that the immunomodulatory effect shown is resulting from the isolated use of LI 4, as occurred with ST36.We suggest comparative research between the ACP and use of EA modulation of immunity. It is necessary also to EA more research in humans, because we observed that most research made in this technique occurs in animals.The modern science advances to each moment, for wide steps, especially with regard to technological resources for evaluation. However the human suffering still persists, especially for the ones that do not have access to sources.As a researcher and expert in acupuncture more than two decades ago, we imagine there is still understandings that underlie the basic theories of TCM, acupuncture with respect to the future will be revealed comprehensible from the viewpoint of immunology.

## Author details

Sandra Silvério-Lopes[1] and Maria Paula Gonçalves da Mota[2]

1 Faculdade de Tecnologia do IBRATE (Instituto Brasileiro de Therapias e Ensino), Curitiba, Brasil

2 Universidade Trás-os-Montes e Alto Douro (UTAD)/Centro de Investigação em Desporto e Desenvolvimento Humano (CIDESD), Portugal

## References


[1] Witt CM, Jena S, Beinkhaus B, Liecker B. Wegscheider K, Willich SN. Acupuncture for patients with chronic neck pain. Pain. 2006;125:107-113.

[2] Silvério-Lopes S, Nohama P. Influencia da freqüência estimulatória envolvida nos efeitos analgésicos induzidos por eletroacupuntura em cervicalgia tensional. Revista Brasileira de Fisioterapia. 2009;13(2):52-158.

[3] Silvério-Lopes S. Electroacupuncture and stimulatory frequencies in analgesia. In: Saad,M(ed.) Acupuncture,concepts and physiology. Rijeka(Croatia): In Tech ; 2011.p69-90.

[4] Macioccia G. A Prática da Medicina Chinesa. São Paulo, Roca; 2009.

[5] Yamamura Y. A arte de Inserir. São Paulo: Roca; 2009.

[6] Coste M, Paugam JY. Acupuncture Tradition et Recherche Moderne. La Nef Chastrusse. 2006.

[7] Liu J, Qin W, Sun J, Sun K, Yuan K, Liu P et al. Distint Brain Networks for Time-varied Characteristics of Acupuncture. Neuroscience Letters. 2010;468:353-358.

[8] Liu P, Zhanh Y, Zhou GY, Yuan K, Qin W, Zhou, Lu et al. Partial Correlation Investigation on the Defaut Mode Network Involved in Acupuncture: An FMRI Study; Neuroscience Letters. 2009;462:183-187.

[9] Kong J, Gollub RL, Rosman IS, Webb JM, Vangel MG, Kirsch I et al. Brain Activity Associated with Expectancy-Enhanced Placebo Analgesia as Measured by Funcional Magnetic Resonance Imaging. The Journals of Neuroscience. 2006;26(2):381-388.

[10] Yongping J, Stefanovic J. The Acupuncture and Treatment of Peripheral Neuropaty in HIV/AIDS. Journal Chinese Medicine. 2002;68:27-29.

[11] Johnston MF, Sánches EO, Vujanovic NL, Li W. Acupuncture May Stimulate Anticancer Immunity via Activation of Natural Killer Cells. Oxford University Press. 2011;1-14.

[12] Mota DDCF,Pimenta CAM. Fadiga em pacientes com câncer avançado:conceito,avaliação e intervenção.Revista Brasileira de Cancerologia.2002,48(4) 577-583.

[13] So RCH, Joseph KFN, Gabriel YFN. Effect of Transcutaneous electrical acupoint stimulation on fadigue recovery of quadriceps. European Journal Applied Phisiology. 2007;100:693-700.

[14] De Lavor,A. Foco nas populações vulneráveis e excluídas.Radis,Comunicação e Saúde.Fundação Oswaldo Cruz. Rio de Janeiro,2012(115);22-23.

[15] Leitão JC, Fernandes C, Campaniço J, Pereira A, Mota P, Bodas AR, Bento T, Vicente J, Cortinhas A. Metodologia de Investigação em Educação Física e Desporto:introdução a revisão sistemática.UTAD,Vila Real(Portugal),2010.

[16] Li YN, Huang YX. The effects of brain gut peptides and cytokines on the acupuncture's modulatory mechanism in the gastrointestinal immunity. Shijie Huaren Xiaohua Zazhi. 2001;9:329-332.

[17] Petti FB, Liquori A, Ippoliti F. Study on cytokines IL2, IL6, IL10 in patients of chronic allergic rhinitis treated with acupuncture. Journal Traditional Chinese Medicine. 2002; 22(2): 104-111.

[18] Tian L, Huang YX, Wen QS, Li YM, Zhao HF, Wang QL. Therapeutic effect and mechanism of electro-acupuncture on rats with ulcerative colitis. World Chinese Journal Digestolology. 2002; 10(8): 916-921.

[19] Karst M, Scheinichen D, Rueckert T, Wagner T, Wiese B, Fink M. Acupuncture has no immediate treatment effect on the neutrophil respiratory burst: a randomized simple-blinded two period crossover study. Brain Behavoir Immunonoly. 2002; 16 (6):813-816.

[20] Mori H, Alishijo K, Kawomura H, Ako T. Unique immunomodulation by electro-acupuncture in humans possibly stimulation of the autonomic nervous systems. Neuroscience Letters. 2002;320:21-24.

[21] Choi GS, Oh SD, Han JB, Bae HS, Cho YW, Yun YS et al. Modulation of natural killer cell activity affected by electroacupuncture through lateral hypothalamic area in rats. Neuroscience Letters. 2002; 329: 1-4.

[22] Karst M, Scheinichen D, Rueckert T, Warner T, Wiese B, Piepenbrock S et al. Effect of acupuncture on the neutrophil respiratory burst: a placebo controlled single blinded study. Complementary Therapies in Medicine. 2003; 11: 4-10.

[23] Tian L, Huang YX, Gao W,Chang Q. Down regulations of electroacupuncture at ST36 on TNFa, in rats with ulcerative colitis. World Journal Gastroenterology. 2003; 9(5): 1028-1033.

[24] Akimoto T, Nakahori C, Aizawa K, Kimura F, Fu-Kubayashi T, Kono I. Acupuncture and responses of immunologic and endocrine markers during competition. Medicine & Science M Sports & Exercice.2003;35(8):1296-1302.

[25] Yu P, Bai H, Chen L, Zhang W, Xia Y, Wu G. Clinical study on therapeutic effect of acupuncture on Behcet's disease. Journal of Tradicional Chinise Medicine. 2003; 23(4): 271-273.

[26] Park MB, Ko E, Ahn C, Choi H, Rho S, Shin MK et al. Supression of IgE production and modulation of Th1/Th2 cell response by electroacupuncture in DNP-KLH immunized mice. Journal of Neuroimmunology. 2004; 151: 40-44.

[27] Ng DK, Chow PY, Ming SP, Hong SH, Lan S, Tse D et al. A double-blind, randomized, placebo-controlled trial of acupuncture for the treatment of childhood. Persistent Allergic Rhinitis Pediatrics. 2004; 114(5): 1242-1247.

[28] Johansen M, Yu GJ, Madden T, Chiang JS. Effect of acupuncture on circulating cytokines in healthy subjects. Medical Acupuncture. 2004;15(2) :19-24.

[29] Magnusson AL, Svensson REBR, Leirvik C. The effect of acupuncture on allergic rhinitis: a randomized controlled clinical trial. The American Journal of Chinese Medicine. 2004;32(1):105–115.

[30] Scognamillo-Szabó MVR, Bechara GH, Ferreira SH, Cunha FQ. Effect of various acupuncture treatment protocols upon sepsis in wistar rats. Annals New York Academy Sciencies. 2004; (1026); 251-256.

[31] Hahm ET,Lee JJ, Lee WK, Bae HS, Min BI,Cho YW.Electroacupuncture enhancement of natural killer cell activity suppressed by anterior hypothalamic lesions in rats.Neuroimmunomodulation 2004 :11-268-272 (2004)

[32] Scognamillo-Szabo MRV, Bechara GH, Cunh FO. Efeito inibitório da acupuntura sobre a migração de neutrófilos para a cavidade peritoneal de ratos. ARS Veterinária. 2005-A;21(1):91-95.

[33] Scognamillo-Szabó MVR, Bechara GH, Ferreira SH, Cunha FQ. Effect of acupuncture on TNF∞, ILβ and IL10 concentrations in the peritoneal escudates of carrageenan-induced peritonitis in rats. Ciência Rural. 2005-B; 35(1): 103-108.

[34] Wang J, Wang Y-K, Yu J, Cao X-D, Wu GC. Electroacupuncture supresses surgical trauma stren-induced lymphacyte apoptosis in rats. Neuroscience Letters. 2005;383:68-72.

[35] Kim CK, Choi GS, Oh D, Han JB, Kim SK, Ahn, HJ et al. Electroacupuncture up-regulates natural killer cell activity identification of genes altering their expressions in electroacupuncture induced up-regulation of natural killer cell activity. Journal of Neuroimnunology. 2005; (168): 144-153.

[36] Kou W, Bell JD, Gareus I, Pacheco-Lopez G, Goebel MV, Spahn G et al. Repeated acupuncture treatment affects leukocyte circulation in healthy ying male subjects : a randomized single-blind two period crossover study. Brain Behavior and Immunity. 2005;19:318-324.

[37] Zhang RX, Lao L, Wang X, Fan A, Wang L, Ren K et al. Electroacupuncture attenuates inflammation in a rat model. The Journal of Alternative and Complementary Medicine. 2005; 11(1): 135-142.

[38] Shen GM, Zhou MQ, Xu GS, Xu Y, Yin G. The modulations of electroacupunture on gastric motility in stressed rats. World Jornal Gastroenterology. 2006;12(38): 6156-6160.

[39] Huang CL, Huang CJ, Tsai PS, Yan LP, Xu HZ. Acupuncture stimulation of ST36 (Zusanli) significantly mitigates acute lung injury in lipopolysaccharide-stimulated rats. Acta Anaesthesiology Scandinavia. 2006;50:722-730.

[40] Yamaguchi N, Takahashi T, Sakura M, Sugita T, Uchikawa K, Sakaiharas S et al. Acupuncture regulates leukocyte subpopulations in human peripheral blood. Advance Access Publications. 2007;4(4):447-453.

[41] Yim YK, Lee H, Hong KE, Kim YI, Lee BR, Son CG et al. Electro-acupuncture at acupoint ST36 reduces inflammation and regulates immune activity in collagen-induced arthritic mice.Evidence Based Evidence Based Complementary and Alternative Medicine. 2007;4(1):51-57.

[42] Lee Y, Kim SK, Kin Y, Lee H, Shiu MK, Hong MC et al. The $\alpha$ adrenoreceptor mediation of the immunomodulatory effects of electroacupuncture in DNP-KLH immunized mice. Neuroscience Letters. 2007;423:149-152.

[43] Arranz L, Guayerbas N, Siboni L, De La Puente M. Effect of acupuncture treatment on the immune function impairment found in anxious women. The American Journal of Chinese Medicine. 2007;35(1):35-51.

[44] Lu W, Hu D, Dean-Clower E, Gilman AD, Legedza ATR, Lee H et al. Acupuncture for chemotherapy induced leucopenia: exploratory meta-analysis of randomized controlled trials. Journal of the Society for Integrative Oncology. 2007; 5(1): 1-10.

[45] Li YM, Zhuang LX, Lai XS, Jiang GH. Effects of electroacupuncture on plasma vasoactive intestinal peptide and substance P in perennial allergic rhinitis patients. Zhen Ci Yan Jiu. 2007; 32(2):136-8.

[46] Huang CL, Tsai PS, Wang TY, Yan LP, Xu HZ, Huang CJ. Acupuncture stimulation of ST36 (Zusanli) attenuates acute renal but not hepatic injury in lipopolysaccharide-stimulated rats. Anesthesia & Analgesia. 2007;104:646-54.

[47] Ye F, Liu D, Wang S, Xu L Effects of electro-acupuncture on T cell subpopulations, NK activity, humoral immunity and leukocyte count in patients undergoing chemotherapy. Journal Traditional Chinese Medicine. 2007 Mar;27(1):19-21

[48] Mao HJ, Wu HH, Bu LL, Zhou YB, Sun J, Sun PL. Relationship between electroacupuncture-induced regulatory effect on leukocytes and the caliber of splenic sinusoid basal lamina eyehole on rabbits. Zhen Ci Yan Jiu. 2008; 33(5): 291-295.

[49] Zhang LJ, Song AF, Wang ZH, LU Y. Effects of the needling method for regulating kidney and smoothinf liver on endocrine and immune functions in the patient with hyperplasia of mammary glands. Zhongquo Zhen Jiu. 2008; 8(9):648-652.

[50] Lai M, Wang SM, Wang Y, Tang CL, Kong LW, Xu XY. Effects of electroacupuncture of Zusanli(ST36), Hegu(LI 4) and or Sanyinjiao(SP9) on immunofunction gastric carcinectomy rats. Zhen Ci Yan Jiu. 2008;33(4):245-9.

[51] Yan J, Zhang H, Chen CT, Yang QY, Liao WF, Chen PG. Effects electroacupuncture at Shangjunu (ST37) on Interleukin 1β and Interleukin-4 in ulcerative colites model rats. Journal of Traditional Chinese Medicine. 2009;29(1):60-63.

[52] Kim SK, Lee Y, Cho H, Koo S, Choi SM, Shin MK et al. A parametric study on the immunomodulatory efffects of electroacupuncture in DNP-KLH imnunized mice. Evidence Based Complementary and Alternative Medicine. 2009 :1-5.

[53] Gao H,Li XZ,Ye WW,Zhou BY,Jin YJ,Qiu Y,Wu JJ. Influence of penetrative needling of Shendao(GV11)on the symtom score and serum IgE content in chronic urticaria patients. Zhen Ci Yan Jiu. 2009 ;34(4) :272-5.

[54] Ferreira AS, Lima JGM, Ferreira TPT, Lopes CMT, Meyer R. Prophylactic effects of short-term acupuncture on zusanli (ST36) in wistar rats lipopoly saccharide induced acute lung injury. Journal of Chinese Integrative Medicine. 2009;7(10):969-975.

[55] Lu W, Matulonis UA, Doherty-Gilman A, Lee H, Dean-Clower E, Rosulek A, et al. Acupuncture for Chemoterapy-induced neutropenia in patients with gynecologia malignancies: a pilot randomized, sham-controlled clinical trial. Journal Alternative Complementary Medicine. 2009; 15 (7); 745-753

[56] Wang J, Zhao H, Mao-Ying QL, Cao XD, Wang YQ, Wu GC. Electroacupuncture downregulates TLR 2/4 and pro-inflamatory cytokine expression after surgical trauma stress without adrenal glands involvement. Brain Research Bulletin. 2009 ; 80(1-2) :89-94.

[57] Wang K, Wu H, Wang G, Li M, Zhang Z, Gu G. The effects of electroacupuncture on TH1/TH2 cytokine mRNA expression and mitogen-activated protein kinase signaling pathways in the splenic T cells of traumatized rats. Anesthesia & Analgesia. 2009 Nov;109(5):1666-73.

[58] Lee HJ, Lee JH, Lee EO, Lee HJ, Kim KH, Kim SH et al. Substance P and beta-endorphin mediate electro-acupuncture induced analgesia in mouse cancer pain model. Journal of Experimental & Clinical Cancer Research. 2009;28-102.

[59] Sena-Fernandes V, França DLM, Souza D, Santos KCM, Sousa RS, Manoel CV et al. Acupuncture at Zusanli (ST36) and SanYinjiao(SP6) points on the gastrointestinal tract : a study of the bioavailability of 99 mtc-sodium pertechnetat in rats. Evidence Basead Complementary and Alternative Medicine. 2010;1-6.

[60] Matsubara Y, Shimizu K, Tanimura Y, Myamoto T, Akimoto T, Kono I. Effect of acupuncture on salivary immunoglobulin A after about of intense exercise. Acupuncture Medicine. 2010;28:28-32.

[61] Karst M, Schneidewind D, Scheinichen D, Juettner B, Bernateck M, Molsberger A, et al. Acupuncture induces a pro-inflamatory immune response intensified by a conditioning-expectation effect. Forschende Komplementarmedizin. 2010; 17:21-27.

[62] Han YF, Gong Z, Huang LQ, Xia X, Zhao WJ. Clinical study on acupuncture for leucopenia induced by chemotherapy. Zhongquo Zhen Jiu. 2010; 30(10): 802-805.

[63] Ouyang BS, Che JL, Gao J, Zhang Y, Li J, Yang HZ et al. Effects of electroacupuncture and simple acupuncture on changes of IL1, IL4, IL6 and IL10 in peripheral blood and

joint fluid in patients with rheumatoid arthritis. Zhongguo Zhen Jiu. 2010; 30(10): 840-844.

[64] Sun H, Zhao H, Zhang J, Bao F, Wei J, Wang D, Zhang Y. Effect of acupuncture at Baihui (GV20) and Zusanli (ST36) on the level of serum inflammatory cytokines in patients with depression. Chinese Acupuncture & Moxibustion Zhonqquo Zhen Jiu. 2010;30(3):195-9

[65] Pavão TS, Vianna P, Pillat MM, Machado AB, Bauer ME. Acupuncture is effective to attenuate stress and stimulate lymphocyte proliferation in the elederly. Neuroscience Letters. 2010;484(1): 47-50.

[66] Silva MD, Guginski G, Werner MFP, Baggio CH, Marcon R, Santos ARS. Involvement of interleukin-10 in anti-inflamatory effect of sanyinjiao (SP6) acupucture in a mouse model of peritonits. Ecam Advance Access. 2010;(29):1-9.

[67] Yuan SY, Qin Z, Liu DS, Yin WQ, Zhang ZL, Li SG. Acupuncture for pelvic pain syndromes (CPPS) and its effect on cytokines in prostatic fluid. Zhong Guo Zhen Jiu. 2011; 31(1): 11-14.

[68] Zijlstra FJ, Ineke VDBL, Frank JPMH, Klein J. Anti-inflamatory actions of acupuncture. Mediators of inflamation.2003(12)59-69.

[69] Chen JX, Ibe BO, Ma SX. Nitric oxide modulation of norepinephrine production in acupuncture points. Life Science. 2006;79(23):2157-64.

[70] Cho ZH, Hwang SC, Wong EH, Son YD, Kang CH, Park, TS et al. Neural substrates experimental evidences and functional hypotesis of acupuncture mechanisms. Acta Neurological Scandinava. 2006;113:370-377.

[71] Ma XM, Li XY, Sakurai T, Pandjaitan M. Evidence of enhanced non-enzymatic generation of nitric oxide on the skin of acupuncture points: an innovative approach in humans. Nitric Oxide. 2007;17:60-68.

[72] Kavoussi B, Ross E. The Neuroimmune Basis the Antinflamatory Acupuncture. Integrative Cancer Therapies. 2007; 6(3): 251-257.

[73] Cabioglu MT, Cetin BE. Acupuncture and immuno modulation. The American Journal of Chinese Medicine. 2008;36(1):25-36.

[74] Peng G. Acupuncture and innate immunity. Zhen Ci Yan Jiu. 2008;33(1):49-52

[75] Roberts J, Huisson A, Dretzke J, Wang D, Hyde C. A systematic review of the clinical effectiveness of acupuncture for allergic rhrinitis. BMC Complementary and Alternative Medicine. 2008; 8 (13):1-10.

[76] Brinkhaus,B,Witt,CM,Jena S,Liecker B,Wegscheider K,Willich SN.Acupuncture in patients with allergic rhinitis:a pragmatic randomized trial. Annals Allergy Asthma Immunology Journal.2008;101(5):535-43.

[77] Lee MS, Pittler MH, Shin BC, Kim JI, Ernst E.Acupuncture for allergic rhnits :a systematic review.Annals of Allergy Asthma Immunology Journal. 2009 ;(102):269-279.

[78] Takahashi T, Sumino H, Kanda T, Yamaguchi N. Acupuncture modifies immune cells. Journal Experimental. Clinical Medicine. 2009;1(1):17-22.

[79] He TF, Yan WJ, Zhang SH, Zhang CY, LB, Chen YF. Electroacupuncture inhibits inflammation reaction by upregulating vasoactive intestinal peptide in rats with adjuvant induced arthritis. Evidence Based Complementary and Alternative Medicine. 2011. Article ID 290489. 8p.

[80] Manni L, Rocco S, Paparo B, Garagna M. Electroacupuncture and nerve growth factor potential clinical applications. Archives Italiannes de Biologie. 2011;149(2): 247-255.

[81] Campos HS. Asma: suas origens, seus mecanismos inflamatórios e o papel do corticosteróide. Revista. Brasileira de Pneumolologia Sanitaria. 2007;15(1):47-60.

[82] Francis L, Gleeson M, Pyne DB, Callister R, Clancy RL. Variations of salivary immunoglobulins in exercicing and sedentary populations. Medicine & Science in Sports & Exercice. 2005;571-578.

[83] Peake JM, Suzuki K, Hordern M, Wilson G, Nosaka K, Coombes JS. Plasma cytokine changes in relation to exercise intensity and muscle damage. European Journal Applied Physiology.2005;10:1007.

[84] Silva WD, Mota I. Bier imunologia básica e aplicada. Rio de Janeiro: Guanabara Koogan, 2003.

[85] Abbas AK, Lichtman AH,Pillai,SHIV. Imunologia celular e molecular. 7.ed. Rio de Janeiro: Elsevier, 2012.

[86] Cooper E.L. Neuroendocrineimmune, Electroacupuncture and Gene Expression. The Journal of Alternative and Complementary Medicine. 2010;7(2)149–150.

[87] Gleeson M. Nutrition interventions to limit exercice-induced immunodepression. In Teixeira AM (ed): Conferences in Exercice Immunology. Centro de Estudos Biocinéticos. Coimbra. 2007; 45-69.

Chapter 4

# Acupuncture Effects on Bladder Activity and State of Vigilance Through GABAergic Neuronal Systems

Yoshimasa Koyama and Hui Wang

Additional information is available at the end of the chapter

http://dx.doi.org/10.5772/55405

## 1. Introduction

It has been reported that acupuncture to sevaral acupoints increases bladder capacity and that it is used effectively for therapy to overactive bladder or for improving the symptoms of nocturnal enuresis [1-3]. Acupuncture to other points can change the state of vigilance or improve insomnia [4-6]. Acupuncture effets are, thus, confirmed in various clinical treatments, however the neural mechanisms mediating these effects remain unknown.

We have shown that acupuncture to the sacral vertebra supresses bladder activity [7], and the same point has an effect to induce the state close to deep sleep in urethane anesthetized rats [8, 9]. During this series of experiments, it became clear that bladder activity had a close relation with brain activity; that is, urinary bladder was more active when the rats were in a light anesthetized condition than in a deep anethetized condition [10]. It can be expected that the same mechanisms mediating acupuncture effects on bladder activity and on the state of vigilance reside in the central nervous system.

In this article, based upon our neurophysiolgical data on the regulation of sleep and wakefulness and of micturition, we would introduce our hypothesis on the neural mechanisms mediating the effects of acupuncture to the sacral vertebra.

## 2. Methods

### 2.1. Animals

Male rats (Sprague-Dawley) were used for the experiments. Rats were anesthetized by intraperitoneal injection of urethane (1.0 g/kg) and additional doses (2 to 5 % of the initial dose) of the same anesthetic were given to maintain an appropriate level of anesthetic. The animals were put in prone position with their heads fixed to a stereotaxic frame. All surgical wounds were infiltrated with 2% lidocaine. Rectal temperature was kept at 37 °C with a heating pad controlled through a feedback circuit. The present study was performed in Fukushima Medical University under the control of the Animal Research Committee in accordance with the Guidelines on Animal Experiments of Fukushima Medical University and the Animal Protection and Management Law of the Japanese Government.

### 2.2. Experimental procedures

Rats were fixed to a stereotaxic instrument in prone posture. To analyze the effects of acupuncture, activity of urinary bladder, electroencephalogram (EEG) and single neuronal activity from the brainstem were recorded.

For recording urinary bladder pressure, a polyethylene catheter (outer diameter, 0.96 mm) was inserted from the dome into the urinary bladder through a small incision in the lower abdominal wall, the catheter was fixed securely and the wound was closed. The catheter had a bifurcation, with one end connected to a pressure transducer (Nihon-Koden, TP400-T) and the other to a syringe filled with physiological saline. The latter was used to inject physiological saline through an infusion pump (Harvard, Pump 11) to the bladder at a rate of 0.2 ml/min until this induced spontaneous bladder contraction (0.4-1.0 ml). For recording electroencephalogram (EEG), stainless steel bolts 1.0 mm in diameter were screwed to the skull overlying the frontal and parietal cortices. Single neuronal activity was recorded through a glass pipette electrode filled with 0.5-M sodium acetate containing 2% Pontamine sky blue. The electrode was penetrated stereotaxically into the brainstem through a hole made in the skull overlying the cerebellum. To avoid penetration of the venous sinus, the electrode was angled posteriorly at 30° and lowered through the cerebellum. Neuronal activity was amplified through a high-impedance amplifier and then a conventional amplifier with a time constant of 0.01 s. Recording sites were marked by ejection of Pontamine sky blue from the recording electrode.

For acupuncture stimulation, an acupuncture needle (diameter 0.3 mm) was positioned almost vertically at the periosteum about 5 mm lateral to the midline of the lumber and sacral vertebrae (L6 to S4) and rotated manually at a speed of about 1.5-2 turns/sec for one minute. The vertebra for stimulation was located by palpation and in some animals the stimulated vertebra was ground by a thick needle and accuracy of the target vertebra was checked after removing the muscle around the vertebrae. It was confirmed that an acupuncture needle inserted to the stimulation points and put there for one minute without rotation had no effect on bladder contractions or neuronal activity. Acupuncture stimulation was judged to affect bladder activity when the relaxation periods (time from the end of a bladder contraction to the beginning of the next contraction after the stimulation) just after the stimulus exceeded twice the average of five relaxation periods before stimulation.

To examine the involvement of the GABAergic system in acupuncture regulation, a dose of 2~4 mg/kg of bicuculline (GABA receptor antagonist, Sigma) was intraperitoneally injected and the effects of acupuncture stimulation were compared with those before the injection. Effects of acupuncture stimulation on neural activity were judged by comparing the mean

http://dx.doi.org/10.5772/55405

firing rate measured for five contraction-relaxation cycles before stimulation with that measured after stimulation. When the mean firing rate after stimulation increased to more than 150% of that before stimulation, it was judged to be excitatory, while when the value was less than 50% of that before the stimulation, it was judged to be inhibitory.

### 2.3. Histology

After the experiment, the animal was deeply anesthetized with pentobarbital, and perfused transcardially with 300 ml of 4% paraformaldehyde in 0.1-M phosphate buffer (pH 7.4). The brain was removed from the skull and post-fixed in the same solution overnight, immersed in 30% sucrose for several hours, and cut on a freezing microtome at 50 μm in the frontal plane. To identify cholinergic neurons, sections were processed for NADPH-diaphorase, a specific marker of brainstem cholinergic neurons [11]. The sections were then counterstained by Neutral Red.

## 3. Results

### 3.1. Relation of bladder activity and state of vigilance

Under urethane anesthesia, rats alternatively exhibited two patterns of electroencephalogram (EEG): larger amplitude slow wave, indicating a state of deep anesthesia and smaller and slightly faster wave, sign of a light anesthesia. During a light anesthesia state, bladder contractions occurred regularly and contentiously, while during a deep anesthesia state,

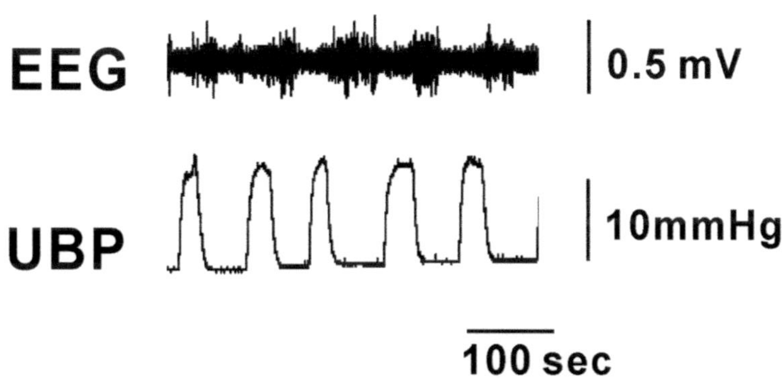


**Figure 1.** Changes in bladder activity and electroencephalogram (EEG) under urethane anesthesia. Under urethane anesthesia, EEG exhibits alternative patterns, large amplitude slow wave and small amplitude faster wave. Urinary bladder contracts when EEG shows smaller amplitude, while it becomes flaccid when EEG shows large amplitude. EEG, electro encephalogram; UBP, urinary bladder pressure.

### 3.2. Micturition center neurons in the brainstem regulating bladder contraction

The brain area regulating micturition was first investigated by Barrington [12], who revealed that a restricted area from the caudal mesencephalon to rostral pons functions as a micturition center and the locus was named, after him, the Barrigton's nucleus. His work was confirmed by electrical or chemical brain stimulation studies [13-15] or neuroanatomical studies showing efferent and afferent connections between the micturition center and the lumbosacral spinal cord [16-19]. We have emphasized that the most effective stimulus site for inducing bladder contraction is restrticted to, as well as the Barrington's nucleus, the area ventral to the ana-

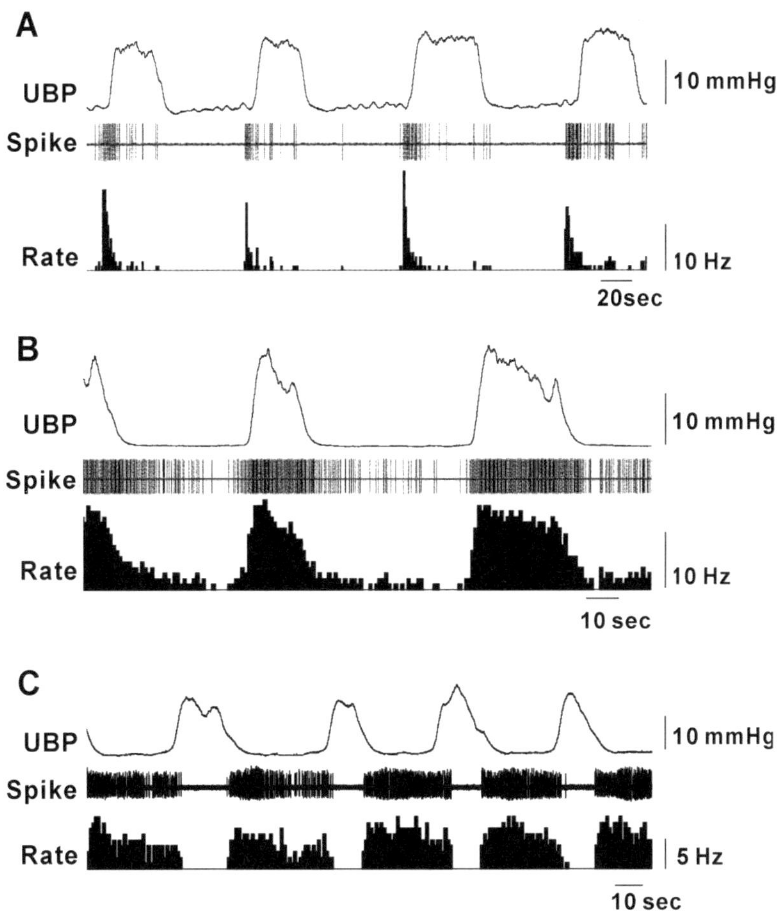


**Figure 2.** Three types of bladder activity-related neurons. A, Type E1 neuron. B, Type E2 neuron. C, Type I neuron. Spike, raw trace of action potentials of the neuron. Rate, firing rate of the neuron.

We have recently revealed, through single neuronal recording studies, that there are three types of neurons in and around the Barrington's nucleus, exhibiting discharges modulated in relation to spontaneous contraction of the urinary bladder (bladder activity-related neurons).

The three types were named Type E1, Type E2 and Type I neurons (Fig. 2). In this study, it was found that Type E1 neurons started to discharge prior to the onset of bladder contraction but the discharge declined before or soon after the onset of contraction, then the neurons became almost inactive at the latter half of the contraction or the following relaxation period (Fig. 2A). Type E2 neurons showed tonic firing during bladder contraction. The rate of firing changed in parallel with bladder pressure (Fig. 2B). In a majority of type E2 neurons, firing started to increase prior to the start of contraction, but the preceding time (the period between onsets of firing and contraction) was clearly shorter than that of type E1 neurons. Type I neurons showed a firing property which was mirror image of Type E2 neurons, that is, they discharged during relaxation; their discharge was suppressed at the rising phase of bladder pressure and was strongly suppressed during the contraction period. The strong suppression of firing occurred soon after the bladder pressure started to rise steeply, but the onset of the decrease of firing seemed to be prior to the start of bladder contraction (Fig. 2C).

When the urinary bladder was extended by infusion of saline, activity of about half of Type E neurons were modulated. Almost all (93%) of Type E neurons showed excitatory response, while

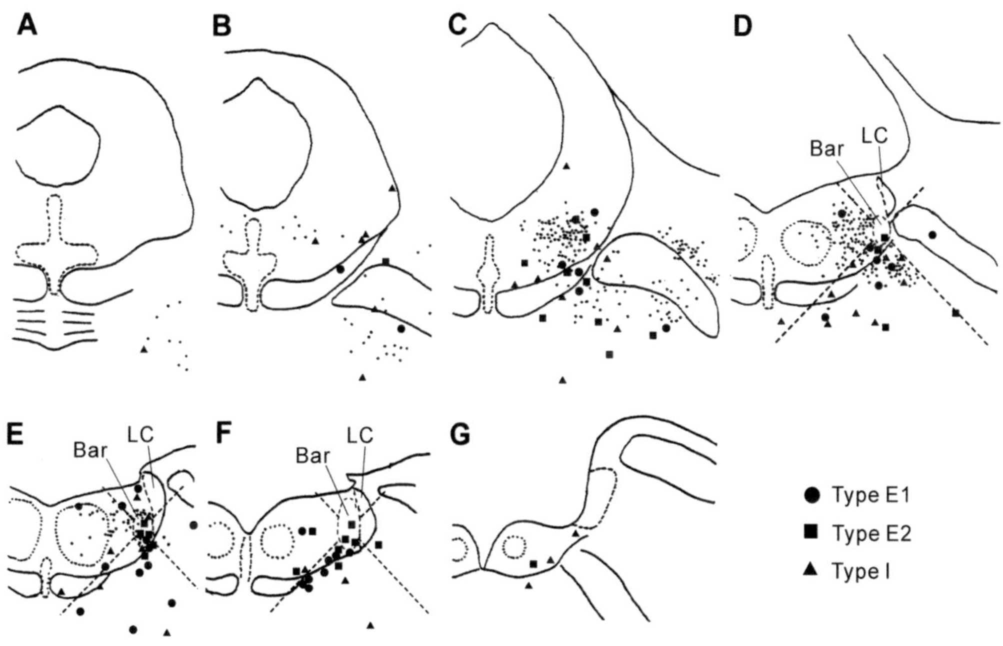


**Figure 3.** Locations of bladder activity-related neurons plotted on diagrams of serial coronal sections at intervals of 300μm. The small dots represent the exact distribution of NADPH-diaphorase-positive (i.e., cholinergic) neurons in the laterodorsal tegmental nucleus (LDT) in one animal. Circles, type E1 neurons. Squares, type E2 neurons. Triangles, type I neurons. Bar, Barrington's nucleus. LC, locus coeruleus.

As shown in Fig. 3, bladder activity-related neurons were located not only in the Barrington's nucleus but also outside of the Barrington's nucleus. Of these, Type E2 neurons were encountered more frequently in the Barrington's nucleus than outside of it. Type E1 neurons were frequently located ventral or ventromedial to the Barrington's nucleus. Type I neurons were distributed in the reticular formation more widely and more distant from the Barrington's nucleus than Type E neurons.

Based on these firing profiles of bladder activity–related neurons, we could draw hypothetical brainstem-spinal circuits regulating bladder activity (see Fig.10). Anatomical studies have demonstrated the neurons in and around the Barrington's nucleus directly project to the spinal (sacral) cord [17,18]. Pseudorabies virus injected into the urinary bladder was retrogradely and transsynaptically transferred to the Barrington's nucleus [19]. Since location of Type E2 neurons looks to correspond to the area where the pseudorabies virus was retrogradely transferred, Type E2 neurons would, directly projecting to the sacral spinal cord, command the bladder contraction (② in Fig. 10). Considering the time course of Type E1 and Type E2 neurons, Type E1 neurons would send excitatory drive to Type E2 neuron to initiate contraction. Different responses (excitation and inhibition) of Type I neurons to bladder distension suggest two populations of Type I neurons. One type would be tonically active during resting period and suppresses Type E neurons. Another type would receive excitatory input from the urinary or spinal level, and would suppress Type E neurons during contraction-relaxation cycles.

### 3.3. Cholinergic and aminergic neurons in the brainstem regulating sleep and wakefulnesss

Based up the pioneering work by Moruzzi and Magoun, it became clear that there were neural populations in the reticular formation of the brainstem that activate the entire cerebral cortex, which they proposed as ascending reticular activating system [21] (Fig. 4A). Recent neuroanatomical and neurophysiological studies have revealed the transmitter phenotype of the neurons which compose the ascending reticular activating system. These neurons, locating in the area extending from caudal mescencephalon to the rostral pontine tegmentum, include the cholinergic neurons in the laterodorsal tegmental nucleus (LDT) and pedunculopontine tegmental nucleus (PPT), noradrenergic neurons in the locus coeruleus (LC) and serotonergic neurons in the dorsal raphe (DR). They send their axons widely to the cerebral cortex, thalamus or basal forebrain, and exert influences on the cerebral cortex directly or through the thalamus or basal forebrain (Fig. 4B). Single neuronal recording studies in animals under natural sleep/waking cycles have revealed that some of the cholinergic neurons in the LDT/PPT are highly active during waking and REM sleep, while the noradrenergic neurons in the LC and serotonergic neurons in the DR are specifically active during waking (Fig. 4C). These neurons are, therefore, considered to be involved in inducing or maintaining wakefulness and are called waking promoting neurons.

The cholinergic and monoaminergic neurons can be discriminated from other phenotype of neurons by the shape of action potentials (spikes) recorded extracellularly or juxtacellularly [22, 23]. The neurons recorded from the LDT that generate spikes of a longer duration with a shoulder at the falling phase of the spike are cholinergic (Fig. 5C). Noradrenergic neurons in the LC and serotonergic neurons in the DR also generate spikes of similar shape. Based on this

http://dx.doi.org/10.5772/55405

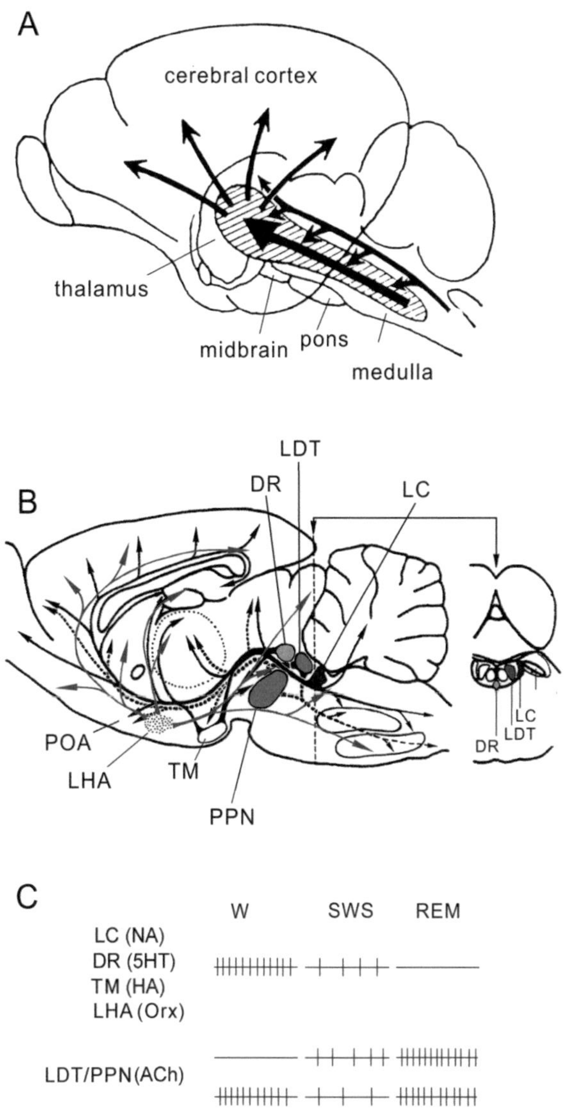


**Figure 4.** A, Schematic diagram of ascending reticular activating system proposed by Moruzzi and Magoun. B, Brain areas and nuclei crucial for regulation of sleep and wakefulness, and the projection of neurons located in these areas. C, Summary of firing of neurons crucial for regulation of sleep and wakefulness during wakefulness (W), slow wave sleep (SWS) and REM sleep (REM). In C, a vertical bar indicates an action potential of the neurons. NA neurons in the LC, 5HT neurons in the DR, HA neurons in the TM and Orx neurons in the LHA are most active during W, decrease their firing during SWS and cease from firing during REM sleep. A population of ACh neurons in the LDT and PPT are active both during W and REM sleep and become less active during SWS, while another population are least active during W and most active during REM sleep. ACh, acetylcholine. DR, dorsal raphe. HA, histamine. LC, locus coeruleus. LHA, lateral hypothalamic area. LDT, laterodorsal tegmental nucleus. NA, noradrenalin. Orx, orexin. POA, preoptic area. PPN, pedunculopontine tegmental nucleus. TM tuberomammillary nucleus. 5HT, serotonin.

finding, the neurons displaying spikes of a shorter duration (brief spikes) are considered to be non-cholinergic and non-monoaminergic.

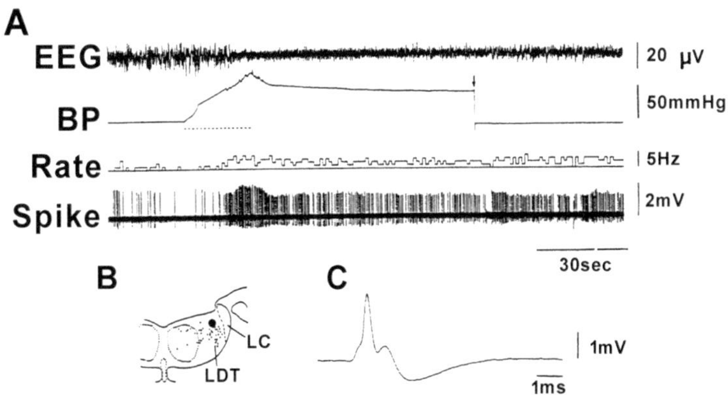


**Figure 5.** Effects of bladder distention on the EEG and the cholinergic neurons in the LDT. A, Changes of EEG and firing rate of the cholinergic LDT neuron after infusion of saline (broken line) into the urinary bladder. Arrow, time of drainage of infused saline (Urinary tract was legated during and after the infusion). B, Recording site. C, Shape of action potential recorded from a site of closed circle (●) in B.

### 3.4. Afferents from the urinary bladder have influences on the vigilance state through the waking promoting neurons

During deep anesthesia, while the animals were showing a large amplitude slow EEG, extension of the urinary bladder by infusion of saline caused activation of the cholinergic LDT neurons (Fig. 5A). Within a few seconds after the increase of firing, the EEG changed to that of light anesthesia [24]. Similar results were obtained from the noradrenergic neurons in the LC [25]. These results suggest that the state of urinary bladder affects the vigilance state by acting on the waking promoting neurons in the brainstem.

### 3.5. Acupuncture effects on state of vigilance and on wake promoting neurons

Acupuncture stimulation to the sacral vertebrae, when given during light anesthesia, induced changes in the state of vigilance; changes in the state from light anesthesia to deep anesthesia [8]. As shown in Fig. 6, when a smaller amplitude and faster EEG was observed, acupuncture stimulation to the sacral vertebra induced a change to a larger amplitude and slower EEG (Fig. 6A).

FFT analysis revealed that the peak frequency before the stimulus appeared in the delta band (1.46~2.44 Hz) and the theta band (3.92~4.9 Hz) (Fig. 6B), while after the stimulus, the peak shifted to the lower frequency delta band (0.98~1.95 Hz) (Fig. 6C). Changes in the EEG pattern occurred from 22 seconds to 31 minutes after the stimulus. The most frequent latency ranged from 100 seconds to 150 seconds. The latencies less than 450 seconds constituted one peak in the histogram of latency distribution and occupied 63% (71/112) of the response after the

http://dx.doi.org/10.5772/55405

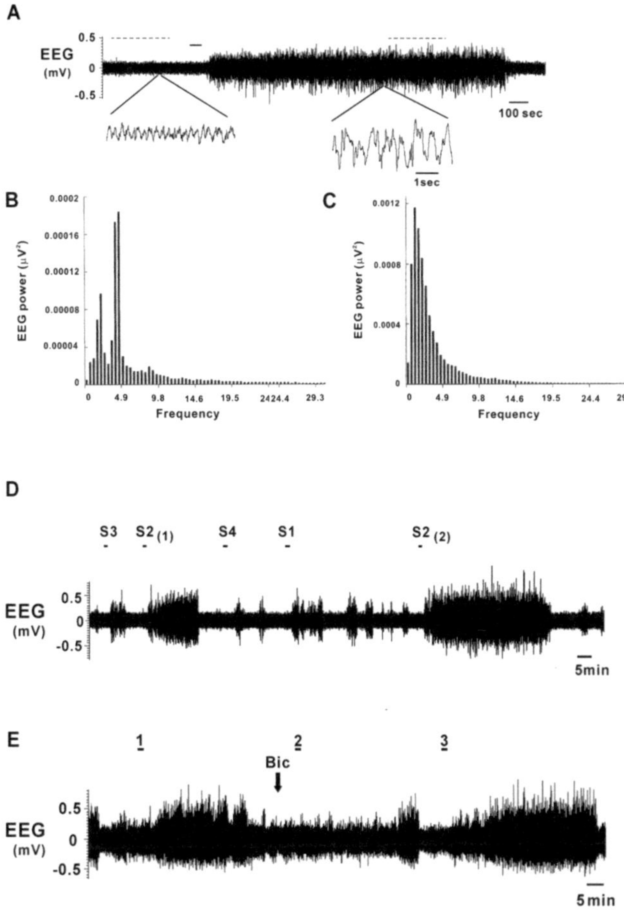


**Figure 6.** Effects of acupuncture stimulation to sacral vertebra on EEG changes. A, EEG change after acupuncture stimulation to sacral vertebra S3 (bar). Time-expanded EEG traces before and after acupuncture stimulation are shown below the contentious recording of EEG. B, EEG power spectrum obtained before the stimulus (broken line on top left) C, EEG power spectrum obtained after the stimulus (broken line on top right). D, Regional differences in effect of acupuncture stimulation to different sacral vertebrae Acupuncture stimulation to S2 ($S2_{(1)}$ and $S2_{(2)}$) was more effective in inducing large-amplitude slow EEG than stimulation to other vertebrae (S1, S3, and S4). E, Effect of intraperitoneally injection of bicuculline (Bic) on stimulus-induced EEG changes. Large-amplitude slow EEG induced by stimulation (bar 1) was not observed after Bic injection (arrow), even when the same stimulus (bar 2) was applied. About 50 min after Bic injection, acupuncture stimulation (bar 3) again induced EEG changes.

stimulus. Under urethane anesthesia, the spontaneous transition of EEG from smaller to larger occurred at mean intervals of about 800 sec. So, in the present experiment, the responses with latency less than 450 seconds were considered to be stimulus evoked, while those with longer latencies to be spontaneous occurring EEG changes. Acupuncture's effect on vigilance state was different across segments. Stimulation to the S2 vertebra induced a longer duration of large amplitude EEG than stimulation to other vertebra (Fig. 6D). When a large amplitude EEG was induced, the state of functions regulated by the autonomic nervous system, including respiration, blood pressure and heart rate were unchanged.

The acupuncture-induced EEG changes were suppressed by intraperitoneal injection of $GABA_A$ receptor antagonist bicuculline (Bic). In Figure 6E, a large amplitude slow EEG induced by stimulation to sacral vertebra S3 (bar 1) was not observed when the same stimulation (bar 2) was applied 5 minutes after Bicuculline injection (arrow). These results suggest that the acupuncture effects on the state of vigilance are mediated through GABAergic neural system.

Changes of vigilance state or its associated physiological changes were induced by acupuncture to several other points: Shenmen, Yongquan, or Neiguan is used in therapy for insomnia

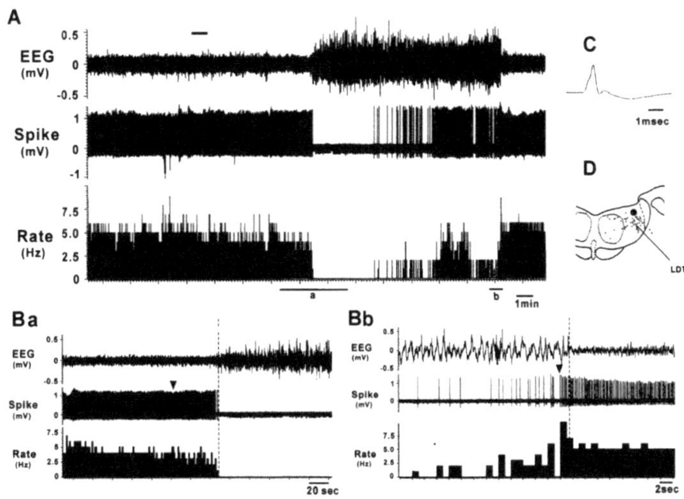


**Figure 7.** Effects of acupuncture stimulation to the sacral vertebra on the EEG and the cholinergic neurons in the LDT. A, Changes of EEG and firing rate of the neuron when the stimulation was given to S3 at the period of a bar on top. Ba and Bb, Time expanded scales of bar a and bar b in A, respectively showing the change of neuronal activity in relation with EEG change. Arrowheads: the start of the change of the neuronal activity. Broken lines: the start of the EEG change. C, shape of the action potential recorded from a site of closed circle (●) in D.

When the acupuncture stimulation induced a large amplitude slow EEG, the activity of the cholinergic neurons in the LDT and the noradrenergic neurons in the locus coeruleus was remarkably suppressed [8,9]. The cholinergic neurons in the LDT (Fig. 7), which showed tonic discharge about 4.7 Hz before the stimulation, decreased and completely stopped firing during the large EEG period. At the later period of large EEG, the firing gradually increased and completely recovered when the small amplitude faster EEG reappeared. In most cases, the decrease in firing started prior to the induction of large EEG, while the increase in firing started prior to the EEG change from large to small amplitude. As shown in Figure 7Ba, the significant decrease of neuronal firing (indicated by triangles), occurred about 43 seconds before the EEG change, while in Figure 7Bb, when the large and slow EEG changed to a smaller and faster one, the increase of firing occurred about 1.6 seconds before the change of the EEG [8]. Similar results were obtained from the noradrenergic LC neurons [9].

http://dx.doi.org/10.5772/55405

Taken together, it can be concluded that acupuncture stimulation to the sacral vertebrae suppress the activity of waking promoting neurons in the brainstem through GABAergic system and, under urethane anesthesia, lead to the changes in the state from light anesthesia to deep anesthesia. Under unanesthetized condition, noradrenergic neurons in the LC and cholinergic neurons in the LDT/PPT have some roles, in addition to sleep-waking regulation, in maintaining arousal level or attention to novel stimuli, in the process of anxiety or pain, learning or reward [29,30]. It is highly probable that acupuncture to the sacral vertebrae has some influences on these higher brain functions.

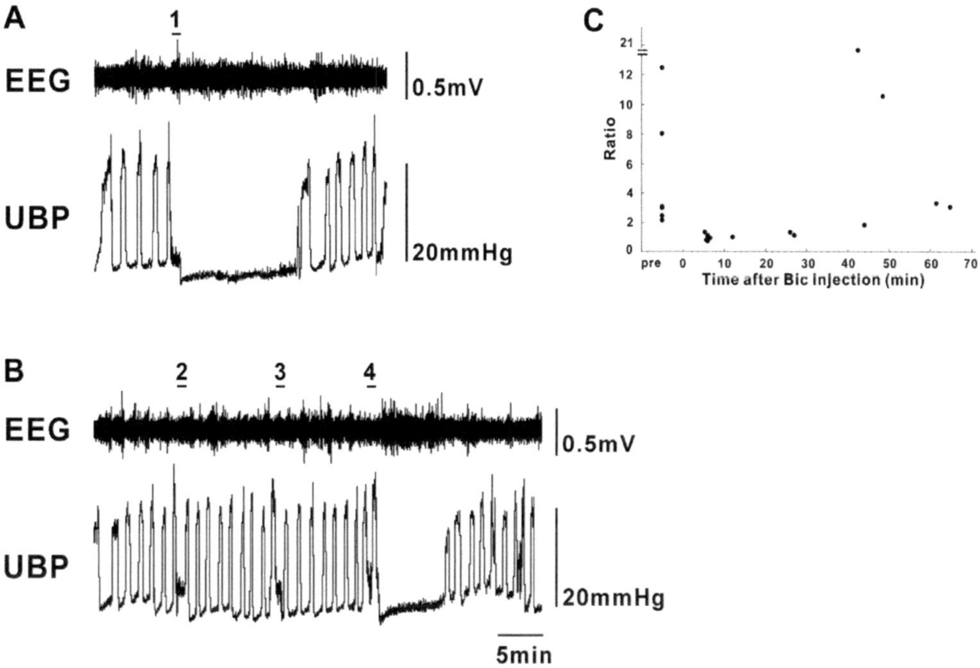


**Figure 8.** Effect of intraperitoneal injection of bicuculline (Bic) on stimulus-induced suppression of bladder activity. A, Bladder activity suppression induced by acupuncture stimulation (bar 1) before Bic injection. B, Bladder activity suppression by acupuncture stimulation after Bic injection. Bars 2, 3, and 4 represent periods of stimulation about 27, 38, and 48 minutes after Bic injection, respectively. C, Time course of changes in "Ratio" values before and after Bic injection. Ratio (vertical scale)indicates the ratio of average relaxation period just after stimulation to that before stimulation, a degree of suppression induced by acupuncture stimulation.

### 3.6. Acupuncture effects on bladder activity and bladder activity–related neurons

When the urinary bladder was exhibiting rhythmical contraction, acupuncture stimulation to the sacral vertebra suppressed the contraction [31]. As shown in Figure 8, the suppression started just after the acupuncture to the S2 vertebra (bar 1) and continued for 13 minutes. The same stimulus induced changes in EEG (Fig. 6), however in this case, no EEG change was observed, meaning that bladder activity is more strongly affected than state of vigilance by acupuncture stimulation to the sacral vertebra. The suppression started within a few minutes after the stimulus and continued from 30 seconds up to 40 minutes. Across several vertebrae (from L6 to S1), acupuncture stimulation to the S2 vertebra suppressed the bladder activity most effectively, while stimulation to the S4 was a least effective. The segmental effects on bladder activity was similar to the effect on state of vigilance. Other aspects of the autonomic nervous system, including respiration, blood pressure, and heart rate were unaffected by the sacral stimulation [31].

The stimulus-induced suppression of bladder activity was blocked by intraperitoneal application of bicuculline (Bic). About 27minutes after Bic injection, the acupuncture stimulation failed to suppress bladder contraction (Fig. 8B, bar 2). The stimulation about 38 minutes after Bic injection also had no suppressive effect on bladder contraction (Fig. 8B, bar 3). Forty-eight minutes after Bic injection, the stimulus again suppressed bladder activity (Fig.8B, bar 4). Figure 8C indicates the time course of stimulus-induced suppression after Bic injection, that is, the ratio of the mean relaxation time after the stimulus to that before the stimulus. When the contractions were suppressed by acupuncture stimulation, the values increased according to the duration of suppression. The value 1.0 indicates that the relaxation time is the same before and after the stimulus, meaning that the stimulus had no effect. Figure 8C indicates that the effects of Bic lasted for about 30 minutes. These results indicate that acupuncture suppression on bladder activity is mediated through $GABA_A$ receptor systems.

When bladder activity was suppressed by acupuncture stimulation, almost all of Type E neurons (both Type E1 and Type E2 neurons) decreased firing. As shown in Fig. 9A, some Type E2 neurons stopped firing just after the acupuncture stimulation simultaneous with suppression of bladder contraction. The neuronal firing recovered when the bladder regained contraction. In other Type E2 neurons, the decrease in firing appeared before the suppression of bladder contraction (Fig. 9B), while in the third class of Type E2 neurons, the rhythmic firing continued after the suppression of bladder contraction (Fig. 9C). In contrast to Type E neurons, some of Type I neurons exhibited an increase in firing after acupuncture stimulation (Fig. 9D). The increase in firing started before the suppression of bladder activity. The firing further increased and, during the suppression period of bladder activity, exceeded the value during the relaxation period of spontaneous contraction before the stimulation. Of 14 type I neurons, 4 exhibited increased firing, 3 exhibited decreased firing and the remaining 7 exhibited no response to acupuncture stimulation.

In total, acupuncture stimulation suppresses Type E neurons and activates half of Type I neurons, leading to suppression of bladder activity. Another half of Type I neurons which were inhibited by acupuncture might be receiving neural inputs from urinary bladder and be working to maintain the basic level of bladder pressure which would be crucial to continue contraction. Time course of suppression in Type E neurons differ among neurons (Fig. 9 A-C). Acupuncture stimulation, therefore, would disturb the synchronous firing in Type E neurons rather than suppress all of the neurons in a similar magnitude, resulting in irregular and insufficient bladder contraction at the beginning of suppression.

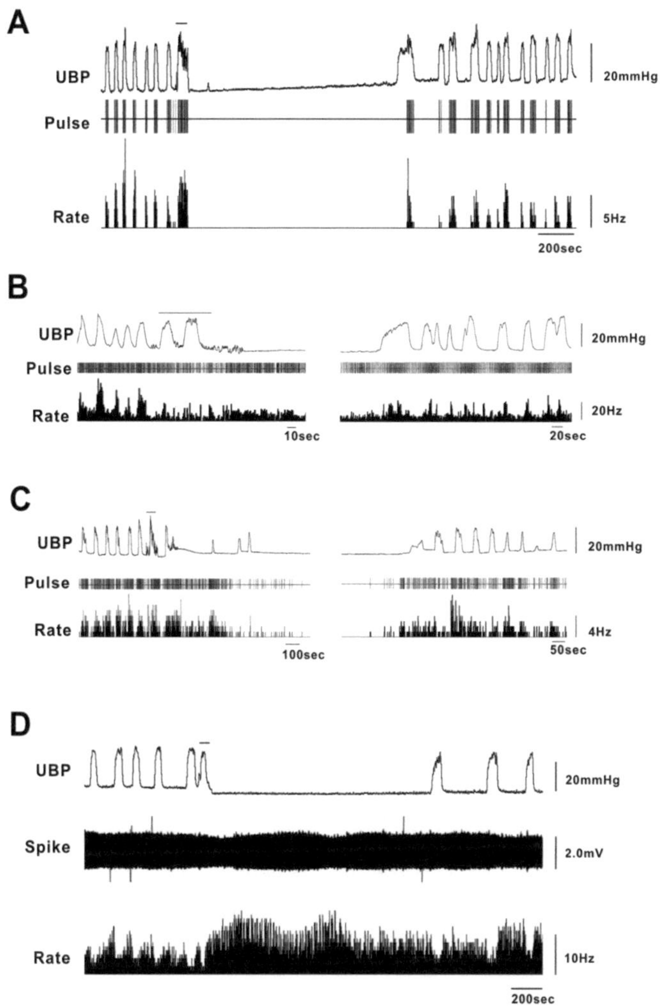


**Figure 9.** Effects of acupuncture stimulation on the bladder activity-related neurons and urinary bladder A to C, Type E2 neurons. D, Type I neuron. See text for detail.

# 4. Conclusion

Acupuncture stimulation to the sacral vertebrae in rats suppressed bladder activity and altered the firing profiles of bladder activity-related neurons in and around the micturition center. Acupuncture stimulation to the sacral vertebrae also affected the state of vigilance by inhibiting the activity of wake-promoting neurons. These effects were blocked by $GABA_A$ receptor antagonist bicuculline.

Since acupuncture stimulation to the sacral segment suppressed overactive bladder in spinal injured patients [32,33], it is highly possible that the acupuncture effect is mediated through the spinal level. However, the present study showed that when acupuncture was applied, a population of bladder activity-related neurons changed firing before the suppression of bladder contraction, suggesting the possibility that the acupuncture effect is mediated through the central nervous system, especially through the brainstem micturition center. In a similar way, suppression of firing in waking promoting neurons occurring before the changes in the state of vigilance suggests that the acupuncture effect is mediated through the waking promoting neurons.

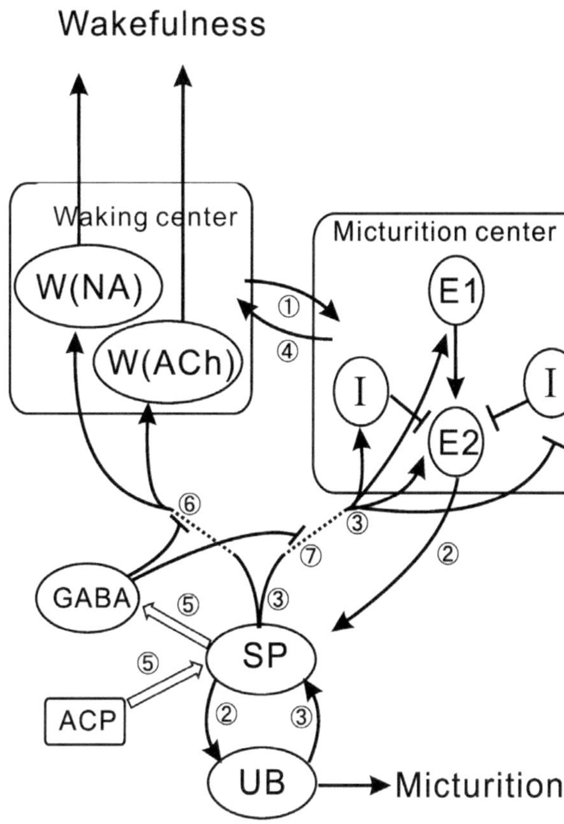


**Figure 10.** Schematic diagram representing neural circuit mediating acupuncture effects on micturition system and waking system. ACh, acetylcholine. ACP, acupuncture. NA, noradrenaline. SP, spinal cord. UB, urinary bladder. W wake-promoting neuron.

### 4.1. Hypothetical neural pathways mediating acupuncture effects on micturition and state of vigilance

Taking these findings in account, we could draw hypothetical schema explaining the neural mechanism mediating acupuncture effects on micturition and state of vigilance (Fig. 10). In summary, as is mentioned in Section 1 and Section 4, the waking center in the brainstem and micturition center in the Barrington's nucleus are mutually excitatory each other (① in Fig. 10). Type E2 neurons in the micturition center exert excitatory drive on urinary bladder (②) and inputs from the urinary bladder have excitatory influences on Type E neurons and a half of Type I neurons, while they have inhibitory influences on another half of Type I neurons (③). They also have excitatory influences on waking promoting neurons in the waking center (④). Acupuncture stimulation to the sacral vertebra causes excitation in GABAergic neurons of somewhere (⑤) which inhibit the pathways activating wakefulness (⑥) or facilitating micturition center (⑦). The location of GABAergic neurons and sites of action of GABAergic inhibition are still unknown (broken lines), and would be a subject of future study.

### 4.2. Clinical implications

The present findings provide a scientific validity for the therapy of overactive bladder in spinal injured patients [32,33] or nocturnal enuresis [1-3]. If the sacral acupuncture is effective for changing the state of vigilance in human, it would lead to a therapy for insomnia or would be useful for putting a patient in sedation.

Acupuncture has been used traditionally in China for thousands of years and is growing prominent in the Western countries. Acupuncture, thus, plays a crucial role in complementary and alternative medicine. To establish a better supported therapy of acupuncture more confirmedly, integration with the Western medicine is indispensable. Further studies to elucidate the neural mechanisms of acupuncture action would be urgently required.

## Acknowledgements

This study was supported by Grants-in-Aid for Scientific Research from the Ministry of Education, Culture, Sports, Science and Technology of Japan.

## Author details

Yoshimasa Koyama[1*] and Hui Wang[2]

*Address all correspondence to: koyamay@sss.fukushima-u.ac.jp

1 Department of Science and Technology, Fukushima University, Fukushima, PRC

2 Department of Physiology, Guiyang College of TCM y, Guiyang City, Guizhou Province, PRC

## References

[1] Honjo, H, Kawauchi, A, Ukimura, O, Soh, J, Mizutani, Y, & Miki, T. Treatment of Monosymptomatic Nocturnal Enuresis by Acupuncture: A preliminary Study. International Journal of Urology (2002)., 9-672.

[2] Bower, W. F, & Diao, M. Acupuncture as a Treatment for Nocturnal Enuresis. Autonomic Neuroscience (2010).

[3] Yuksek, M. S, Erdem, A. F, Atalay, C, & Demirel, A. Acupressure versus Oxybutinin in the Treatment of Enuresis. Journal of International Medical Research (2003). , 31(6), 552-556.

[4] Kim, Y. S, Lee, S. H, Jung, W. S, Park, S. U, Moon, S. K, Ko, C. N, Cho, K. H, & Bae, H. S. Intradermal Acupuncture on Shen- men and Nei-kuan Acupoints in Patients with Insomnia after Stroke. American Journal of Chinese Medicine (2004). , 32-771.

[5] Lin, Y. Acupuncture Treatment for Insomnia and Acupuncture Analgesia. Psychiatry and Clinical Neuroscience (1995). , 49-119.

[6] Tsay, S. L, Cho, Y. C, & Chen, M. L. Acupressure and Transcutaneous Electrical Acupoint Stimulation in Improving Fatigue, Sleep Quality and Depression in Hemodialysis Patients. American Journal of Chinese Medicine (2004). , 32-407.

[7] Tanaka, Y, Koyama, Y, Jodo, E, Kayama, Y, Kawauchi, A, Ukimura, O, & Miki, T. Effects of Acupuncture to the Sacral Segment on the Bladder Activity and Electroencephalogram. Psychiatry and Clinical Neuroscience (2002). , 56-249.

[8] Wang, H, Tanaka, Y, Seki, H, Jodo, E, Kayama, Y, Kawauchi, A, Miki, T, Otsuki, M, & Koyama, Y. Acupuncture Stimulation to the Sacral Segment Affects State of Vigilance in Rats. Neuroscience Research (2007). , 57-531.

[9] Wang, H, Koyama, Y, Jodo, E, & Kayama, Y. Suppressive Effect of Acupuncture Stimulation to the Sacral Segment on the State of Vigilance and the Brainstem Cholinergic Neurons. Fukushima Journal of Medical Science (2006). , 52(2), 125-134.

[10] Yamao, Y, Koyama, Y, Kawauchi, A, Jodo, E, Kayama, Y, & Miki, T. Are Micturition Systems Influenced by Sleep-arousal System? Psychiatry and Clinical Neuroscience (2000). , 54(3), 259-261.

[11] Vincent, S. R, Satoh, K, Armstrong, D. M, & Fibiger, H. C. NADPH-diaphorase: A Selective Histochemical Marker for the Cholinergic Neurons of the Pontine Reticular Formation. Neuroscience Letters (1983). , 43-31.

[12] Barrington FJFThe Effect of Lesion of the Hind- and Midbrain on Micturition in the Rat. Quarterly Journal of Experimental Physiology (1925). , 15-81.

[13] Nishizawa, O, Sugaya, K, Noto, H, Harada, T, & Tsuchida, S. Pontine Micturition Center in the Dog. Journal of Urology (1988). , 140-872.

[14] Yamao, Y, Koyama, Y, Kawauchi, A, Kayama, Y, & Miki, T. Discrete Regions in the Laterodorsal Tegmental of the Rat Regulating the Urinary Bladder and External Urethral Sphincter. Brain Research (2001). , 912-162.

[15] Mallory, B. S, Roppolo, J. R, & De Groat, W. C. Pharmacological Modulation of the Pontine Micturition Center. Brain Research (1991). , 546-310.

[16] Blok, B. F, & Holstege, G. Direct Projections from the Periaqueductal Gray to the Pontine Micturition Center (M-region). An anterograde and Retrograde Tracing Study in the Cat. Neuroscience Letters (1994). , 166-93.

[17] Ding, Y. Q, Takada, M, Tokuno, H, & Mizuno, N. Direct projections from the Dorsolateral Pontine Tegmentum to Pudendal Motoneurons Innervating the External Urethral Sphincter Muscle in the Rat. Journal of Comparative Neurology (1995). , 357-318.

[18] Holstege, G, Griffiths, D, De Wall, H, & Dalm, E. Anatomical and Physiological Observations on Supraspinal Control of Bladder and Urethral Sphincter Muscles in the Cat. Journal of Comparative Neurology (1986). , 250-449.

[19] Nadelhaft, I, & Vera, P. L. Central Nervous System Neurons Infected by Pseudorabies Virus Injected into the Rat Urinary Bladder Following Unilateral Transection of the Pelvic Nerve. Journal of Comparative Neurology (1995). , 359(3), 443-56.

[20] Seki, H, Kayama, Y, Kawauchi, A, Miki, T, & Koyama, Y. Urinary Bladder-Associated Activity and Neurotransmitters of the Micturition Center Neurons. In: the 36th Annual Meeting of Society for Neuroscience, October (2006). Atlanta, GA, USA., 14-18.

[21] Moruzzi, G, & Magoun, H. W. Brain Stem Reticular Formation and Activation of the EEG. Electrocephalographic Clinical Neurophysiology (1949). , 1-1155.

[22] Koyama, Y, Honda, T, Kusakabe, M, Kayama, Y, & Sugiura, Y. In Vivo Electrophysiological Distinction of Histochemically-Identified Cholinergic Neurons Using Extracellular Recording and Labelling in Rat Laterodorsal Tegmental Nucleus. Neuroscience (1998). , 83-1105.

[23] Takahashi, K, Kayama, Y, Lin, J. S, & Sakai, K. Locus Coeruleus Neuronal Activity During the Sleep-Waking Cycle in Mice. Neuroscience (2010). , 169(3), 1115-1126.

[24] Koyama, Y, Imada, N, Kawauchi, A, & Kayama, Y. Firing of Putative Cholinergic Neurons and Micturition Center Neurons in the Rat Laterodorsal Tegmentum During Distention and Contraction of Urinary Bladder. Brain Research (1999). , 840-45.

[25] Imada, N, Koyama, Y, Kawauchi, A, Watanabe, H, & Kayama, Y. State Dependent Responsiveness of the Locus Coeruleus Neurons to Bladder Distention. Journal of Urology (2000). , 164-1740.

[26] Luo, Y. F, Gao, X. Z, & Wei, J. Acupointology. Shanghai Science and Technology Publishing House, Shanghai (1998).

[27] Sun, P, Li, L, & Si, M. Comparison Between of Acupuncture and Epidural Anesthesia in Appendectomy. ZhenCi YanJiu (1992). , 17-87.

[28] Lou, Z, Sun, W, Liu, Y, & Tong, Z. Effect of Electro-Acupuncture on Cortical and Hippocampal EEG in Adjuvant Arthritis Rats. ZhenCi YanJiu (1992). , 17-129.

[29] Vankov, A, Hervé-minvielle, A, & Sara, S. J. Response to Novelty and Its Rapid Habituation in Locus Coeruleus Neurons of the Freely Exploring Rat. European Journal of Neuroscience (1995). , 7(6), 1180-1187.

[30] Sara, S. J. The Locus Coeruleus and Noradrenergic Modulation of Cognition. Nature Review Neuroscience (2009). , 10(3), 211-223.

[31] Wang, H, Tanaka, Y, Kawauchi, A, Miki, T, Kayama, Y, & Koyama, Y. Acupuncture of the Sacral Vertebrae Suppresses Bladder Activity and Bladder Activity-Related Neurons in the Brainstem Micturition Center. Neuroscience Research (2012). , 72(1), 43-49.

[32] Kitakoji, H, Terasaki, T, Honjo, H, Odahara, Y, Ukimura, O, Kojima, M, & Watanabe, H. Effect of Acupuncture on the Overactive Bladder. Japanese Journal of Urology (1995). , 86-1514.

[33] Cheng, P. T, Wong, M. K, & Chang, P. L. A therapeutic trial of acupuncture in neurogenic bladder of spinal cord injured patients--a preliminary report. Spinal Cord (1998). , 36(7), 476-480.

Chapter 5

# Plausible Biomedical Consequences of Acupuncture Applied at Sites Characteristic of Acupoints in the Connective-Tissue-Interstitial-Fluid System

Peter Chin Wan Fung

Additional information is available at the end of the chapter

http://dx.doi.org/10.5772/53901

## 1. Introduction

### 1.1. Acupuncture as one major branch of Traditional Chinese Medicine (TCM)

Traditional Chinese Medicine (TCM) has been in existence for several thousand years, based on the general philosophy that the physiological states of a healthy body are kept balanced. Pathogenesis occurs when such a balance is upset. There have been more and more studies using modern biomedical techniques and animal models on the clinical benefits of herbal TCM in the recent two decades. Fruitful developments have been made on the analysis of the biochemical ingredients of the herbs considered. However, standardization of ingredients of the herbs, the concept of "complex recipe" and a modern theory of herbal TCM described in terms of modern western medicine conception, are still issues of discussion while herbal TCM progresses.

Acupuncture is a part of TCM and the theory of acupuncture mechanism was put forth initially based on a series of hypotheses, conjectures in view of the numerous clinical examples accumulated. Using modern biomedical knowledge to understand the TCM meridians, to practice acupuncture, and to study the benefits of acupuncture seem to be somewhat more readily accepted (compared to herbal TCM) in the west [1]. Zhou et al [2] found 761 English articles published in the year 2006 directly related to acupuncture from various countries, 208 Chinese articles according to Medline search. There are also many other articles and books written in Chinese language published in institutional journals. Thus, English and Chinese are the two main languages for articles and books related to acupuncture research in number.

### 1.2. The types of acupuncture research carried out internationally

#### *1.2.1. Clinical acupuncture research*

Clinical data/reports have been collected with a long history in China on the benefits of treating various disorders of health, using the TCM concept of "energy flow" along the meridians, and certain basic principles stated in classics (without direct verification). Some such books incorporating new concepts in biomedical science also appear in the recent two decades or so. These writings have been published mainly in the Chinese language [3-4]. There are also clinically oriented books written by acupuncturists in acupuncture centers/institutes of western countries, Japan and Korea. Those written in English are focused more on using various modalities of acupuncture as means to treat pains [5-6]. Some of these writings use the concept of triggered points rather than TCM acupoints, and the benefits of acupuncture are usually associated entirely with signals transmitted through the nervous systems [7].

#### *1.2.2. Basic evidence-based acupuncture research*

The fast development of biomedical science with new techniques and concept has helped to inject enthusiasm and good attempts/results from scientists globally using animal models, in vitro experimentations, or clinical settings to analyze the following general issues: (I) the anatomical characteristics of the meridian channels/acupoints; (II) to investigate on how the acupuncture signals could be transmitted from the acupoint to other parts of the body, and via the meridian channels; (III) the plausible physiological consequences of acupuncture in action; these consequences include both biophysical and biochemical aspects.

#### *1.2.3. Accumulation of a huge data base from biomedical science/engineering research which is indirectly related to the mechanism of acupuncture in action*

For a long time, biochemical force is considered to be the most fundamental force in cell signaling involved in physiological processes, and in initiating cellular response to external stimuli. However, research during the last 20 years on cell signaling and cellular structure reveals that mechanical sensors (integrins with the focal adhesion complexes and mediators) exist at the cell membrane to bridge the extra-cellular matrix (ECM) and cytoskeletal elements in transmitting mechanotransduction signals. Then cytoskeletal elements build up prestress and contractile structures, joining the nucleus to the cytoskeletal base of the mechanical sensor unit. Mechanical stimulation initiates a cascade of cytoskeletal remodeling. Thus, the cell nucleus, via mechanotransduction, can react directly to a wide range of mechanical stresses. It has also been found that mechanotransduction, which exists between adjacent cells, and between extracellular fluid and cells, plays even more fundamental roles than biochemical interactions [8-11].

In fact, mechanotransduction is a key fundamental concept to physiology, ensuing the organism's structural stability and development. A lot of new experimental data, new conceptual knowledge, plus consequential deductions related to mechanotransduction have been published based on modern knowledge of biophysics and biochemistry. These results provide important clues to the understanding of the basic acupuncture mechanism.

### 1.3. Objectives of this chapter and the settings in presentation

Based on the remarks mentioned in Sections 1.2 (B and C), I would review first briefly in Section 2 the basic knowledge of mechanotransduction via solid and fluid objects for convenience of more in-depth discussion about plausible consequences of acupuncture in later sections of this chapter. Evidence and reasons on the occurrence of the meridians/ acupoints in the connective-tissue- interstitial fluid (CTIF) system is presented in Section 3; the typical anatomical features of acupoints are briefly highlighted. Section 4 starts with a description on the initial response of the CTIF system when manual acupuncture is applied to a typical acupoint in the CTIF system. Section 5 is devoted to a discussion on the plausible consequence of acupuncture when the mechanical stimulus reaches the ECM of cells building the blood vessels, with support from results of some clinical studies and in vivo animal investigation. Note that an acupoint is found to be near nerve endings and nerves. Various types of neural signals are found to be triggered with evidence from laboratory and clinical studies. Therefore a brief analysis on the neural aspects of mechanotransduction is carried out in Section 6. In Section 7, the evidence on the existence of fluid flow along channels (which are not blood flows) correlating to the TCM meridian channels is presented. The importance of maintaining a proper flow of the interstitial fluid to health is emphasized. The issue on whether acupuncture could help to keep the homeostasis of such fluid flow in the body is discussed in Section 7. Section 8 is catered for a brief discussion on the degranulation of mast cells, which have been found to be near typical acupoints. The plausible release and activation of transforming-growth-factor-β (TGFβ) upon unfolding of an abundant protein, the fibronectin in the ECM of fibroblasts is discussed. Since TGFβ activates local stem cells specification, and mast cells sustain fibroblasts, the release and activation of TGFβ and mast cell degranulation are discussed together as part of the function group for immunity and wound repair processes in Section 8. The plausible consequences of acupuncture described in Sections 4-8 is summarized with the help of a flow chart in Section 9. This section also presents some frontier issues and new ideas for future acupuncture research. Section 10 concludes this chapter. Unless otherwise stated, acupuncture refers to manual acupuncture, as this chapter is focused on the consequences of acupuncture arising from mechanotransduction.

## 2. Basics of mechanotransduction, relevant to discussion in this chapter

### 2.1. Tensegrity of living organism on earth and mechanotransduction

Any living organism living on the massive earth is subjected (a) to the gravitational force which manifests as a mechanical pull on every part of the body continuously, and (b) frequently to external mechanical and other forms of stimuli from other objects.

Research during the past two decades on cell signaling and cellular structure indicates that (1) external stimuli of mechanical or electrical nature control many fundamental biochemical interactions; (2) tissues are composed of a network of "connected" cells and proteins, rather than individual cells plus proteins in a body fluid. Putting these two observations and recalling the two "disturbances" (a) and (b) on organisms on earth just stated above, one is inclined to consider that a special architecture system must be at work in each living entity particularly suitable for transmission of mechanical signals, if it is to remain as that entity. Such an architecture system is one important basis for allowing acupuncture signals to be transmitted to certain parts of the body. Ingber and other workers have realized the importance of this living architecture and developed the tensegrity model of a cell [12].

Mechanical signals are inferred to be transmitted through mechanotransduction in principle to various parts of the body based on the hierarchy (systems within systems) nature of the body, with connective tissues (CT) embedding other tissues/organelles/organs. The mechanical forces involved in mechanotransduction through the body are mainly tensile and compression for solids, and shear stress (which is the friction force of fluid flow acting on the surface of cells) and pressure for fluids [13].

Note that mechanosensitive ion channels, which are also "fundamental components" for processes of mechanotransduction, were discovered long ago (1950) among neurons [14]. Mechanosensitive channels were documented in various other cells in the 1980s [15]. During that time, the tensegrity concept was not brought in from architecture.

### 2.2. Mechanical signals at the cell membrane can cascade a series of signals reaching the cell nucleus – Integrin starts the story

Integrins, being composed of alpha and beta subunits with various combinations, are cell membrane receptors which can bind to proteins in the ECM with specificity [16]. There is ample evidence that the basic mechanism of ECM- cytoskeletal elements connection is mediated by integrin clustering [8, 11]. When the integrins are stimulated mechanically, they connected intracellular proteins like focal adhesion kinase (FAK), Src-family kinases. Activation of these kinases triggers off a series of pathways associated with cytoskeletal remodeling. In particular, it was demonstrated that the stress-induced mechanical strain stimulated conformational activation of $\alpha$ – and $\beta$- integrins of NIH3T3 cells [17]. Such activation was mediated by phosphoinositol 3-kinase and was followed by new integrin ligand binding to ECM proteins, which then mediated c-Jun NH2-terminal kinase (JNK), initiating a series of cellular responses without upsetting the existing integrin-ECM binding. In general, responding to mechanical stimulation, there is growth of focal adhesion, leading to a stress-dependent increase in cytoskeletal (CSK) stiffness. The CSK stiffness changes because there is rearrangement of the microfilaments (MF), microtubules (MT) and intermediate filaments (IF). Since these structures join the nucleus surface after such CSK remodeling [11], expressions of different genes are affected to produce the relevant proteins to maintain the cell integrity and initiate the necessary physiological processes [18].

### 2.3. Intercellular communication through mechanotransduction – Connexin plays one key role

Various connexin proteins build up gap junction proteins between adjacent cells [19]. It has already been known, based on analysis of synchronous contraction of myocardial cells, that the gap junction proteins participate in the transfer of mechanical stimulation, indicating that mechanotransduction can be "passed on" between adjacent cells of a tissue/organ [20]. In the same work, it was shown that electrical synaptic transmission between nerve cells depended also on the integrity of gap junctions. Instead of building a passive gateway for the transportation of electric charge and relatively small molecules, the connexin protein Cx43 has been found to bind directly or indirectly to some intracellular proteins like caveolin, 20-β-catenin, tubulin, src which have various functions, supporting the idea that gap junctions take part also in mechanotransduction [21]. The correlation between activation of connexin and acupoints will be followed up in Section 9.

### 2.4. Intra and inter-cellular calcium ions oscillations are involved in the mechanotransduction processes of many cell types, including fibroblast

Many biochemical pathways involving different secondary messengers occur consequentially to a simple mechanical stimulus at a cellular mechanical sensor [22, 23]. First, there is ample evidence that intra-cellular $Ca^{2+}$ oscillations and inter-cellular $Ca^{2+}$ waves are involved in the mechanotransduction processes of many cell types, including fibroblasts, though the term mechanotransduction might not formally be put in all the articles at that time [24-27].

Recent studies also identify changes in cellular $Ca^{2+}$ concentration to be one major step of translating mechanical forces and deformation at the cell membrane into biochemical signals [28]. Note that Inositol 1 4, 5-Trisphosphate (IP3) - dependent or independent pathway may be involved in these $Ca^{2+}$ activities in various cells [29, 30].

The question of how intracellular $Ca^{2+}$ concentration $[Ca^{2+}]_i$ oscillations could affect mitochondrial functions has been investigated. It was demonstrated in [31] that IP3-dependent intracellular $[Ca^{2+}]_i$ oscillations were transmitted to the mitochondria of hepatocytes, based on the fact that $Ca^{2+}$ regulates some calcium-sensitive mitochondrial dehydrogenases (CSMDHs). This finding suggests that the mitochondria are tuned to oscillating $[Ca^{2+}]_i$ signals and different ranges of frequency are related to different potential activities of CSMDHs. As the function of the mitochondria is a very important aspect of cells and tissues, the expected consequence is a cascade of physiological cellular events. On the other hand, the characteristics of these intra-cellular and inter-cellular calcium activities are dependent on the amount of extracellular calcium ions (in the "extracellular calcium store") associated with the stimulated cells [32]. Moreover, variation in cytoplasmic $Ca^{2+}$ activities was found to correlate with those of nuclear calcium. In fact, it was demonstrated that cytoplasmic calcium and nuclear calcium activities control gene expressions in different ways [33, 34]

In vitro experiment [27] using 3T3 fibroblasts demonstrated that stretching forces applied through the flexible substrates (mimicking the CT) would induce increase in intracellular $Ca^{2+}$ concentration due to influx from extracellular calcium store [27]. These fibroblasts (then) showed cytoskeletal contractility, an aspect crucial to transmission of acupuncture signal through the CTIF system. The correlation between calcium concentration and acupoints will be discussed in Section 9.

## 3. The CTIF system as platform for acupuncture signals to cause biomedical effects via mechanotransductions of various kinds

### 3.1. Crucial characteristics of the CTIF system relevant to providing means for transmission of acupuncture signals

Connective tissue (CT) is the most abundant tissue of the body. The components in CT are the collagen fibers of various types [35], glycoproteins like fibronectin, laminin, tenascin, elastin and various subclasses of proteoglycans. Among these sub-classes, hyaluronan is the dominant glycosaminoglycan serving as the backbone for the assembly of other glycosaminoglycans in the CT. These proteins form different networks (with different combination of components) in the extra-cellular matrix (ECM) associated with different tissues/organs "wrapped" by the CT [36, 37].

The interstitial fluid serves to transport nutrient proteins, ions, oxygen and water from the capillaries to the general tissues for their functions. It also removes cellular excreta, unused proteins to the lymphatic system as well as transports $CO_2$ from the tissues to the venous capillaries. The proteoglycans of CT form extremely thin fibrils which interact with the surrounding interstitial fluid (IF) to form a gel-like ground substance [38, 39], allowing slow flow for proper distribution of nutrients and processing of excreta.

The connective tissue interstitial fluid (CTIF) system forms a body frame with connected layers which embeds the neurovascular tracts, connects tunicae around the visceral organs, and extends to form the periosteum, nourishing the bones [38-41]. Nerve fibers are densely populated around acupoint sites in the CTIF system. These nerve fibers innervate blood vessels, lymphatic vessels, with different types of endings serving as specific or polymodal nociceptive receptors [42]. The residence cells in the CTIF system are lymphocytes, macrophages, adipocytes, plasma cells, eosinophils, fibroblasts, chondroblasts, osteoblasts, stem cells and mast cells [43]. Fibroblasts sustain collagen fibers [44] while mast cells upkeep the proliferation of fibroblasts [45]. The "organ/adherent cells" are defined here to be those forming part of the "non-CTIF" tissue/organ like blood/lymphatic vessel cells, nerve cells, visceral organ cells.

Without reference to special particulars of the acupuncture mechanism, some earlier studies already indicated that fibroblasts throughout the connective tissues system were connected among themselves [46, 47]. It was found that fibroblasts in different tissues grown in cell culture were seen to contact one another with gap junctions at contact points [48-50]. Moreover, many cryptic binding sites of the fibronectin modules have been identified; these binding sites are hidden when the fibronectin proteins are in the folded state. Unfolding the fibronectin by mechanotransduction through the CTIF system could unfold the modules into fibrils, releasing some of the already bound growth factors as well as exposing other binding sites to take part in biochemical activities; see review of [51].

### 3.2. Early evidence of the involvement of connective tissues (CT) during acupuncture in action, up to year 2000

According to the TCM classics [52a], which was written a few thousand years ago, it was hypothesized, based on clinical experience using acupuncture, that "..... the twelve meridians go through regions between muscles, are deep and cannot be seen...... ". Now we know that in between the muscle spindles are connective tissues with deposited proteins, as part of the CTIF system. So the correlation of the connective tissues with the meridians was already hinted/stated in ancient Chinese classics. A series of research work starting from 1980s leads to the analysis on the anatomical structure of the acupoint sites (of cadavers) and it was found that acupoints of the "earth positions" [52b, 52c] were three-dimensional spaces being close to nerve endings or branches of nerves, blood vessels and lymphatic vessels; these regions or "spaces" referred to always include also one type of connective tissues or another within the CTIF system [53-55]. Direct verification that acupoints are actually within the CTIF system was not directly reported until science and technology developed to that stage around 1990s.

In 1992, it was reported in [56] that after sparrow-pecking and twisting manipulation of acupuncture needles to acupoints BL23, BL24, BL25 of human subjects until de qi was felt, some transparent materials were found to be attached to the needles by microscopic analysis. The materials contained collagen fibers, elastic fibers, fibroblasts, mast cells, macrophages and adipocytes. In another study [57], based on morphological analysis of five cadavers, the 3D structure of the acupoint SP6 was found to contain nervous, vasculature structures embedded in connective tissues. Dang et al in [58] used three cadavers and inserted needles to 11 acupoint sites of the Lung Meridian. In doing so, the acupuncturist also cast the needle to each acupoint on a healthy male volunteer until de qi, and carried out computerized tomography x-ray examination of the needle position, to be compared with that exercised on the cadavers. Nine out of the eleven acupoints of the Lung Meridian were found to be on the periosteum layers of the related bones. Using three cadavers, the investigators [59] carried out an anatomical analysis of all the acupoints of the GB meridian channel below the head and found that from GB20 to GB44, 18 acupoints were mainly associated with the periosteum and interosseous membrane, the other 7 were related to fascia, epineurium of the nerve and articular capsule of the knee. All these anatomical structures are in fact connective tissues of one form or another. Fei et al employed a video microscope [60] to examine the specimens around the acupoint ST36 of cadavers and discovered that the anatomic structure of capillaries, nerve plexus and lymphatic ducts formed a complex structure with connective tissues as basis. They also analyzed the anatomy structure of 73 acupoints along three different meridians of three cadavers and reported that all these acupoint sites were associated with connective tissues. Other similar characteristics have been reported along the acupoints of the Stomach Meridian [61]. So many acupoints were found to be within layers of connective tissues in, at least, all these studies.

### 3.3. Evidence of the involvement of connective tissues during acupuncture in action, starting from the twenty-first century

To probe the mechanism of acupuncture signal transmission, Langevin's group produced a series of works, demonstrating that connective tissues of rat abdominal wall explants would wind around a rotating needle but not around an inserted one [62]. The suction force and torque experienced by an acupuncturing needle in vivo during de qi were measured quantitatively by the machine they built. It was demonstrated that fibroblasts in the stated explants would change the morphology from the "quiescent" round shape to elongated one when the collagen fibers whirled around the (acupuncture) needle. In 2003, Ding et al [63] repeated the above-stated force and torque measurement with a simpler machine. Comparing fig.6 of [62] and fig.8b of [63], it appears that fig.8b gives an additional feature ("vibrating-like" wave, representing relaxation) to verify the involvement of elastic anatomical tissues during the relaxation part of one complete action of winding and unwinding in the in vivo experiments of subjects.

Later, more than 80 % of acupoints were found to coincide with intermuscular or intra-muscular connective tissue planes of postmortem tissue sections of the arm [64]. Images were obtained from a digital data set derivable from 8556 slices of a female cadaver [65]. Likewise, similar images were obtained from 9232 slices of a male cadaver [66]. Based on such datasets, 3D images were obtained to generate the frames of the connective tissues for the whole female and male bodies [41]. They located the positions of acupoints according to TCM on such frames and reported that for one body, 361 acupoints were all located in various types of connective tissues, with a maximum of 204 in the intermuscular (loose) septa.

Further, it was demonstrated in [67] that needle-rotation-induced morphological change in mouse fibroblasts explants was inhibited by inhibitors of actomyosin activity, Rho kinase and Rac signaling. Analyzing these intracellular biochemical pathways, that "tension-induced signaling by acupuncture would lead to cytoskeletal remodeling of fibroblasts" was considered to be directly verified in the explants experiments. These changes in cell shape required the presence of both intact microtubules and microfilaments, implying an active, cytoskeletal-dependent mechanism.

## 4. Response of the CTIF system to acupuncture at a typical acupoint in the loose connective tissue layer

### 4.1. Fibroblasts in their quiescent state are not isolated, intact cells; traction of fibroblast can trigger rapid global self-organization of the collagen matrix system

It was shown that slow local motion of collagen fibers driven by fibroblasts induced rapid global self-organization of collagen gel (in minutes) in in vitro experiments [68]. Later, another in vitro study showed that fibroblasts in their quiescent state formed a whole body-like network, with their processes in close proximities [69], implying that fibroblasts are not really "isolated" cells. It has been demonstrated by another group that fibroblasts interact with 3D relaxed collagen matrices to form dendritic type of extensions without the alignment of cytoskeletal microtubules [70]. However, at a high tension state (typical of cells on "coverslips" in in vitro settings of such types of experiments, or consequence of acupuncture rotation in the loose connective tissue), cells spread with lamellipodial extensions, requiring the function of microtubules, meaning that the fibroblasts are exerting attraction force (back) to the ECM matrix if the mechanical stimulus is strong enough. It has also been found further that migration of fibroblasts can remodel the architecture of the collagen matrix both locally and globally [71], substantiating and adding more to [68]. All these studies demonstrate that there is a strong mechanical coupling between the fibroblasts and elements of the connective tissues system, as a basis of transmitting mechanical signals through the CTIF system, particularly when the tension of the collagen fibers reach a certain magnitude.

### 4.2. The rapid global self-organization of the collagen matrix system is initiated by fibronectin fibrils formation

Despite the experimental discovery of the rapid self-organization of the collagen matrix as a phenomenon, stated in Section 4.1, a scientific link is still missing as to understand the basic mechanism on how such organization could occur rapidly to distances much greater than cell size. Note that a number of proteins are attached to the ECM of cells with specifications (Section 3.1). Among them, fibronectin (Fn) is produced by most cell types into their ECM [72]. Using fluorescence resonance energy transfer techniques, it has been found only several years ago in [73] that traction force of cells could stretch an initially nodular assembly of Fn (with quaternary structure) to many times its initial length. It is noted that the unfolding of Fn played an import role to outside-in and inside-out mechanotransduction due to cell traction or when mechanical stimulus arrives the membranes of cells. Thus, the in vitro experiments suggests that in vivo acupuncture in action causes not only morphological changes of fibroblasts, but also (as a consequence) an anatomical change-unfolding of Fn, leading to formation of Fn fibrils in the collagen matrix. The CTIF system is thus mechanically well connected for efficient mechanotransduction. Whether other proteins like laminin or tenascin (Section 3.1) would participate in a different or similar way to assist mechanotransduction is still a future research project. Now we understand at least Fn plays one key role in global self-organization by forming fibrils.

### 4.3. Inter- and intra-muscular connective tissue cleavage planes favor mechanotransduction to longer distance – suggestive of high efficiency of mechanotransduction through the meridian channels

A high correlation between inter- and intramuscular connective tissue cleavage planes and acupoints (around 80 %) and meridians (around 50 %) was found via analysis of cadaver sections [64]. Though the exact percentages different in other studies [41, 58, 60], by far the majority acupoints were found in the loose and other types of connective tissues, including that building up the periostia to join the bones. To set up in vitro models of the intermuscular plane, type 1 collagen was cast in circular gels of different radii, elliptical gels with quantified major and minor axes, matching the large and small circular gels respectively [74]. Collagen was also cast in planar gels with constraint on two sides. Acupuncture needles were inserted into the gel specimens and rotated by motors, mimicking acupuncture in action. It was found that rotation in planar gels with constraint on two sides, elliptical gels, circular gels generated the strongest, less strong and weakest alignment of collagen fibers respectively. With fibroblasts in the gel specimens, the phenomenon of durotaxis was demonstrated [39]. In other words, fibroblasts followed alignment of collagen fibers, with denser population along stronger alignment. Result of such in vitro experiment, in view of the special anatomical characteristics of acupoint sites, supports the notion that efficiency of mechanotransduction through the acupoints and meridian channels is relatively high, compared to non-acupoints, when induced by acupuncture action.

## 5. On the issue of peripheral blood vessel dilation resulting from acupuncture

### 5.1. Recent revisit to the long standing question – Why would muscle compression on blood vessels trigger immediate vessel dilation?

Biomedical scientists have been trying for years to explain the daily-experienced occurrence of the immediate increase in blood flow to skeletal muscles at the onset of exercise.

In 2006, rat soleus arteries were isolated and pressure compressions were applied in a series to the vessels [75]. It was found that dilation of these arteries was elicited by brief periods of compression mimicking extravascular contractions, substantiating the stated daily experience at the onset of exercise. Scientists still have to find out more about the mechanism behind the phenomenon of "self-regulatory type" of dilation.

### 5.2. Recent discovery: Unfolding of fibronectin fibrils in the ECM of vessel cells as one key clue for Nitric Oxide-mediated local dilation

Using intravital microscopy in in vivo animal experiment, it was reported for the first time [76] that fibronectin (Fn) fibrils in the CT near blood vessel would transduce mechanical signals from contracting skeletal muscle to trigger a fast, specific and reversible local vessel dilation mediated by nitric oxide, the commonest vessel dilator. The active part of the Fn fibrils was found to be type III-I of Fn. Moreover, Fn, administered intravenously, was found to assemble quickly into elongated, branching fibrils in the extracellular matrix of intact cremaster muscle, showing active polymerization of Fn in areas adjacent to blood vessels. These two sets of experiments indicated that unfolding of the fibronectin fibrils of adult connective tissue plays a dynamic role in regulating both vascular responses and vascular tone. Though the experiment was meant to find out why exercise caused vessel dilation, the important result of these studies is that mechanotransduction, when reaching the ECM of vessels could cause unfolding of Fn, triggering biochemical events leading to nitric oxide (NO)-mediated vasodilation (various aspects of NO generation are discussed also in Section 9.4). This series of studies put forth the notion that blood vessels have self-regulating system to tone the dilation in response to external mechanical disturbance, for survival of the organism.

### 5.3. Direct evidence of acupuncture-induced local vessel dilation

In a clinical setting, the levels of NO and the protein Interleukin-2 (IL-2) contents of peripheral blood were reported to be significantly higher in 42 subjects after warm needling at ST36 [77]. Using animal models, it was demonstrated [78] that electro-acupuncture at ST36 reduced blood pressure by activation of two nitric oxide Synthases (eNOS and nNOS, Section 9.4). In another clinical study with 20 subjects, it was demonstrated that acupuncture would cause enhanced release of NO locally, leading to improved blood circulation. In particular, NO concentration in the plasma from the acupunctured arm was significantly higher after acupuncture. Blood flow in the palmar subcutaneous tissue of the acupunctured arm was also increased [79]. Moreover, acupuncture was performed at LU7 of 56 subjects [80], and the skin blood flow was found to be raised along the track from LU7 to LU5, using a laser Doppler flowmeter.

### 5.4. The observation of infrared radiant tracks along the TCM meridians on the skin during acupuncture and the recent discovery of adenosine triphosphate (ATP) enhancement at acupoint region after acupuncture

A number of studies have been carried out to measure the temperature of different parts of the skin (particularly the limbs) after acupuncture was applied to a diversity of acupoints of human subjects and animals, using thermograms with resolution about o.1 degree Celcius [4, 81, 82]. Infrared radiant tracks were detected along lines correlating with various TCM meridian channels on the skin during acupuncture. Later, specimens along and away from outside of these infrared radiant tracks of animal models were taken and it was found that both the P substance and ATPase were higher with statistical significance along the meridian lines [83]. In another animal study [84], points along the Du meridian were taken as test points and points 2.5 cm sideway to the test points were taken as reference. The oxygen partial pressure $PO_2$ values in the deep tissues along these test points were found to be significantly higher than that of the reference points. The above results suggest that higher metabolism rate was the source of the infrared radiant tracts observed on the skin, subsequent to acupuncture action.

Recently, it was found in a mice model that acupuncture at ST 36 triggers an increase in the ECM concentrations of ATP, ADP, AMP and adenosine. Abundance of these basic units of bio-energy indicates occurrence of high metabolism rate [85]. The appearance of infrared radiant tracks on the skin part of the meridians can be interpreted as enhancement of blood flow through the blood vessels (arising from activation of eNOS or non-NOS enzymes which cause vessel dilation) along the meridian channels during/after acupuncture, leading to a higher metabolic rate.

## 6. Transmission of the acupuncture signals through mechanotransduction from connective tissues to the nervous system

### 6.1. Acupoints are close to various types of nerve receptors

It has been hypothesized/inferred with evidence as stated in [39, 60, 86, 87] that acupoints are close to high density sites of polymodal and specific nociceptive receptors, neurovascular structure, lymphatic vessels, and mast cells. In fact, high density of nerve endings was also found at many acupoint sites of rat models recently [88]. All peripheral nerve fibers are embedded by various CT layers (endoneurium, perineurium, epineurium) with epineurium forming the outermost layer. Thus acupuncture applied at the acupoint sites which are embedded in the CTIF system would send mechanical signals readily to the mechanical nerve sensors close to the acupoints. Upon receiving mechanical stimulation, the mechanical receptors of nerve cells would have some of the cations and $Ca^{2+}$ activated [89]. The in-flux and out-flux of the associated ions leads to the appearance of the action potentials which propagate as signals through the nerve fibers. Evidence-based result suggests that mechanotransduction originated from acupuncture could send signals through the skin, as well as through reflexes carried out by nerves deeper down, to be briefly specified below.

### 6.2. Acupuncture could initiate signals via mechanotransduction to travel along the skin level of the meridian channels based on animal model studies

In a series of study, 125-I-tyrosine was injected to animal models [90-92]. The epidermis and dermis part of the skin was exposed to x-ray films for weeks. Longitudinal distributed lines with rich sympathetic substance (neurotransmitters) were found on the skin. These lines were inferred to be correlated to the skin parts of the known TCM meridian channels. Acupuncturing at ST36 was demonstrated to relief pain of the rabbit model, but injection of inhibitors of neurotransmitters or cutting the part of the skin en route the Stomach Meridian at the back of the animal model abolished the analgesic effects. These studies provide evidence that acupuncture could cause signals to be transmitted along meridian channels at the skin level. The signals propagate as if jumping over nerve endings. Other independent studies [93] documented that evoked potential could be transmitted across skin nerve endings of the Urinary Bladder Meridian of the bullfrog model using electrophysiology technique. So far neural transmission was interpreted as axon reflex along the skin employing hairy animal models in the above four references. More detailed analysis is needed to make more concrete statement on the stated skin-phenomenon associated with the application of acupuncture to "non-hairy animal models".

### 6.3. Acupuncture leads to "external-internal connection" (a TCM concept) by way of somato-visceral organ reflexes based on animal models studies

In Chinese medicine the external-internal connection has been emphasized for several thousand years [52c]. In modern biomedical science language, the function of visceral organs is regulated by the autonomic nervous system and the function of the skin and skeletal muscle is regulated by the somatic nervous system. Since specific muscles are connected to a visceral organ/system in general, the somatic nervous system also participates in the regulation of the visceral organ. Thus the external (acupuncture at sites near nerve sensors) and internal (visceral organs function) connection via the somato-visceral organ reflexes are explainable physiological pathways [94-96]. As the somato- and visceral-nerve fibers are connected to one or more spinal cord segments, and eventually to the brain, the organization centers of the somato-visceral organ reflexes can be at the spinal cord segment(s) or the brain [94]. As noted in [96], the somato-visceral reflexes can be mediated through four major pathways: (i) the axon reflex which has no direct automatic involvement but performs as if there is automatic activation; (ii) the spinal reflex characteristics of segmental organization; (iii) the medullary reflex which is integrative in nature; (iv) supra medullary reflex which is related to hormonal secretion like sweating and regulation of cerebral blood flow.

### 6.4. Acupuncture induces immunity-mediated or neurogenic inflammation around the region of stimulus

Some somato-visceral neurons, having their cell bodies in the dorsal root ganglia, behave as afferents as well as efferents by releasing neuropeptides from their peripheral terminals. These peptides induce a cascade of changes, collectively called "neurogenic inflammation", specified by two general events [97]: (i) Antidromic vasodilaton (ADV), the increased blood flow seen in tissues on stimulation of the sensory dorsal roots. (ii) Plasma extravasation.

The C and A delta neuron endings with abundant nociceptive receptors are hypothesized with evidence to be acupoint sites [39, 60, 86, 87], and they are being involved in such inflammation. Antidormic vasodilatoin (ADV) is only clearly seen when C-fibers or some of Aδ fibers are excited [97, 98]. What our body system tries to do is "reasonable" and obvious microvessels (particularly the capillaries) dilate, and increase the permeabilities of the vessel walls so that blood flow is increased together with enhanced exudation of plasma to the injured site where acupuncture was applied. During this time more leukocytes, which are activated by the hormones, are released from the nociceptive sensory receptors. These leukocytes can migrate from the blood to the interstitial site, and together with the "residence" immune cells of the CTIF (macrophages, eosinophil, .....), they carry out their basic immunity duties, while the excreta are being carried away by relatively larger fluid volume to the lymphatic vessels to be processed at the lymph nodes. That acupuncture would lead to neurogenic inflammation has already been analyzed in [87]. Though acupuncture-induced neurogenic inflammation could bring benefits (details like pain treatment are outside the scope of in this chapter), the effect must be regulated/fine-tuned. For example, manual acupuncture has been documented to modulate capsaicin-induced edema, a phenomenon within the general concept of neurogenic inflammation [99, 100]. Concerning the fine-tuning aspect, there is evidence that the nervous system can regulate the inflammatory response reflexively in real time [101]. To find out the modality of acupuncture that could regulate neurogenic inflammation by stimulating selective and reversible reflexive neural systems is perhaps another topic of acupuncture research in the future.

### 6.5. Acupuncture can trigger signals through afferent nerve fibers to reach the brain – MRI demonstrations

Using magnetic resonance imaging (MRI) technique, investigations have been carried out to analyze the parts of the brain being activated in response to acupuncture or electroacupuncture applied at acupoints and non-acupoints. It was found that acupuncture stimulation of acupoints has specific effects on cortical neuronal activity, but not so for non-acupoints [102]. The integrated response of the human cerebellar system to acupuncture stimulation at ST36 was found to be correlated with the psycho-physical response [103]. There was evidence suggesting that chronic pain patients responded to acupuncture differently than healthy normal subjects, through a coordinated network including hypothalamus and amygdala [104]. However, a recent study points out that nonferromagnetic needles need to be used during acupuncture if MRI measurement is to be carried out [105]. I would note that the magnetic field inside a MRI tube is typically ~ 15, 000 gauss, whereas the earth's magnetic field is around 0.5 gauss. The magnetic field at the point of acupuncture application has to be well-shielded during MRI scanning, if the needle is ferromagnetic, for obvious scientific reasons. Therefore, I could not comment on the MRI results unless proper needles are used in this type of studies or proper magnetic–shielding is clearly specified in the report.

Another alternative is to employ real time source imaging analysis using multi-channel electroencethalogram (EEG) to analyze the brain function [106] during acupuncture in action. It might be possible to make more concrete statement on how the brain responds in real time to the action of acupuncture employing this new neural imaging technique using dipole source analysis in the future.

### 6.6. Mechanotransduction induces release of vasodilatory neuropeptides from nerve endings, a very recent study

Acupuncture was applied to acupoint Hegu (L14) of subjects, while the frequency content of skin blood flow signals was measured using Laser Doppler flowmetry (LDF) simultaneously [107]. It was demonstrated that needling L14 significantly increased blood perfusion at the acupoint, but not at nearby non-acupoint sites. Based on a wavelet transform analysis technique of the LDF data [108], it was inferred that the resultant blood flow increase was caused by the release of vasodilatory neuropeptides from nerve endings, which subsequently interact with sympathetic vasoconstriction neurons. Thus apart from more direct NO-mediated vessel dilation triggered by mechanical signals applied to vessel cells discussed in the last section, acupuncture could induce vessel dilation through interaction with nerve endings.

## 7. Acupuncture may influence the flow characteristics of the interstitial fluid, leading to biomedical consequences

### 7.1. Evidence of the interstitial fluid flows correlating with some TCM meridian channels using radioactive tracers

Starting from 1960, Chinese researchers began to inject radioactive materials in acupoints and recorded the radiation using scintillation counter outside the test body. The first formal report released to the public appeared in [109]. Tiberiu et al then [110] recorded the radioactive trace to follow from UB61 to UB67, away from the heart [110]. It was found also in [110] that there was a "stationary time interval" during which propagation did not proceed at all and this interval varied among individuals and among meridians, having a mean of 37.28 s. Later, radioactive material was injected into acupoints of the extremities (fingertips and those around the ankles) of 94 volunteers. The longest radioactive track detected was identified to be along the Spleen Meridian, to a length of 85.87 cm and the shortest propagation path was 33.21 cm, correlating to the Large Intestine Meridian [111-113]. These authors concluded that the flows were not along blood vessels.

### 7.2. Evidence of fluid flow along channels of low dynamical resistance in animal models using pressure transducers

While the existence of the interstitial fluid is well established in physiology, fluid pressure measurement in vivo was progressed very slowly due to experimental difficulty. Guyton [114] and Levick [115] developed two basic methods [116] using mechanical transducers connected to special needles which were inserted to sites of investigation in vivo. Analyzing signals obtained from the transducers give information on the relative pressure of the interstitial fluid. Zhang modified these methods and to measure the fluid pressure and discovered that many sites of relative low fluid dynamic resistance existed in the subcutaneous connective tissue layers of animals (rabbits, pigs ) and humans [117, 118]. From such series of studies, he inferred that the meridians were interstitial fluid channels flowing with different speeds at different sites, substantiating the existence of flows correlating with some TCM meridians and general characteristics of "uneven flow rates" discovered in the radioactive tracer experiments.

### 7.3. Can acupuncture influence the flow characteristics of the interstitial fluid in the CTIF system?

It is well-known in classical physiology that the IF flow characteristics are controlled by the hydrostatic pressure $P_{if}$ of IF, the colloid osmotic pressure (Starling's law) as well as the lymphatic draining strength. While the vasculature system is well studied, the features of IF flow and variations of $P_{if}$ transports are relatively un-explored. If there is a difference of $P_{if}$ between two adjacent points in the interstitium, IF tends to flow to balance such a pressure difference. Since gravity also acts on the IF, at any instance, the $P_{if}$ in different parts of the interstitium are different, and the values of $P_{if}$ depends on the posture of the body [119]; a recent revisit has been paid to analyze how would the interstitium operate as a dynamic interface for water and solute distribution over the body [120]. As the IF flows through a complicated structure of fibers, proteins, cells in the interstitium, intuition argues that the CT structure would influence IF flow characteristics. If a subject is to remain in the (healthy) physiological state, the IF must have the proper flow speeds at various sites for healthy distribution of nutrients and drainage of excreta (Section 3.1). There is evidence that the integrins of the residing cells and growth factors in the CTIF together play active role tending to keep IF homeostasis [121, 122]. On the other hand, it is documented in [123] that $P_{if}$ in (breast) tumor is increased, caused by tumor-associated angiogenesis, and the IF flow speed becomes faster. Such rise in $P_{if}$ inhibits pharmaceutical chemicals to reach the target tumor; moreover, cancer cells might be driven to the lymphatic vessels nearby. The aspects on how physical force of the flowing IF would regulate tumor invasion were analyzed in [124]. The issue on the synergies between lymph drainage and flow- induced mechanotransduction in stroma of cancer cells is being studied very recently [125]. Thus controlling proper $P_{if}$ seems to be important for health, but biomedical scientists are still in the "infancy state" of IF research. When we rotate a needle back and forth during acupuncture, in addition to sending mechanical signals along the CTIF system, intuition seems to support the idea that there is a redistribution of tension among the collagen fibers affected. Since the collagen fibers of the CT are embedded in the IF, acupuncture gives room for the IF to redistribute the $P_{if}$ also. Thus I hypothesize that acupuncture serves as a toning process of the IF flow, tending to keep homeostasis of $P_{if}$ along the meridian channels (see a related article [126]). Further research along this line is also important, keeping in mind that $P_{if}$ rise in tumor is the consequence of a pathological process.

## 8. Acupuncture causes mast cell degranulation as an immunity response, and may cause release of transforming -growth- factor-β from ECM of fibroblasts, as activators for local stem cell lineage specification

### 8.1. Mast cells degranulation induced by acupuncture action

Mast cell densities were found to be higher around acupoints than nearby non-acupoints [127-131]. There is evidence that mast cells interact with connective tissue matrix components through integrins [132]. Interaction of nerve cells and mast cells [133-135] causes degranulation of the latter, releasing part (as a "piecemeal" release) or all of the large number of enclosed biochemical molecules which are involved in physiological and pathophysiological events [136]. These biomolecules include serotonin, proteases, heparin, granulocyte, macrophage, colony-stimulating factor (GM-CSF), leukotrienes, interleukins, transforming growth factors (TGF), tumor necrosis factor-$\alpha$ (TNF$\alpha$), calcitonin, nerve growth factor (NGF), stem cell factor (SCF), substance P, histamine, prostaglandin, thromboxane, and other peptides like fibroblast growth factor (FGF) [45, 136, 137]. Such biomolecules, working separately or cooperatively, are involved in (1) allergy response, (2) acquired immunity, (3) innate immunity, (4) maintaining the life of sensory neurons, (5) inflammation, (6) supporting the growth of T cells and various tissues, (7) metabolic rate, (8) noxious stimuli response, (9) blood vessel tone regulation, (10) fibroblast growth, (11) wound healing, and (12) osteoblast formation.

There is direct evidence that acupuncture could cause degranulation of mast cells via mechanotransduction [130, 131]. Thus mast cells can be considered as mediators of the effector function of acupuncture. Note also that in classical physiology, mast cells are linked mainly to allergy response. However, as pointed out in [136], "why does an extraordinary cell type spend its life from the bone marrow through the circulation system, to the skin and lungs

http://dx.doi.org/10.5772/53901

aveola and just waiting for a few allergy antigens?" Also, according to more recent acupuncture research, why do more mast cells migrate along channels correlating with the TCM meridians? [39] Why are there so many "biomedical ingredients" or contents inside this cell type? [137] The interesting issue is: a mast cell degranulates under certain conditions (like increase of tension of collagen fibers attached to ECM of mast cell, via acupuncture) as a "grand sacrifice for life" and the empty shell seems to recycle after use and the story repeats [136]. I conjecture that, in the future, bridging acupuncture research and biomedical research of the functions of mast cell subset $MC_{tc}$ (here the subscripts t, c stand for tryptase and chymase respectively), which resides in the connective tissue, would give clues to extensive answers of the above interesting questions, relating closely to immunity, wound healing and other physiological aspects.

### 8.2. Unfolding of the fibronectin (Fn) fiber fibrils associated with fibroblasts could activate and release transforming grow factors during wound healing, with stem cells specification playing a plausibly crucial role

Mesenchymal stem cells (MSC) are far away from their orginal source (bone marrow) and are "wandering" near various tissues/organs in the CTIF system for repair after injury, reinforcement of growth when necessary [138]. Upon activation, they differentiate into skeletal myocytes, smooth muscle cells, adipocytes, osteoblasts, chondrocytes and even neurons [139] and the substrate's mechanical property like elasticity is one key factor that decides which phenotype each stem cell is deveolped into [140]. It has been found also [141] that TGF-β can activate the differentiation of these adult stem cells. Since the transforming growth factor molecules are secreted (by various cells, including degranulation of mast cells) into the CTIF system in the dormant/latent state [142] in the midst of glycoproteins (fibronectin, laminin, ...), it is intriquing to ask under what conditions will the TGF-β molecules be activated. We have already discussed the evidence of cell-mediated unfolding of the Fn fibrils and the subsequent exposure of cryptic binding sites of blood vessel cells in Section 4 and [143, 144]. Now cellular Fn is synthesized by many cells, including fibroblasts, endothelial cells, chondrocytes, synovial cells and myocytes [145]. Some recent study [146] indicates that there are Fn cryptic binding sites which can be specifically bound by TGF-β. The above cited series of studies provide the possible/plausible linkage between mechanotransduction plausible arising from acupuncture, and the release of activated TGF-β in specification of stem cells for normal growth, repair/wound healing.

Along this line of logic, first note that latent transforming-growth-factor-β-binding protein (LTBPs) are ECM glycoproteins which play the major role of storing latent TGF-β in the ECM. In vitro study [147] indicated that Fn fibrils and their continous presence were required for controlled storing of LTBP1 in the ECM of fibroblasts. Since TGF-β plays important roles in a wide range of cellular processes (including apoptosis and proliferation), it is important to find out whether Fn-activated TGF-β is controlled, at least in in vitro injury/healing model experiment. In fact, in a very recent study of liver injury, it has been shown that fibronectin protects excessive liver fibrosis by controled local activation of TGF-β [148, 149]. The maneuvering process of acupuncture, either by piston-like action or rotation, automatically extends the fibronectin network and tones the mechanical tension of other fibers, and that one consequence is the activation of TGF-β in the CTIF. The activated TGF-β molecules under the control of Fn fibrils may activate adult stem cells for proper healing [141]. Moreover, Fn matrices have been shown to act as storage of various growth factors which regulate cellular proliferation [72, 150]. Future research on whether acupuncture type of mechanotransduction would trigger release and/or activate some of these growth factors, for tissue/organ homeostasis, wound repair is an important project.

## 9. Discussions – Summary of the plausible consequences of acupuncture and some frontier issues in future acupuncture research

### 9.1. The emergence of the meridians as a natural system of communication of all multi-cell organisms

After a cell has completed its first mitosis into two and more cells, a system of communication must have existed to cater for the coordination of the function of a group of cells, and morphogenic development as a whole, before the nervous system is built up. Mechanical forces, including that derived from fluid flow in the embryo play crucial roles [151] in these functions. The mesoderm at a later stage develops mainly into the largest tissue of the body--the connective tissue system. Thus the CTIF system is a natural platform for communication, with the nervous system joining in at a later stage; those parts which can carry signals most efficiently, become the natural meridians channels. With the development of the blood and lymph circulations, nerve systems, immune system of various cells......, there are stations through which various types of signals can be sent/relayed with better efficiency to other parts of the body for survival of the organism. Acupoints have been hypothesized as such functional sites along the natural communication network [39]. Therefore, it is not too surprised to find from in vitro experiment that the CTIF network is mechanically connected once fibroblasts exert traction on the collagen fibers due to mechanotransduction, of which the action of acupuncture is one example. I would further note that the expression of the protein connexin 43 (Cx43) around acupoint ST36 and other acupoints along the stomach meridian was found to be higher than that of non-acupoints, suggesting that intercellular communication through the stomach meridian is more efficient than that through nonacupoint sites; see Section 2.3 & [152]. Moreover, two recent studies showed that manual acupuncture at ST36 influenced the pain thresholds of acid-induced and heat-induced pain in Cx43 heterozygous gene knockout mice [153, 154]. Having analyzed above, I would remark that some of the acupoints could also be morphological centers developed from embryo, as proposed in [155].

### 9.2. Summary of the plausible consequences of acupuncture action at a typical acupoint: acupuncture represents a micro-injury or micro-massage the consequences of which should be able to be explained by biomedical knowledge in principle

Referring to Fig.1, the number at each box indicates the section number for which the process is discussed. We start with the box 3.3, marked "acupuncture at acupoint". This block joins via a solid arrow to the left box number 4.1, which represents fibroblasts cytoskeletal remodeling. The solid arrow signifies that such a statement is suggested and supported by either in vitro or in vivo experiment. The dotted arrow towards another box is only speculative/hypothesized, without direct experimental support so far. An arrow together with a question mark from box 3.3 to box 9.5 indicates that, whether such a possibile connection exists, is still an open question, awaiting further research to give clue to an answer. The dotted double-headed arrow joining boxes 7.3 and 9.5 represents a speculation that the two processes might be related. With some relevant basics introduced in Sections 2 & 3, following the discussions presented from Sections 4-8, the float chart is self-explanatory.

Acupuncture is a micro-injury with certain specific procedures. Manual acupuncture in action should in principle be able to be explained by evidence-based medical science. However, the effects of acupuncture as a whole are the complex physiological consequences of all types of mechanotransduction events (with different time scales) triggered by the needling action. Therefore, the acupuncture mechanism cannot be deduced by a simple sequence of experiments or a simple theory. Reviews bridging advancements in sections 1(B and C) might serve to help in probing the mystery existing over several thousand years. When we understand more about such "bridges" (of which this chapter is only one small example), we can attempt to explain step by step, but gaining progress continuously, more specifically the reasons behind the consequences of acupuncture.

### 9.3. The mystery of calcium concentration at acupoints

Employing the proton induced X-ray emission (PIXE) technique, the calcium content at various sites of the connective tissues of the lower limbs of 7 cadavers was measure [60]. The calcium concentration at a typical known acupoint was reported to be several tens higher than that of the non-acupoints which were along the same meridian, but was 100~200 times higher than that of non-acupoint, non-meridian sites. A needle shape electrode was built selectively catered for $Ca^{2+}$ detection by another group [156]. The relative $Ca^{2+}$ concentrations were found to be higher at five acupoints, as well as two mid-points between two known adjacent acupoints of the ST meridian as compared to sites of control (certain distances away). Correlation between relatively high calcium concentrations and various acupoints (as compared to non acupoints) have also been reported by other groups [157-160]. Above stated research results suggest that there are (extra-cellular, Section 2.4) calcium stores at, or near the acupoint sites. Note that a number of acupoints are found in the periosteum [58]. I hypothesize that there are also high concentrations of calcium stores at or near these acupoints because from basic physiology, we learn that there is continuous calcium transport from the bone back to the circulation system, while new stem cells, i.e. osteoblasts are migrating along the periosteum to build new bone in our daily life [38].

Incidentally, it is amazing to find experimentally that in the biological world the calcium waves can be frequency-modulated or amplitude-modulated to transmit information and be detected in cells [161-163], similar to radio signal communication. Whether different frequency of manual and electrical acupuncture stimulus could be "decoded" in a quantitative way by relevant cells will be an interesting topic. Thus there are intriquing aspects relating calcium activity and acupuncture

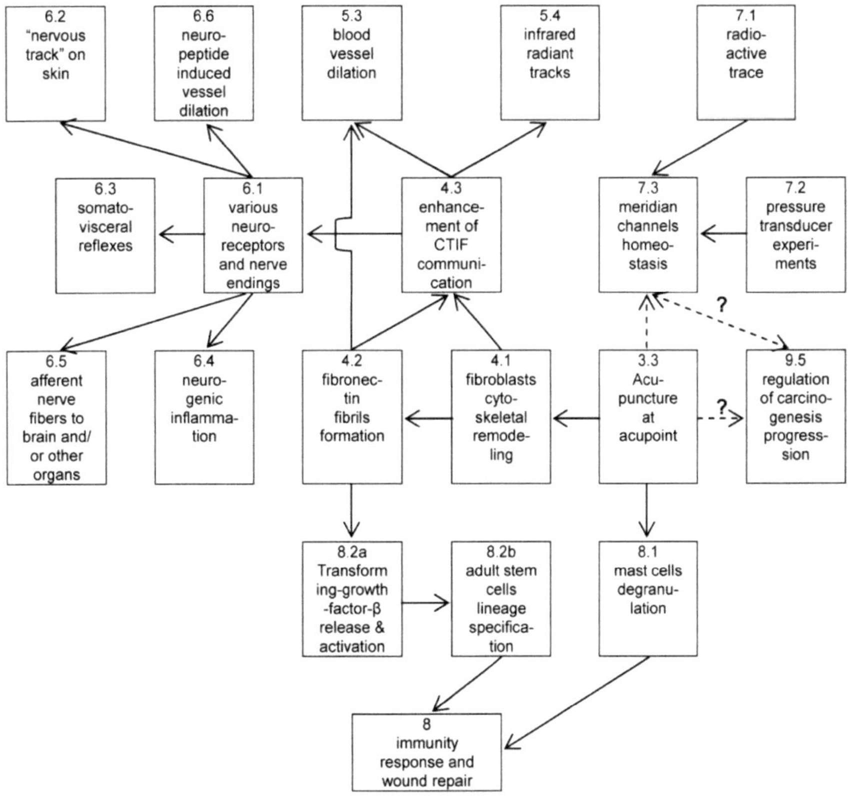


**Figure 1.** Some plausible biomedical consequences of acupuncture. Solid arrows represent deductions supported by either *in vivo* or *in vitro* experiments. Dotted arrows represent proposal/speculation, to be verified. Dotted arrow with question mark represents open questions. The dotted double-headed arrow joining boxes 7.3. and 9.5 represents a suggestion that two processes are related. The number in a box refers to the section number in the text where more details can be found. The basic of these processes are introduced in section 2 and.3.

## 9.4. The double-edge nature of nitric oxide and Hot/Cool concept in TCM in relation to the activation of different isoforms of the nitric oxide synthase

One very important function of $Ca^{2+}$ is its combination with the calcium-calmodulin protein in the inner cell membrane to activate nitric oxide synthase (NOS) which catalyzes the substrate L-arginine to produce nitric oxide that can propagate through (lipid) cell membrane and through intra- and extra-cellular fluid. There are three isoforms of NOS, i.e., endothelial form eNOS, inducible form iNOS and neuronal form nNOS. The first one is active in endothelial and other cells to produce NO for (blood, lymph) vessel dilation and is continuously needed for living. The enzyme iNOS is activated when the immunity system is alarmed and produces a large amount of NO (with time scale around hours) that combines with superoxide in the mitochondria to form peroxinitrite $(ONOO)^-$ which is supposed to be detrimental to membrane of alien cell. However, over expression of iNOS is very harmful to our body, playing important roles in various types of pathogenesis [164, 165]. Therefore iNOS inhibitor can be used as drug to treat organ transplant rejection [166]. On the other hand, nNOS is expressed in neuronal cells and catalyzes (L-arginine) to produce NO also to act mainly as neural transmitter. Thus NO is a double-edge molecule: not enough NO from eNOS would cause hypertension; too much NO from iNOS would trigger a harmful auto-immune response (rejection of donor organ in case of transplantation); too much NO from nNOS would cause too much neural transmission, upsetting the nervous system. Too much iNOS activation may be associated to "Hot" type of disease in immune response; and too much nNOS activation may be related also to the "Hot" syndrome in nervous system; too much eNOS may be related to the "Cool" aspect of food causing hypotension, in the nomenclature of TCM. Whether a specific type of acupuncture modality would specifically enhance one specific isoform of the stated three enzymes is a challenging question which may or may not have a specific answer.

### 9.5. Can acupuncture modulate the routes of carcinogenesis?

Various cell types, including the epithelial cell, embryo fibroblasts, vascular smooth muscle cells, were cultured on Fn-coated hydrogel-based substrata which mimicked the physiological stiff CT. Starting from the basics of cell cycle analysis, it has been found that tension transmitted through integrin receptors to the cytoskeleton cooperates with the cyclins to control the $G_1$ phase of these cells types [167]. In another study, there is evidence that CT matrix stiffness controls the ability of ectopically expressed cyclin $D_1$ to go through the S phase entry during breast cancer progression [168]. Moreover, atomic force microscopy and fluorescence imaging in mice model indicates that comparable enhancement in arterial tissue stiffness occur at sites of cell proliferation in vivo [167].

On the other hand, TGF-β can regulate a diversity of cellular functions like proliferation, motility and differentiation with distinct specificity in different cell types. We have noted in section 8 that Mast cells liberate TGF-β during degranulation (e.g. via acupuncture) and unfolding of fibronectin could activate TGF-β which is often in its latent state. In most non-transformed epithelial cells, TGF-β induces apoptosis as a mean to avoid tumorigenesis. However, more rigid substrates in an in vitro study of epithelial cells treated with TGF-β induced epithelial-mesenchymal transition, leading to cell proliferation instead [169], showing double-edge nature. During the recent few years, a lot of works, with a few examples stated above, have been published on the profound influence of the mechanical properties of the ECM, together with the participation of proteins, cytokines on (organ/adherent) cell fate, carcinogenesis of tissues [170-173]. In all these studies, the stiffness of the ECM in the micro-environment is the major focus of attention. Note that in addition to TGF-β, other growth factors, like fibroblast growth factors (FGFs), the insulin-like growth factors (IGFs), and the epidermal growth factor (EGF) are also kept in the ECM of different cells; see discussion in [146]. Note that each organ is enclosed by a CT network and fibroblasts have abundant Fn in their ECM. That micro-mechanical stimulation or micro-massage from the action of acupuncture, on the ECM of the relevant cells might interfere the progress of carcinogensis is not far- fetched. In fact, it has even been shown that the malignant phenotype of parenchymatous cells is reversible by correction of the altered cues of the ECM [174].

## 9.6. On "bio-thixotropy", warm bianstone meridian-massage and moxibustion

For a homogenous substance, thixotropy may be considered as the ability of a semisolid gel to liquefy when stirred or shaken (or heated) and to return to its semi-hardened state after the external influence is taken away. Paint is one such homogeneous chemical example.

In the living world, and in the macroscopic scale, there was in vivo evidence of changes in short-range stiffness of muscles and tendons arising from compression force induced by a force transducer probe [175]. The result was interpreted as thixotropy property of muscles and CT building the tendons. There was also clear evidence that respiratory muscles of normal subjects also showed thixotropy property during respiration cycles [176]. Denaturation of type I collagen fibrils was reported to be a heat absorbing process accompanied by a change in heat capacity [177]. The fascia system was invoked also to possess thixotropy property to explain the beneficial effects of warm-up exercise and body massage [178]. I would remark that in view of the complicated structure of the CTIF stated above in this chapter, the CTIF is not a homogenous system, and the "bio-thixotropy" property in the microscopic scale (< microns ) has yet to be defined and to be analyzed with grater details in the future.

On the other hand, DNA, cell membrane, collagen fibers, even muscles are found to have properties of liquid crystals [179-181]; they can change phase subjected to change in temperature (plus other parameters). The "bio-thixotropy" property of living tissues could therefore occur upon change in phase of the living liquid crystals. In short, the collagen fibers in the CTIF would become more pliable, more liquid-like upon heating, for example, by warm bianstone massage along the meridians or moxibustion; note that bianstone acupressure was practiced even before needle acupuncture. Upon cooling, the collagen fibers would have been "toned", as a speculation. It is also tempting to speculate that pretreatment with warm bianstone meridian-massage before needle acupuncture might provide a better platform of mechanotransduction along the meridian channels in the CTIF system.

## 9.7. Limitations of this chapter

(a) In this chapter, acupuncture, unless otherwise stated, refers to manual acupuncture only. Electro-acupuncture is outside the general scope of this chapter. The liquid crystal properties of living tissues certainly bring high complexity in electrical and optical communications within our bodies and deserve concerted effects of research in the future. (b) A number of plausible consequences are deduced based on in vitro experiments only here, with some verified by in vivo animal studies and / or clinical results. In order to expedite the accumulation of evidence-based knowledge, and progress of acupuncture research, this approach is inevitably workable according to the author, else we are leaving behind numerous results of in vitro experiments obtained in biomedical science research alone; these results are in fact related (though in many cases indirectly) to the consequences of acupuncture at this stage. (c) Other growth factors, in addition to TGFs are indeed kept in the CTIF system but have not been discussed here at this moment. Detailed consequences of mast cells degranulation, cells migration have not been analyzed here. Further review and research are necessary to bring in these aspects and might contribute further to understand better the consequences of acupuncture in action.

http://dx.doi.org/10.5772/53901

## 10. Conclusion – Acupunture research is important for modern medicine, east and west

There are ex vivo and in vitro experiments to support the notion that piston-like or rotation type acupuncture at a typical acupoint activates the CTIF system which forms a mechanically well connected communication network. Recent in vitro experimental analysis indicates that mechanotransduction can be transmitted more efficiently along intra- and inter-muscular cleavage planes of the activated CTIF system, where most of the acupoints are found to be located, supporting the hypothesis [39] that the mechanical signals from acupuncture can be transmitted to the ECM of other residence cells (like mast cells) as well as ECM of organ/adherent cells (like cells of blood, lymph vessels, nerves). A large number of plausible biomedical events take place as explained in Sections 4-9; a schematically representation of some crucial events is presented in the flow chart of Section 9.2. Acupuncture is a micro-injury or micro-massage, the consequence of which should, in principle, be explained by evidence-based biomedical science. Therefore building bridges between results of the works stated in Section 1.2 (B and C) with reference to acupuncture research is important in modern medicine, east and west.

## Acknowledgement

Part of the work was completed during the affiliation of the author to the Department of Medicine (LKS Faculty of Medicine), University of Hong Kong. The present affiliations are the Centre on behavioral health (Faculty of Social Sciences) and Department of Electrical and Electronic Engineering (Faculty of Engineering), University of Hong Kong. Thanks are addressed to my brother Mr. Benjamin Fung for his long enduring help and Miss Peggy Lee as well as Miss Celia Chor for their very helpful assistance in preparing this manuscript.

## Author details

Peter Chin Wan Fung[1,2,3]

1 Centre on Behavioral Health (Faculty of Social Sciences), University of Hong Kong, PRC

2 Department of Electrical and Electronic Engineering (Faculty of Engineering), University of Hong Kong, PRC

3 Department of Medicine (LKS Faculty of Medicine), University of Hong Kong, Hong Kong, PRC

## References


[1] National Institute of Health (USA): Acupuncture. NIH Consensus Statement Online 1997, 15:1-34.

[2] Zhou D, Liu YY, Li GL, Guo Y, Summarization and analysis on acupuncture-related articles embodied in medline data-base in 2006. Zhongguo Zhenjiu (Chinese Acupuncture and Moxibustion), 2008, 28(2): 151-155.

[3] Sun GJ, Acupuncture (Advance Level Series of Traditional Chinese Medicine). People's Health Publisher, Beijing, 1998.

[4] Li DZ, Li XZ, Probing the Secrets of Meridians in Traditional Chinese Medicine – Investigation of Transmissions through the Meridians and the Mechanism of External Treatment of Diseases. People's Liberation Army Publisher, Beijing, 2003.

[5] Filshie J, White A, Medical Acupuncture, a Western Scientific Approach. Churchill, Livingstone, 1998.

[6] Stux G, Berman B, Pomerantz B, Basics of Acupuncture. Springer-Verlag, New York, 5th edition, 2003.

[7] Dung HC, Clogston OP, Dunn JW, Acupuncture: an anatomical approach. CRC Press, 2004.

[8] Chen CS, Marksich M, Huang S, Whitesdies GM, Ingber DE, Geometric control of cell life and death. Science, 1997, 276: 1425-1428.

[9] Orr AW, Helmke BP, Mechanism of mechanotransduction. Developmental Cell, 2006, 10:11-20.

[10] Wells RG, The role of matrix stiffness in regulating cell behavior. Hepatology, 2008, 47: 1394-1400.

[11] Wang N, Tytell JD, and Ingber DE, Mechanotransduction at a distance: mechanically coupling the extracellular matrix with the nucleus. Nature Reviews/Molecular cell Biology, 2009, 10:75-82.

[12] Ingber DE, Tensegrity: the architectural basis of cellular mechanotransduction. Annual Review of Physics, 1997, 59:575-99.

[13] Chen CS, Mechanotransduction-a field pulling together? Journal of Cell Science, 2008; 121:3285-3292

[14] Katz B, Depolarization of sensory terminal and the initiation of impulses in the muscle spindle, Journal of Physiology (London), 1950, 111:261-282.

[15] Sachs F, Mechanical transduction in biological systems, CRC Critical Reviews in Biomedical Engineering, 1988, 16:141-169.

http://dx.doi.org/10.5772/53901

[16] Sastry SK, Burridge K, Focal adhesions: a nexus for intracellular signaling and cytoskeletal dynamics. Experimental Cell Research, 2000, 261(1):25-36

[17] Katsum A, Naoe T, Matsushita T, Kaibuchi K, and Schwartz MA, Integrin activation and matrix binding mediate cellular responses to mechanical stretch. The Journal of Biological Chemistry, 2006, 280(17):16546-16549.

[18] Bershadsky AD, Balaban NQ & Geiger B, Adhesion-dependent cell mechanosensitivity. Annual Review of Cell & Development Biology, 2003; 19:677-695.

[19] Nicholson BJ, Gap junctions-from cell to molecule. Journal of Cell Science, 2003, 116:4479-4481.

[20] Kumar NM, Gilula NB, The gap junction communication. Cell, 1996, 84:381-388.

[21] Delma M, Coombs W, Sorgen P, Duffy HS, M. Taffet SM, Structural bases for the chemical regulation of Connexin43 channels. Cardiovascular Research, 2004, 62(2): 268-275.

[22] Gianatti F and Ruoslahti E, Integrin signaling. Science, 1999, 285:1028-1032.

[23] Janmey PA, McCulloch CA, Cell mechanics: Integrating cell responses to mechanical stimuli. Annual Review of Biomedical Engineering, 2007, 9:1-34.

[24] Charles AC, Merrill JE, Dirksen ER, Sanderson MJ, Intercellular Signaling in Glial Cells: Calcium Waves and Oscillations in Response to Mechanical Stimulation and Glutamate. Neuron, 1991, 6:983-992.

[25] Demer LC, Wortham CM, Dirksen ER, Sanderson MJ, Mechanical stimulation induces intercellular calcium signaling in bovine aortic endothelial cells. American Journal of Physiology, Heart and Circculation Physiology, 1993:H2094-H2102.

[26] Glogauer M, Arora P, Yao G, Sokholov I, Ferrier J and McCulloch CA, Calcium ions and tyrosine phosphorylation interact coordinately with actin to regulate cytoprotective response to stretching. Journal of Cell Science, 1997, 110:11-21.

[27] Munevar S, Wang YL, and Dembo M, Regulation of mechanical interactions between fibroblasts and the substratum by stretch-activated $Ca^{2+}$ entry. Journal of Cell Science, 2004, 117:85-92.

[28] Jaalouk DE & Lammerding J, Mechanotransduction gone awry. Nature Reviews Molecular Cell Biology, 2009, 10:63-73.

[29] Rooney TA, Renard DC, Sass EJ, Thomas AP, Oscillatory Cytosolic Calcium Waves Independent of Stimulated Inositol 1, 4, 5-Trisphosphate Formation in Hepatocytes. The Journal of Biological Chemistry, 1991, 266(19):12272-12282.

[30] Boitano S, Dirksen, ER, Sanderson MJ, Intercellular Propagation of Calcium Waves Mediated by Inositol Trisphosphate. Science, 1992, 258: 292-295.

[31] Hajnoczky G, Gao E, Nomura T, Hoek JB, Thomas AP, Multiple mechanisms by which protein kinase-A potentiates inositol 1, 4, 5 – Trisphoshate induced $Ca^{2+}$ mobilization in permeabilized hepatocytes. Biochemistry Journal, 1993, 293:413-422.

[32] Putney JW and Bird GS, Cytoplasmic calcium oscillations and store-operated calcium influx. Journal of Physiology, 2008, 586(13):3055-3059.

[33] Hardingham GE, Sangeeta C, Johnson CM, Badling H, Distinct functions of nuclear and cytoplasmic calcium in the control of gene expression. Nature, 1997, 385:260-265.

[34] Dolmetsch RE, Xu K, Lewis RS, Calcium oscillations increase the efficiency and specificity of gene expression. Nature, 1998, 392:933-936.

[35] Aumailly M and Gayraud B, Structure and biological activity of the extra-cellular matrix. Journal of Molecular Medicine, 1998, 76:253-265.

[36] Iozzo RV, Matrix proteoglycans: from molecular design to cellular function. Annual Review of Biochemistry, 1998, 67: 609-652.

[37] Schwarzbauer JE and Sechler JL, Fibronectin fibrillogenesis: a paradigm for extracellular matrix assembly. Current Opionion in Cell Biology, 1999, 11:622-627.

[38] Marieb EN, Human Anatomy and Physiology, 4th Ed., Addison Wesley Longman, Menlo Park, 1998, p.119-138.

[39] Fung PCW, Probing the mystery of Chinese medicine meridian channels with special emphasis on the connective tissue interstitial fluid system, mechanotransduction, cells durotaxis and mast cell degranulation. BioMed Central, Chinese Medicine, 2009, 4:10 (6 pages).

[40] Page KE, The role of the fascia in the maintenance of structural integrity. Academy of Applied Osteopathy Yearbooks, 1952; 70.

[41] Yuan L, Yao DW, Tang L, Huang WH, Jiao PF, Lu YT, Dai JX, Zhang H, He ZQ, Zhong SZ, A study on morphological basis of Chinese acupuncture and moxibustion from digital human body. Jiepou Xuebao (Acta Anatomica Sinica) 2004; 35:337-343.

[42] Kawakita K, Gotoh K, Role of polymodal receptors in the acupuncture mediated endogenous pain inhibitory systems, in (Edit) Kumazawa T, Kruger L, Mizumura K.: The Polymodal Receptor: A gateway to Pathological Pain., 1996:507-523, Elsevier, Amsterdam, The Netherlands.

[43] Majno G, Joris I: Cells, Tissues and Disease: Principles of General Pathology. Oxford University Press, New York, USA, 2004:342-629.

[44] Narayanan AS, Page RC, Swanson J, Collagen synthesis by human fibroblasts. Regulation by transforming growth factor-beta in the presence of other inflammatory mediators. Biochemistry Journal, 1989, 260(2):463-469.

[45] Metcalfe DD, Baram D, Mekori YA, Mast cells, Physiological Reviews, 1997, 77:1033-1079,

[46] Novotny GEK, Gommert-Novotny E, A simple procedure for demonstrating the overall morphology of fibroblasts in routine histological preparations of adult tissues, using silver impregnation. Journal of Microscopy, 1990, 159:99-107.

[47] Novotny GEK, Gnoth C, Variability of fibroblast morphology in vivo: a silver impregnation study on human digital dermis and subcutis. Journal of Anatomy, 1991, 177:195–207.

[48] Tanji K, Shimiz T, Satou T, Hashimoto S, Bonilla E, Gap junctions between fibroblasts in rat myotendon. Archives of Histology and Cytology, 1995, 58:97-102.

[49] McNeilly M, Banes AJ, Benjamin M, Ralphs JR, Tendon cells in vivo form a three dimensional network of cell processes linked by gap junctions. Journal of Anatomy, 1996, 189:593–600.

[50] Ko K, Arora P, Lee W, McCulloch C, Biochemical and functional characterization of intercellular adhesion and gap junctions in fibroblasts. American Journal of Cell Physiology, 2000, 279:C147–C157.

[51] Wang JHC, Bhavani PT, Lin JS, & Im HJ, Mechanoregulation of gene expression in fibroblasts, Gene, 2007, 391(1-2):1-15

[52] (a) Miraculous Pivot (revised translation) In Huangdi's Internal Classic. Beijing: People's Health Publishing House, 1980: chapter 10. (b) Miraculous Pivot (revised translation) In Huangdi's Internal Classic. Beijing: People's Health Publishing House, 1980:155-173. (c) Miraculous Pivot (revised translation) In Huangdi's Internal Classic. Beijing: People's Health Publishing House, 1980:249-250.

[53] Yuchi J: Discussion of the relationship between meridians and connective tissues. Nanjing Zhongyi Xueyuan Xuebao, 1986, 2:36-37.

[54] Yen ZG, The anatomy foundation of commonly used acupoints, Publisher of the Shanghai Chinese Medicine School, page 5-120, 1988.

[55] Du XJ, The relation of connective tissue to meridian. Zhongguo Zhenjiu (Chinese Acupuncture and Moxibustion), 1989, 9(6):53-54.

[56] Kimura M, Tohya K, Kuroiwa K, Electron microscopical immunohistochemical studies on the induction of "Qi" employing needling manipulation, The American Journal of Chinese Medicine, 1992, 20(1):25-35.

[57] Yu AS, ZhaoYX, Yan ZG, Li XL, Guan XF, Morphological observation of the spatial region around the acupoint Sanyinjiao SP6 (as translated by the author), Zhongguo Zhenjiu (Chinese Acupuncture and Moxibustion), 1997, 17(1):42-44.

[58] Dang RS, Chen EY, Shen XY, and et al. "Relation of connective tissue to the acupoints of the lung meridian", Shanghai Zhenjiu (Shanghai Journal of Acupuncture and Moxibustion), 1997; 16(4):28-29.

[59] Chen EY, Shen XY, Dang RS, Cheng HS, Cai DH, He WS, Fei L, A relation between connective tissue and accumulation of calcium with points on GB channel below

head. Shanghai Zhenjiu (Shanghai Journal of Acupuncture and Moxibustion), 1998, 17(2):36-37.

[60] Fei L, Cheng HS, Cai DH, Yang SX, Xu JR, Chen EY, Dang RS, Ding GH, Shen XY, Tang Y, Expeimental investigation and scientific demonstration of the materialistic foundation of meridians and their functional specialties. Kexue Tongbao (Science Report), 1998, 43:658-672.

[61] Shen XY, Dang RS, Chen EY, Cheng HS, He WQ, Cai DH, Ding GH, Fei L, Relation of acupoints of the stomach channel with structure of connective tissue and accumulation of calcium, Zhenci Yanjiu (Acupuncture Research), 1998, 10:595-597.

[62] Langevin HM, Churchill DL, Fax JR, Badger GJ, Garra BS, Krag MH, Biomechanical response to acupuncture needling in humans. Journal of Applied Physiology, 2001; 91:2471-2478.

[63] Ding GH, Shen XY, Dai JH et al, Research and development on the dynamic system from detecting the force of acupuncture needle during the acupuncture process in clinical practice of traditional Chinese medicine. Journal of Biomedical Engineering, 2003, 20(1):121-124.

[64] Langevin HM, Yandow JA, Relationship of acupuncture points and meridians to connective tissue planes. The Anatomical Record (New ANA.), 2002, 269:257-265.

[65] Zhong SZ, Yuan L, Tang L, Huang WH, Dai JX, Li JY, Liu C, Wang XH, Hong HW, Li H, Luo SQ, Qin D, Zeng SQ, Wu T, Zhang MC, Wu KC, Jiao PF, Lu YT, Chen H, Li PL, Gao Y, Wang T, Fan JH, Research report of experimental database established of digitized virtual Chinese No.1 female, Journal of The First Military Medicine University, 2003, 23(3):196-209.

[66] Yuan L, Tang L, Huang WH, Li JY, Dai JX, Liu C, Wu T, Wang XH, Hong HW, Zhang MC, Jiao PF, Lu YT, Wu KC, Li PL, Fan JH, Gao Y, Wang QZ, Wang LJ, Wu L, Zhang L, Li XA, Chen YH, Ouyang J, Zhong SZ, Construction of data set for virtual Chinese male No.1, Journal of First Military Medicine University, 2003, 23(6):520-523.

[67] Langevin HM, Bouffard WA, Badger GJ, Churchill DL, Howe AK, Subcutaneous tissue fibroblast cytoskeletal remodeling induced by acupuncture: evidence force mechanotransduction based mechanism. Journal of Cellular Physiology, 2006, 207:767-774.

[68] Sawhney RK, Howard J, Slow local movements of collagen fibers by fibroblasts drive the rapid global self-organization of collagen gels. The Journal of Cell Biology, 2002, 157(6):1083-1092.

[69] Langevin HM, Cornbrooks CJ, Taatjes DJ, Fibroblasts form a body-wide cellular network. Histochemistry and Cell Biology, 2004, 122:7-15.

[70] Rhee S, Jiang H, Ho CH, Grinnell F, Microtubule function in fibroblast spreading is modulated according to the tension state of cell-matrix interactions. Proceedings of National American Society, USA, 2007, 104(13):5425-5430.

[71] Miron-Mendoza M, Seemann J, Grinnell F, Collagen fibril flow and tissue translocation coupled to fibroblast migration in 3D collagen matrices. Molecular Biology of the Cell, 2008, 19(5):2051-2058.

[72] Sottile J, Hocking D C & Swiatek P J, Fibronectin matrix assembly enhances adhesion-dependent cell growth. Journal of Cell Science, 1998, 111 (Pt 19), 2933–2943

[73] Smith ML, Gourdon D, Little W, Kubow KE, Eguiluz RA, Luna-Morris S, & Vogel V, Force-induced unfolding of fibronectin in the extracellular matrix of living cells. PLoS, Biology, 2007, 5(10): e268.

[74] Julias M, Buettner HM, and Shreiber DI, Varying assay geometry to emulate connective tissue planes in an in vitro model of acupuncture needling. Anatomical record (Hoboken), 2011, 294(2):243-252.

[75] Clifford PS, Kluess HA, Hamann JJ, Buckwalter JB, & Jasperse JL, Mechanical compression elicits vasodilatation in rat skeletal muscle feed arteries. The Journal Physiology, 2006, 572:561-567.

[76] Hocking DC, Titus PA, Sumagin R, & Sarelius IH, Extracellular matrix fibronectin mechanically couples skeletal muscle contraction with local vasodilation. Circulation Research, Integrative Physiology, 2008, 102:372-379.

[77] Li S, Chen K, Wu Y, Jiao J, Tao L, Effects of warm needling at zusanli (ST 36) on NO and IL-2 levels in the middle-aged and old people. Journal of Traditional Chinese Medicine, 2003, 23(2):127-8.

[78] Kim DD, Pica AM, Duran RG, Duran WN, Acupuncture reduces experimental renovascular hypertension through mechanisms involving nitric oxide synthases. Microcirculation, 2006, 13(7): 577-585.

[79] Tsuchiya M, Sato EF, Inoue M, Asada A, Acupuncture enhances generation of nitric oxide and increases local circulation. Anesthesia & Analgesia, 2007, 104(2):301-7.

[80] Kuo TC, Chen YJ, Kuo HY and Chan CF, Blood Flow Effect of Acupuncture on the human meridian. Medical Acupuncture, 2010, 22(1):33-40.

[81] Zhang D, Fu WX, Wang SY, Ma HM, Wang YC, Comparison of phenomenon of high-thermal lines along channels induced by different acupuncture-moxibustion methods, Zhongguo Zhenjiu (Chinese Acupuncture and moxibustion), 2000, 6:349-353

[82] Zhang D, Application of infrared thermography in studies of acupuncture mechanisms and meridians. Zhongguo Zhenjiu (Chinese Acupuncture & Moxibustion), 2004, 24(1):37-42.

[83] Ma CH, Tan LH, Yue XJ, Relationship between the change of temperature and activity of Na+/K+-ATPase and content of SP in the tissues along the running course of meridians in rabbits. Zhenci Yanjiu (Acupuncture Research), 2002, 27(3):220-225

[84] Xu XY, Hu XL, Wu BH, Observation on the oxygen partial pressure in deep tissues along Du meridian, Zhenci Yanjiu (Acupuncture Research), 2002, 27(4):252-255.

[85] Goldman N, Chen M, Fujita T, Xu Q, Peng W, Liu W, Jensen TK, Pei Y, Wang F, Han X, Chen JF, Schnermann J, Takano T, Bekar L, Tieu K, & Nedergaard M, Adenosine A1 receptors mediate local anti-nociceptive effects of acupuncture. Nature Neuroscience, 2010; 13:883-888.

[86] Kumazawa T, The polymodal receptor-bio-warning and defence mechanisms. In: The Polymodal Receptor: A gateway to Pathological Pain, edited by Kumazawa T, Kruger L, Mizumura K, Amsterdam, The Netherlands: Elsevier, 1996:3-20.

[87] Kawakita K, Okada K, Mechanisms of action of acupuncture for chronic pain relief-polymodal receptors are the key candidates. Acupuncture Medicine, 2006, 24(Suppl):S58-S66.

[88] Liu K, Li AH, Wang W, Xie YK, Dense innervation of acupoints and its easier reflex excitatory character in rats, Zhenci Yanjiu (Acupuncture Research), 2009, 34(1):36-42.

[89] Cho H, Koo JY, Kim SS, Park SP, Yang Y, Oh U, A novel mechanosensitive channel identified in sensory neurons. European Journal of Neuroscience, 2006, 23(10): 2593-2550.

[90] Liu LY, Zhang H, Zhang GF, The actions of receptor alpha, beta and M at channels and the regularity of acupuncture analgesia. Zhongguo Zhongyi Zhazhi (China Journal of Basic Medicine in Traditional Chinese Medicine), 1998, 4(10):51-55.

[91] Liu LY, Pan J, Zhang H, Yang LM, The morphological structure of the skin along the meridian and the transmitting mechanism of arrector pili muscle-sympathetic axon reflex. Zhenci Yanjiu (Acupuncture Research), 2002, 27(4):62-269.

[92] Liu LY, Zhang H, Pan J, Development of sympathetic substance lines on the skin and its relation with meridian essence. Zhenci Yanjiu (Acupuncture Research), 2003, 23(1):23-26.

[93] Zhu DN, Shen XL, Wang T, Hu JB, Trigger of excitatory transmission of skin-nerve endings in "Urinary Bladder Channel" of bullfrog's back. Shanghai Zhenci Zhazhi (Shanghai Journal of Acupuncture), 1998, 17(1):30-32.

[94] Kametani H, Sato A, Sato Y, Ueki K, Reflex facilitation and inhibition of gastric motility from various skin areas in rats. In integrative Control Functions of the Brain, Volume 1. Edited by Ito M. Tokyo: Kodansha Scientific, 1991:285-287.

[95] Sato A, Sato Y, Sugimoto H, Tervi N, Reflex changes in the urinary bladder after mechanical and thermal stimulation of the skin at various segmental levels in cats. Neuroscience, 1977, 2:111-117.

[96] Sato A: Neural mechanisms of autonomic responses elicited by somatic sensory stimulation. Neuroscience and Behavioral Physiology, 1997, 27(5):610-621.

[97] Lynn B, Neurogenic inflammation. Journal of Pharmacological and Biophysical Research, 1988, 1(4):217-224.

[98] Gee MD, Lynn B and Cotsell B, The relationship between cutaneous C fiber type and antidromic vasodilatation in the rabbit and the rat. Journal of Physiology, 1997, 503(1):31-44.

[99] Ceccherelli F, Gagliardi G, Matterazzo G, Visentin R, Giron G, The role of manual acupuncture and morphine administration on the modulation of capsaicin-induced edema in rat paw. A blind controlled study. Acupuncture and Electro-Therapeutics Research; The International Journal, 1996, 21:7-14.

[100] Donnerer J, Holzer-Petsche U, The inhibition of neurogenic inflammation, in Inflammation in Health and Disease (Ed. by Jancso G), Elsevier B.V., Amsterdam, 2009, p. 169-188.

[101] Tracey KJ, The inflammatory reflex. Nature, 2002, 420:853-859.

[102] Fang JL, Krings T, Weidemann J, Meister IG and Thron A, Functional MRI in healthy subjects during acupuncture: different effects of needle rotation in real and false acupoints. Neuroradiology, 2004, 46(5):359-362.

[103] Hui KK, Liu J, Marina O, Napadow V, Haselgrove C, Kwong KK, Kennedy DN, Makris N, The integrated response of the human cerebro-cerebellar and limbic systems to acupuncture stimulation at ST36 as evidenced by fMRI. Neuroimage, 2005, 27(3):479-496.

[104] Napadow V, Kettner N, Liu J, Li M, Kwong KK, Vangel M, Makris N, Audette J, Hui KK, Hypothalamus and amygdala response to acupuncture stimuli in carpal tunnel syndrome. Pain, 2007, 130(3):254-266.

[105] Beissner F, Noth U, & Schockert T, The problem of metal needles in acupuncture-fMRI studies. Evidence-Based Complementary and Alternative Medicine, 2011; 2011, article ID 808203, 5 pages.

[106] Wong TKW, Fung PCW, Chua SE, McAlonon GM, Abnormal spatiotemporal processing of emotional facial expressions in childhood autism: dipole source analysis of event-related potential. European Journal of Neuroscience, 2008, 28(2):407-416.

[107] Hsiu H, Hsu WC, Hsu CL and Huang SM, Assessing the Effects of Acupuncture by Comparing Needling the Hegu Acupoint and Needling Nearby Nonacupoints by Spectral Analysis of Microcirculatory Laser Doppler Signals. Evidence Based Complementary and Alternative Medicine, 2011; 2011, article ID 435928 (9 pages).

[108] Chao PT, Jan MY, Hsiu H, Hsu TL, Wang WK, Lin Wang YY. Evaluating microcirculation by pulsatile laser Doppler signal. Physics in Medicine and Biology, 2006; 51(4): 845–854.

[109] Gu HS, Experimental study of NaI trace along the pericardium meridian. Zi Ran Zha Zhi (Journal of nature), 1980; 3(9):681.

[110] Tiberiu R, Gheorghe G, Popescu I, Do meridians of acupuncture exist? A radioactive tracer study of the bladder meridian. American Journal of Acupuncture, 1981, 9(3): 251-256.

[111] Meng JB, Gao HH, Wang P, Tian JH, Liu YL, Preliminary study of propagation through meridians using radioactive trace technique. Zhenci Yanjiu (Acupuncture Research), 1987, 12(1):77-81.

[112] Meng JB, Study on the propagation along meridians of 12 healthy normals using radioactive X-stroboscopic photography techniques. Zhenci Yanjiu (Acupuncture Research), 1989, 14 (supplement):1.

[113] Li RW, Wen S, Meng JB, Gao HH, Chang BQ, Tian JX, Zhang SW, Analysis of the linear migration of the radionuclide along meridians in perfused extremities of monkey. Zhenci Yanjiu (Acupuncture Research), 1992, 1:67-70.

[114] Guyton AC, Scheel K, Murphere D, Interstitial fluid pressure:III. Its effect on resistance to tissue fluid mobility. Circulation Research, 1966, 19:412-419.

[115] Levick JR, The influence of intra-articular hydrostatic pressure on trans-synovial fluid movement and on capsular expansion in rabbit knee joints. Journal of Physiology, 1979, 289:69-82.

[116] Fadnes HO, Reed RK, Aukland K, Interstitial fluid pressure in rats measured with a modified wick technique. Microvascular Research, 1977, 14:27-36.

[117] Zhang WB, Tian YY, Li H, Zeng YJ, Zhuang FY, Research on the method to continuously detect flow resistance and below epidermal low resistive point. Sheng Wu Wu Li Xue Bao (Acta Biophysica Sinica), 1998; 14(2):373-379.

[118] Zhang WB, Jing Luo Shi Shui Tong Dao (Meridians and collaterals are the water passages). Military Medical Science Publisher, Beijing, second edition, 2009, pp:105-136

[119] Husmann MJ, Barton M, Amann-Vesti BR, Franzeck UK, Postural effects on interstitial fluid pressure in humans. Journal of Vascular Research, 2006; 43(4):321-326.

[120] Bhave G and Neilson EG, Body fluid dynamics: back to the future, Journal of the American Society of Nephrology, 2011, 22(12):2166-2181.

[121] Wiig H, Rubin K, Reed RK, New and active role of the interstitium in control of interstitial fluid pressure: potential therapeutic consequences. Acta Anaesthesiologica Scandinavica, 2003; 47(2):111-121.

[122] Rubin K, Liden A, van Wieringe T & Reed RK, Control of interstitial fluid homeostasis: roles of growth factors and integrins. Vascular complications in Human disease, 2008, Section 2, 105-115.

[123] Polecheck WJ, Charest JL & Kamm RD, Interstitial fluid influences direction of tumor cell migration through competing mechanisms. Proceedings of National Academy of Sciences USA, 2011, 108(27):11115-11120.

[124] Shieh AC and Swartz MA, Regulation of tumor invasion by interstitial fluid flow. Physical Biology, 2011, 8:015012 (8 pages).

[125] Swartz MA, Lund AW, Lymphatic and interstitial flow in the tumour microenvironment: linking mechanobiology with immunity. *Nature Reviews Cancer,* 12:210-219 (March 2012).

[126] Zhang WB, Aukland K, Lund T, Wiig H, Distribution of interstitial fluid pressure and fluid volumes in hind-limb skin of rats: relation to meridians? Clinical Physiology, 2000, 20(3):242-249.

[127] Zhong Am, Wu JL, Hu YL, Study of correlation between the mast cell and acupoint. Shijie Zhenjiu Zazhi (World journal of acupuncture), 1994, 4:53-58.

[128] Deng Y, Zeng T, Zhou Y, Guan X, The influence of electroacupuncture on the mast cells in the acupoints of the stomach meridian, Zhenci Yanjiu (Acupuncture Research), 1996, 21(3):68-70.

[129] Li M, Shi J, Liu XC, Wang LN, Zhang J, Li LL, Guan XM, Effects of electroacupuncture on the number of subcutaneous mast cells in and beside the acupoint and the inflammatory pain focus in the rat. Zhongguo Zhenjiu (Chinese Acupuncture and Moxibustion), 2003, 23:597-601

[130] Yu XJ, Ding GH, Yao W, Zhang R, Huang M, The role of collagen fiber in "Zusanli (ST36) in acupuncture analgesia in the rat. Zhongguo Zhenjiu (Chinese Acupuncture and Moxibustion), 2008, 28:207-213.

[131] Zhang D, Ding G, Shen X, Yao W, Zhang Z, Zhang Y, Lin J, Gu Q, Role of mast cells in acupuncture effect: a pilot study. Explore (NY), 2008, 4:170-177.

[132] Dastych J, Wyczolkowska J, Metcalfe DD, gE-crosslinking alters the avidity of an alpha-5 containing integrin receptor on murine mast cell for fibronectin. Journal of Allergy and Clinical Immunology, 1994, 93:379.

[133] Wiesner-Menzel L, Schulz B, Vakilzadeh F, Czarnetzki BM, Electron microscopical evidence for a direct contact between nerve fibres and mast cells, Acta Dermato-Venereologica, 1981, 61(6):465-469.

[134] Blennerhassett MG, Tomioka M, Bienenstock J, Formation of contacts between mast cells and sympathetic neurons in vitro, Cell Tissue Research, 1991, 265(1):121-128.

[135] Johnson D, Krenger W, Interaction of mast cells with the nervous system – recent advances. Neurochemistry Research, 1992, 17(9):939-951.

[136] Maurer M, Theoharides T, Granstein RD, Bischoff SC, Bienenstock J, Henz B, Kovanen P, Piliponsky AM, Kambe N, Vliagoftis H, Levi-Schaffer F, Metz M, Miyachi Y, Befus D, Forsythe P, Kitamura Y, Galli S, What is the physiological function of mast cells? Experimental Dermatology, 2003, 12(6):886-910.

[137] Gordon JR, Burd PR, Galli SJ, Mast cells as a source of multifunctional cytokines. Immunology Today 1990, 11(12):458-464.

[138] Turksen K, Adult stem cells, Humana Press, Totowa NJ, USA, 2004.

[139] Hofstetter CP, Schwartz EJ, Hess D, Widentalk J, El Manira A, Prockop DJ, Olson L, Marrow stromal cells form guiding strands in the injured spinal cord and promote recovery. Proceedings of National Academy of Sciences USA, 2002, 99:2199-2004.

[140] Engler AJ, Sen S, Sweeney HL, Discher DE, Matrix elasticity directs stem cell lineage specification. Cell, 2006, 126:677-689.

[141] Tenney RM, Discher DE, Stem cells, microenvironment mechanics, and growth factor activation. Current Opinion in Cell Biology, 2009, 21:630-635.

[142] Sinha S, Nevett C, Shuttleworth CA, Kielty CM, Cellular and extracellular biology of the latent transforming growth factor-beta binding proteins. Matrix Biology, 1998, 17(8-9):529-545.

[143] Mao Y, Schwarzbauer JE, Fibronectin fibrillogenesis, a cell-mediated matrix assembly process. Matrix Biology, 2005, 24:389–399.

[144] Klotzsch E, Smith ML, Kubow KE, Muntwyler S, Little WC, Beyeler F, Gourdon D, Nelson BJ, Vogel V, Fibronectin forms the most extensible biological fibers displaying switchable force-exposed cryptic binding sites. Proceedings of National Academy of Sciences USA, 2009, 106 (43):18267-18272.

[145] Wing ST & Kim WS, Plasma and cellular fibronectin: distinct and independent functions during tissue repair. Fibrogenesis & Tissue Repair, 2011; 4:21.

[146] Wells RG & Discher DE, Matrix elasticity, cytoskeletal tension and TGF-Beta : The insoluble and soluble meet. Science Signaling, 2008; 1(10):pe13

[147] Dallas SL, Sivakumar P, Jones CJ, Chen Q, Peters DM, Mosher DF, Humphries MJ, Kielty CM, Fibronectin regulates latent transforming growth factor-beta (TGF beta) by controlling matrix assembly of latent TGF beta-binding protein-1. Journal of Biological Chemistry, 2005 May 13; 280(19):18871-80.

[148] Kawelke N, Vasel M, Sens C, von Au A, Dooley S, and Nakchbandi IA, Fibronectin protects from excessive liver fibrosis by modulating the availability of and responsiveness of stellate cells to active TGF-β. PLoS One. 2011; 6(11):e28181.

[149] Hayashi H, Sakai T, Biological Significance of Local TGF-β Activation in Liver Diseases. Frontier Physiology, 2012, 3:12.

[150] Bourdoulous S, Orend G, MacKenna DA, Pasqualini R & Ruoslahti E, Fibronectin matrix regulates activation of RHO and CDC42 GTPases and cell cycle progression. Journal of Cell Biology, 1998, 143:267–276.

[151] Patwari P & Lee RT, Mechanical control of tissue morphogenesis. Circulation Research, 2008, 103:234-243.

[152] Zheng CH, Huang GY, Zhang MM, Experimental Study on Connexin43 Expression in "Zusanli" (ST36) with Fluorescence Dual-label Technique in Rats. Zhenci Yanjiu (Acupuncture Research), 2005, 30(4):221-224.

[153] Yu WC, Huang GY, Zhang MM, Wang W, Influence of connexin 43 gene knockout on the analgesic acupuncture in visceral pain mice. Zhenci Yanjiu (Acupuncture Research), 2008, 33(1):3-6.

[154] Huang GY, Zheng CH, Yu WC, Tian DS, and Wang W, Involvement of connexin 43 in acupuncture analgesia. Zhongguo Yi Xue (Chinese medicine journal), 2009, 122(1): 54-60.

[155] Shang C, Singular point, organizing center and acupuncture point. American Journal of Chinese Medicine. 1989; 17:119-127.

[156] Guo Y, Xu TP, Wang XY, Zhang YJ, Miao WF, Hu LM, Zhang CX, Chen JS, Jiang P, The correlative study between action of meridians and collaterals and $Ca^{2+}$ in peripheric meridians. Zhenci Yanjiu (Acupuncture Research), 1998, 4:247-250.

[157] Miao WF, Guo Y, Zhang YJ, Xu TP, The influence of changing the $Ca^{2+}$ concentration of the point Quze (PC3) on the curative effect of puncturing Neiguan (PC6) in experimental arrhythmic rabbits. Zhenci Yanjiu (Acupuncture Research), 1993 (3):243-245.

[158] Zhang YJ, Wang XY, Sh LP, Miao WF, Xu TP, Zhang CX, Influence of changing $Ca^{2+}$ concentration in Neiguan (PC6) on the effect of acupuncture treating experimental arrhythmic rabbits. Zhenci Yanjiu (Acupuncture Research), 1995, (2):63-67.

[159] Hu LM, Zhang YJ, Zhang CX, The changes of $Ca^{2+}$ in points along the pericardium channel and the influence of acupuncturing Neiguan. Zhenci Yanjiu (Acupuncture Research), 1998 (4):251-253.

[160] Guo Y, Ma DM, Zhang CX, Hu LM, Yuan YJ, Wang GJ, On the concentration of Calcium element in Zusanli (ST36) in rabbits, Shanghai Zhenci Zha Zhi (Shanghai Journal of Acupuncture and Moxibustion), 2003, (7):26-27.

[161] Gu X, Spitzer NC, Distinct aspects of neuronal differentiation encoded by frequency of spontaneous $Ca^{2+}$ transients. Nature, 1995, 375:784-787.

[162] Berridge MJ, The AM and FM of calcium signaling. Nature, 1997, 386:759-760.

[163] Politi A, Gaspers LD, Tomas AP, Hofer T, Models of $IP_3$ and $Ca^{2+}$ oscillations: frequency encoding and identification of underlying feedbacks. Biophysical Journal, 2006, 90:3120-3133.

[164] Fung PCW, Lam SK, Diseases, nitric oxide and related potent therapy, Medical Progress, 2001, July issue:19-22.

[165] Zhu W & Fung PCW, The roles played by crucial free radicals like lipid free radicals, nitric oxide and enzymes NOS & NADPH in C $Cl_4$ induced acute liver injury of mice, Free Radical Biology & Medicine, 2000, 29(9):870-880.

[166] Lui SL, Chan LY, Zhang XH, Zhu W, Chan TM, Fung PCW, Lai KN, Effect of mycophynolate mofetil on nitric oxide production and inducible nitric oxide synthase gene expression during renal ischemia-reperfusion injury, Nephrology Dialysis transplantation, 2001, 16(8):1577-1582.

[167] Klein EA, Castagnino P, Kothapalli D, Yin L, Byfield FJ, Xu T, Levental I, Hawthome E, Janmey PA, & Assoian, Cell Cycle Control by Physiological Matrix Elasticity and In Vivo Tissue Stiffening. Current Biology, 2009, 19(18):1511-1518.

[168] Bartkova J, Lukas J, Muller H, Lutzhoft D, Strauss M, Bartek J, Cyclin D1 protein expression and function in human breast cancer. International Journal of Cancer, 1994, 57:353–361.

[169] Leight JL, Wozniak MA, Chen S, Lynch ML, and Chen CS, Matrix rigidity regulates a switch between TGF-β1–induced apoptosis and epithelial–mesenchymal transition, Molecular Biology of Cell, 2012; 23(5):781–791.

[170] Bissell MJ, Kenny PA, Radisky DC, Microenvironmental regulators of tissue structure and function also regulate tumor induction and progression: the role of extracellular matrix and its degrading enzymes. Cold Spring Harbor Symposia on Quantitative Biology, 2005, 70:343-356.

[171] Whitehead J, Vignjevic D, Futterer C, Beaurepaire E, Robine S, Farge E, Mechanical factors activate beta-catenin-dependent oncogene expression in APC mouse colon. HFSP Journal, 2008, 2(5):286-294.

[172] Butcher DT, Alliston T, Weaver VM, A tense situation: forcing tumour progression. Nature Reviews Cancer, 2009, 9:108-122.

[173] Levental KR, Yu H, Kass L, Lakins JN, Egeblad M, Erler JT, Fong SF, Csiszar K, Giaccia A, Weninger W, Matrix crosslinking forces tumor progression by enhancing integrin signaling. Cell, 2009, 209:891-906.

[174] Noguera R, Nieto, Tadeo I, Farinas F, Alvaro T, Extracellular matrix, biotensegrity and tumor microenvironment. An update and review. Histology and Histopathology, 2012, 27(6):693-705.

[175] Axelson HW & Hagbarth KE, Human motor control consequences of thixotropic changes in muscular short-range stiffness. Journal of Physiology, 2001, 535(1): 279-288.

[176] Homma I & Hagbarth KE, Thixotropy of rib cage respiration muscles in normal subjects. Journal of Applied Physiology, 2000; 89:1753-1758.

[177] Tiktopulo EL & Kajava AV, Denaturation of type I collagen fibrils is an endothermic process accompanied by a noticeable change in the partial heat capacity, Biochemistry Journal, 1998, 37(22):8147-52.

[178] Evanko S, Extracellular matrix and the manipulation of cells and tissues, IASI Yearbook (International Association of Structural Integrators), 2009, pages 61-68.

[179] Ho MW, Bolton JP, Knight D, Quantitative image analysis of birefringent biological material, Journal of Microscopy, 1997, 187(1):62-67.

[180] Martin R et al, Liquid crystalline ordering of procollagen as a determinant of 3-D extracellular matrix architecture, Journal of Molecular Biology, 2000, 301(1):11-17.

[181] Stewart GT, Liquid crystals in biology. I. Historical, biological and medical aspects, Liquid Crystals, 2003; 30(5):541-557.

Section 2

# New Developments in Acupuncture

Chapter 6

# High-Tech Equipment for Moxibustion in Modern Medicine

Takashi Seki, Junnosuke Okajima, Akiko Kikuchi,
Shin Takayama, Masashi Watanabe,
Hiroko Kusuyama, Ayane Matsuda,
Soichiro Kaneko, Tetsuharu Kamiya, Atsuki Komiya,
Minami Fujiwara, Nobuo Yaegasi,
Tomoyuki Yambe and Shigenao Maruyama

Additional information is available at the end of the chapter

http://dx.doi.org/10.5772/53802

## 1. Introduction

### 1.1. Social background and medical needs

Japan is a super-aging society; year after year, the number of persons older than 65 years of age increases. Because they are frail, elderly persons require treatment methods that best suit their condition. Traditional medicine, which has been handed down and culled throughout history, is one such candidate treatment. Until recently in Japan, moxibustion therapy was provided in most households (Yamaoka, 2001). In recent years, hyperthermia treatment has spread widely in the field of orthopaedics, rehabilitation, and cancer treatment. Typically, medical sites require safe, sanitary treatment methods.

### 1.2. Characteristics and current practice of moxibustion

Moxibustion is widely used in East Asian countries and has long been a common feature of traditional East Asian medicine (Freire et al., 2005). Moxibustion, which entails the burning of moxa (mugwort), is a very important traditional treatment method that has been practiced from ancient times.

In the clinical practice of moxibustion, different treatment methods—for example, direct moxibustion wherein the moxa is applied directly to the skin, material-mediated (indirect) moxibustion wherein a material is placed between the skin and the moxa, and moxibustion with warming needles (Moxa needle) whereby moxa is applied via needle insertion of the skin —are selected and applied based on the condition of the patient (Beijing Digital Museum of TCM, 2012).

In Japan, there are laws regulating the practice of massage, finger pressure, acupuncture, and moxibustion. At present, there are 85 vocational colleges and 5 universities in Japan (Ido no nippon Editorial office, 2008) and more than 84,629 licensed moxibustion practitioners. The number of qualified moxibustion practitioners is almost equal to the number of physicians in Japan (Ministry of Health, Labour and Welfare-Japan, 2009). There are 71 schools in every prefecture that provide acupuncture and moxibustion training to persons who are visually impaired. For the visually impaired, moxibustion treatment is a challenging skill to learn because the risk of burn injury to patients exists, even in the case of general practitioners (Ministry of Education, Culture, Sports, Science and Technology-Japan, 2006). Simple moxibustion kits can be purchased by anyone in Japan at a drugstore or on the Internet (Sennenq, 2012).

### 1.3. Scientific research on moxibustion treatment

If, as seems to be the case, moxibustion treatment can be applied in modern medical settings, then it is possible to anticipate greater treatment efficacy. It has been reported that treating acupoint ST25, located on both sides of the umbilicus, with moxibustion helps the intestines become active and improves their function (Tabosa et al., 2004). We have successfully proved that heating the umbilicus increases the volume of blood flow in the superior mesenteric artery by using a heat conduction treatment device that we developed (Takayama et al., 2010, 2011; Seki et al., 2011). Heating the affected area with moxibustion can remedy the condition of acute lymphangitis. It has also been suggested that moxibustion enhances immune function and is an effective way to promote the blood flow of an animal's brain (Shen et al, 2006). However, there is little research that has quantitatively evaluated moxibustion treatment (Kim et al., 2011). Thus, it is critical to conduct a scientific evaluation of moxibustion treatment.

### 1.4. Issues related to moxibustion treatment

#### *1.4.1. Difficulty of temperature control and invasiveness*

It is vital to precisely control the temperature in a scientific evaluation of moxibustion treatment; however, this is quite difficult to do. Moxibustion is invasive because it poses the risk of a burn injury or leaving a scar on the skin, and women in particular would worry about the scar left on their skin. It is said that the skin tissue will degenerate and exhibit low-temperature burns when the temperature exceeds 44°C (Jiang et al., 2002).

It is difficult to ensure safe treatment unless the practitioner has been trained, because the temperature control depends on the experience of the doctor or practitioners of moxibustion in clinical practice. Moreover, patients whose skin has lost the ability to sense temperature are at risk for easily experiencing a burn injury. There is not only the risk posed by the lack of temperature control, but there is also the fact that, due to the impossibility of quantitative temperature control, the optimum temperature for moxibustion treatment and the relationship between temperature and treatment efficacy of moxibustion treatment have not been sufficiently debated.

#### *1.4.2. Unsanitary*

Moxibustion treatment is difficult to use in the hospital setting because of the copious amount of fumes emitted, and there was a case in which a patient with asthma experienced an asthma attack in a hospital because of moxibustion fumes. The use of moxibustion requires adequate management of the fumes emitted at hospitals where patients with diverse maladies are being treated.

#### *1.4.3. Procuring equipment and user-friendliness*

It is difficult to obtain adequate quality moxa in certain areas. Moreover, practicing moxibustion treatment on-site at clinics is time- and effort-intensive.

## 2. Purpose

The purpose of this research was to develop a treatment device that is safe; is capable of controlling temperature; does not emit fumes; can be substituted for indirect moxibustion, direct moxibustion, and moxa needle; and thereby evaluate such functions. The purpose of advanced temperature control is to prevent the risk of burning, provide appropriate treatment for each patient, contribute to scientific research on moxibustion treatment and achieve high treatment efficacy as a result.

In this research, we developed a thermo-control device that is capable of controlling temperature by using heat conduction and radiant heat. We have applied this device to many patients in clinical practice and have confirmed its treatment efficacy. Typical cases have been described further.

## 3. Methods and results

### 3.1. Device we developed

Our requirements for the device were (1) that it should not emit fumes and (2) be capable of precise temperature control, preventing the temperature from exceeding a certain level for safety. We developed three types of devices with heat conduction and one type with radiation heat (Figure 1).

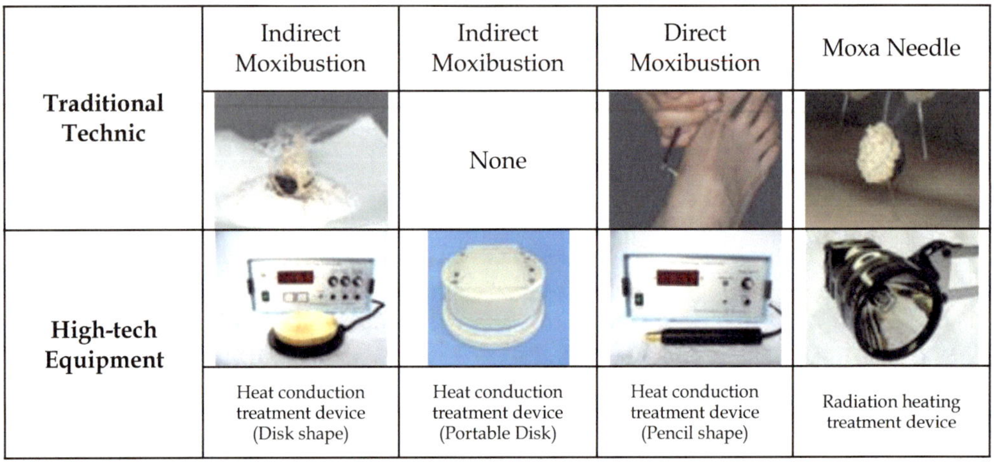


**Figure 1.** List of traditional technic and developed devices.

The following text includes information on device configuration and characteristic performance, as well as cases that are adaptable to basic clinical research and intractable cases.

### 3.2. Heat conduction treatment devices

#### *3.2.1. Heat conduction treatment device: disc shape*

We developed the hyperthermia control device using a heating disc with temperature control to replace the salt-mediated moxibustion (Maruyama et al., 2011).

##### *3.2.1.1. Traditional treatment that can be replaced: indirect moxibustion*

Problems

The problems of indirect moxibustion include its heating characteristic and the difficulty of controlling its temperature, as well as the great amount of fumes it emits. As shown in Figure 2A, it was difficult to control the temperature and the salt-mediated moxibustion emitted a great amount of fumes. Figure 2B shows the distribution of skin temperature after salt-mediated moxibustion is removed. This indicates a non-uniform distribution of temperature, in which the skin temperature at the centre of the area where salt-mediated moxibustion was applied is high and the skin temperature of the surrounding area is low.

##### *3.2.1.2. Configuration*

The heating disc is 100 mm in diameter and made of copper and coated gilding (Figure 3A). As shown in Figure 3B (disc-shaped configuration drawing), the present device is composed of a heating disc and a control device. A thermistor is used for measuring the temperature. The control device is capable of controlling the preset temperature and heating rate. Equipped with proportional control, this device is able to control the temperature without exceeding the

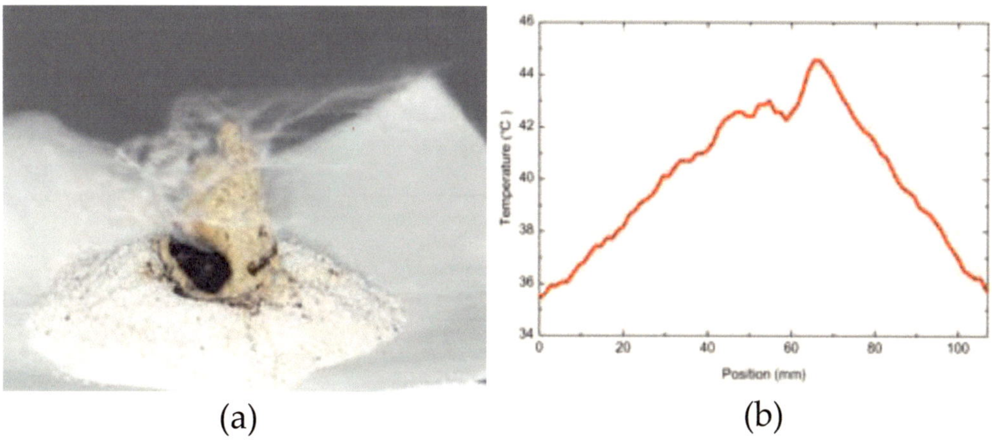


**Figure 2.** a) Indirect (Salt-mediated) moxibustion. (b) Temperature distribution after the moxibustion is removed.

preset temperature and thus decreases the risk of burn injury. In addition, use of copper, which has a high thermal conductivity rate, as the material for the heating disc can make the temperature on the heating surface uniform.

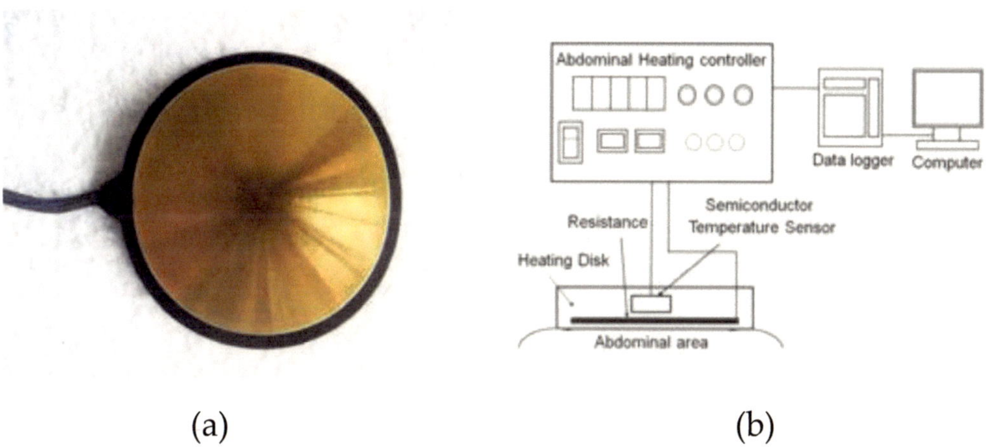


**Figure 3.** a) A picture of the heating disc. (b) The configuration drawing of the disc shape device.

*3.2.1.3. Performance*

Heating characteristic

Advanced temperature control within 0.1°C units.

Principle of temperature control

On/off control is used to control the preset temperature and heating rate. Heat is produced by applying a certain voltage to an electrical resistance, while the temperature is controlled by switching the heater power source on/off. Adjusting proportional gain (Kp) and using the on/off switch enables the controller to raise the temperature to the preset temperature within 0.1°C units. By changing the interval for on/off, it is possible to adjust the heating rate.

Figure 4 shows the formula of proportional control to determine the average of heat quantity. $T_0$ indicates the preset temperature.

$$\bar{\dot{Q}}(t) = K_P\left[T(t) - T_0\right]$$

**Figure 4.** The formula of proportional control.

## Heating rate and achieving temperature

Figure 5A shows that when the four heating rates raised the temperature to the preset temperature of 42°C, all of the rates successfully raised the temperature without exceeding the preset temperature and stayed at the determinate temperature.

## Distribution of the temperature on the heating disc

Figure 5B indicates the six temperature measurement points on the heating disc. Figure 5C shows the temperature change at each measuring point after application of heat in thermally insulating condition and indicates that the temperature at all six points changed in a nearly uniform manner.

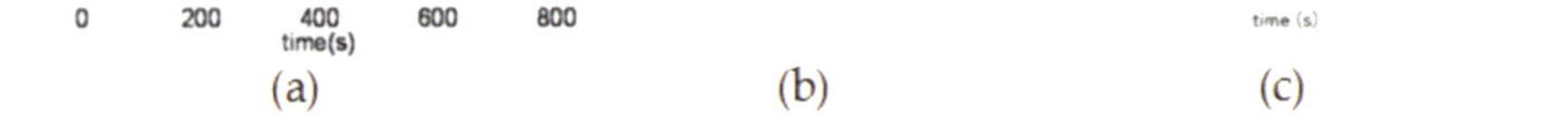


**Figure 5.** a) Change over time in the temperature of the heating disc. (b) Position of thermocouple. (c) Temperature distribution on the surface of the heating disk.

## Temperature distribution on the skin

The distribution of skin temperature after being heated by the heat conduction treatment device on the abdomen is shown in Figure 6A. Temperature was measured using an infrared imaging device (manufactured by NEC Avio Infrared Technologies Co., Ltd., TVS-500). The temperatures within a 10-cm diameter heated by the disc were nearly consistent, which clearly shows the difference between the temperature distribution of the disc and the temperature distribution of the salt-mediated moxibustion, as seen in Figure 2B. Figure 6B is a thermography image of the same areas.

Also, the heating disc is made light enough so that patients feel comfortable when the disc is placed on their abdomens.

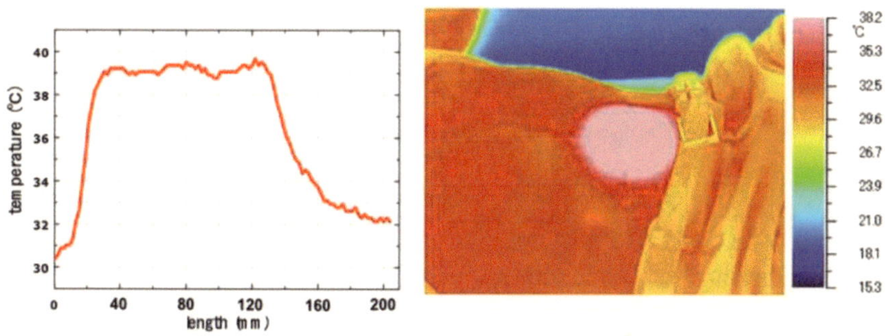


(a) (b)

**Figure 6.** a) Temperature distribution on the skin surface after the heating controller was operated on the abdominal area and then removed. (b) Thermography image of the abdominal area.

### *3.2.2. Heat conduction treatment device: disc shape (portable type)*

We developed the disc-shaped contact-type heating controller in a portable format so patients can easily apply it at home and to enlarge the range of applications of the device. Evaluations were then conducted.

#### *3.2.2.1. Traditional treatment that can be replaced: indirect (material-mediated) moxibustion*

Problem

Indirect moxibustion cannot be applied while the patient is moving or unless placed on a level surface. Thus, such a treatment lacks portability.

#### *3.2.2.2. Configuration*

Unlike the first device, this device can be used while the patient is moving; thus, its usability has a wider range. This device is portable and enables easy, high-level, safe thermal treatment at home at a low cost. Figure 7A depicts the exterior of the device, and Figure 7B shows the configuration of the device.

#### *3.2.2.3. Performance*

The temperature control circuit uses lithium-ion batteries (NP-120 × 2) and is rechargeable. It takes three to four hours to charge the batteries, and the battery duration provides about 20 minutes of use per charge.

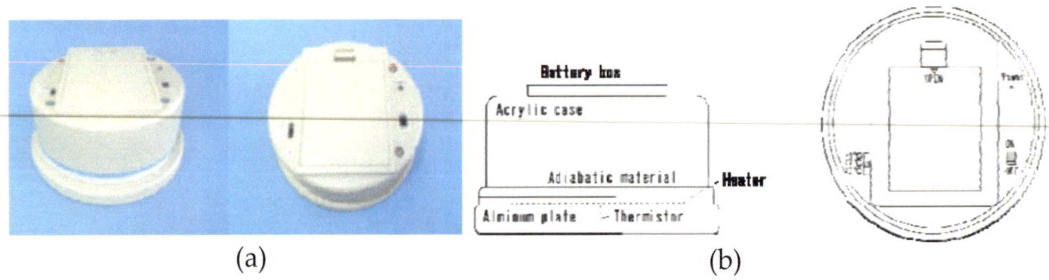


**Figure 7.** a) A picture of the portable disc. (b) The configuration drawing of the portable disc.

The thermistor is used to detect the temperature, and after amplifying the temperature signal by error amplification and amplification, the heater attached to the aluminium plate is run through the constant current circuit of Power MOSFET. It heats up quickly at a low temperature through the rapid heating circuit and controls the temperature at approximately the pre-set temperature. The temperature can be set between 41°C and 45°C, within 1°C units. The thermostat is used to protect the aluminium plate from overheating.

Heating characteristics

It can achieve the targeted temperature and the temperature distribution on the skin. Figure 8A shows the change in temperature after putting the heater into contact with the skin after about 20 minutes when the heater heats up to near body temperature, under the following conditions: pre-set temperature of 42°C, surrounding temperature of 21.4°C, and humidity of 66.7%. This indicates that when the heater made contact with the skin, the temperature decreased slightly but quickly recovered and maintained a constant temperature. The highest temperature achieved was 42.4°C, with a temperature difference of only 0.2°C between the centre and the periphery.

Research has confirmed that the preset temperature can be maintained at other pre-set temperatures (data not shown). Figure 8B shows the time change after removing the device and the change of skin temperature distribution after the device heated the skin. This indicates that the heated surface maintained a nearly uniform temperature after heating. Figure 8C, 8D shows an image and picture of thermography of the abdominal area after it was heated by the same device. The thermography also confirmed that the treated part was uniformly heated. As a result, this device is deemed to be capable of having the same hyperthermic effect as the stationary type.

Safety

The duration time is limited to prevent overheating in the patient. Once the treatment is finished using the device, it can no longer be used unless it is charged again. By limiting the function in this way, human errors, such as patients excessively heating their skin, can thus be prevented.

http://dx.doi.org/10.5772/53802

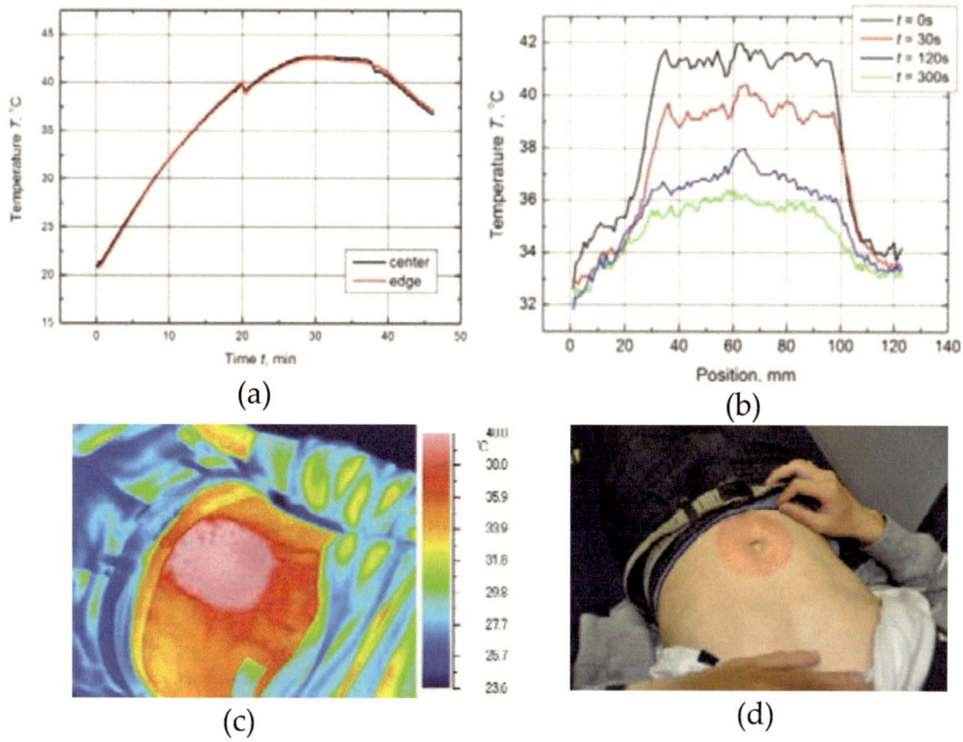


**Figure 8.** a) Change in temperature of the portable heating disc over time. (b) Time change of temperature distribution around the abdominal area after heating. (c)(d) Image and picture of heat around the abdominal area after it was heated.

### *3.2.3. Heat conductive treatment device: pencil shape*

#### *3.2.3.1. Traditional treatment that can be replaced: direct moxibustion*

Problem

Direct moxibustion requires more experienced clinical practice than material-mediated moxibustion to be safe and effective. Also, the moxa used in direct moxibustion must be smaller and easier to harden than the moxa used in indirect moxibustion. Figure 9 is a picture of direct moxibustion.

#### *3.2.3.2. Configuration*

The configuration of the pencil shape is the same as the disc shape, and the heating part is made of copper and coated with gilding. The heating part, which makes contact with the skin, can be replaced with different sizes. Figure 10 shows the configuration and a picture of the pencil-shaped device.

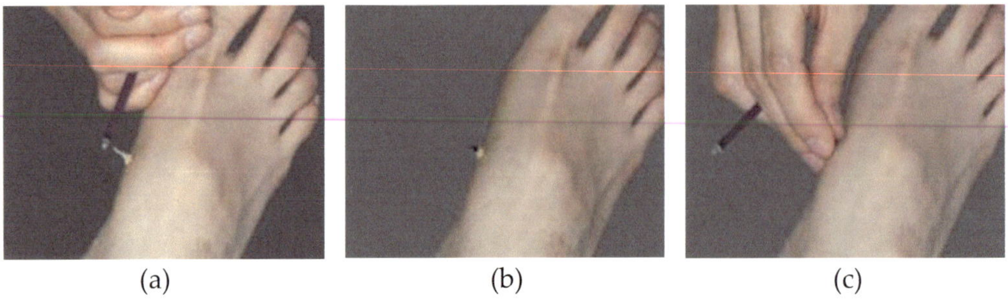


**Figure 9.** The procedure of direct moxibustion.

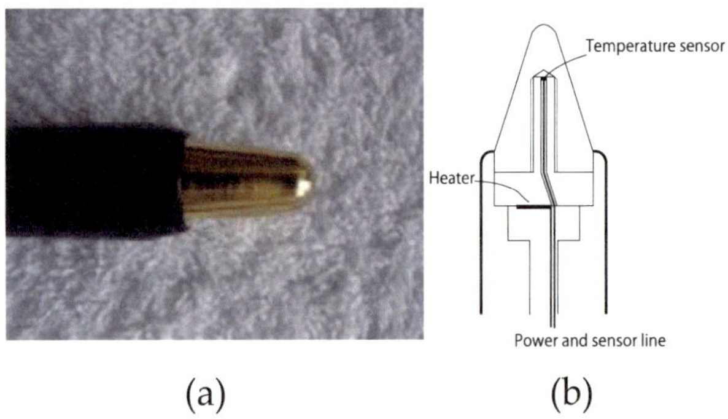


**Figure 10.** a) A picture of the pencil-shaped device. (b) The configuration drawing of the pencil-shaped device.

*3.2.3.3. Performance*

The pencil-shaped device has the same control as the disc-shape device.

### 3.3. The radiation heating treatment device

We developed this radiation heating treatment device to replace Moxa needle. This device is able to control the temperature to prevent the risk of burn injury and also distributes a consistent temperature over the applied area of the body (Maruyama et al., 2012).

*3.3.1. Traditional treatment that can be replaced: Moxa needle*

Problem

Moxa needle is shown in Figure 11A. It is difficult to control the temperature. The only way to prevent the temperature from becoming too high is to remove the moxa burning at the top of the needle or to block the radiating heat by placing a piece of paper between the skin and the moxa. Moxa needles are inserted into the patient's body, followed by moxa on the needles, which is then ignited. Therefore, if the patient moves his or her body during treatment and the burning moxa falls on the skin, the patient may experience a burn injury. The risk of burning moxa falling onto the skin occurs when the temperature is being adjusted.

As shown in Figure 11B, a 3-mm-thick silicon rubber membrane with a thermal conductivity of 0.23 W/(m K) is adhered to an 8-mm-thick copper plate. The rubber has an emissivity of ($\varepsilon$) 0.95, which is close to the emissivity of the human body. We used ethanol to prevent air bubbles from forming within the bond between the rubber and the copper plate. We monitored the rubber membrane surface temperature $T_{upper}$ using infrared thermography (TVS-500, manufactured by Nippon Avionics Corporation). At the time, the temperature of the copper plate was maintained at 37.0°C in the thermostat bath. We ensured that the lower surface of the rubber membrane made complete contact with the copper plate and that the temperature $T_{lower}$ was 37.0°C, i.e., equivalent to the temperature of the copper plate. We stuck an acupuncture needle into the rubber membrane and burned the moxa laced on the needle.

Figure 11C shows the distribution of temperature caused by kyutoshin heating of the rubber membrane surface. The figure indicates the temperature distribution when the temperature is at its highest (20 seconds after igniting the moxa) during the burning of the moxa. This graph depicts a certain line on the horizontal axis, which delineates an image taken with an infrared thermograph. This indicates that the temperature at the centre had reached the level that causes burn injuries, while at the same the temperature of the surrounding area remained low.

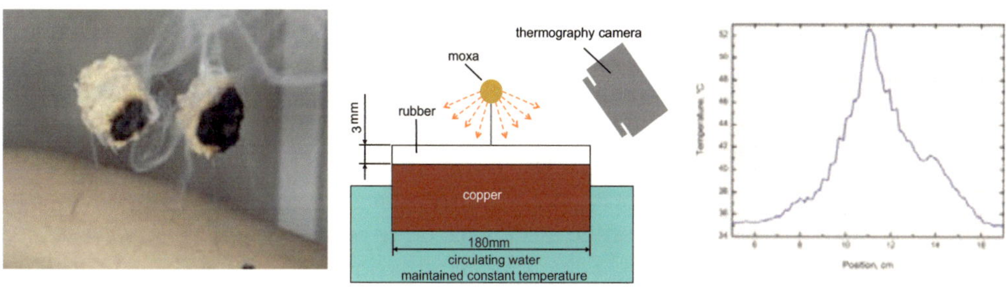


(a) (b) (c)

**Figure 11.** a) Moxa meedle. (b) Measuring the heating characteristics of moxa needle. (c) Temperature distribution of the rubber membrane heated by moxa needle.

### 3.3.2. *Configuration*

We used a halogen lamp with a rated power of 75 W (J12V75W-AXS, manufactured by Mitsubishi Electric Osram), available on the market, as the light source. However, we controlled the radiation intensity by using the power supply device adjustably with a power load lower than the rated power. We used a remodelled Maglite 4-Cell D Flashlight (manufactured by Mag Instrument, Inc.) as the reflection mirror. The reflection mirror is a parabolic mirror, which makes it possible to emit near-parallel light by adjusting the light source to the focal point position of the parabolic mirror. A fan (ICFAN E232190, RED(+), 0410N-12, DC12V, 0.09A manufactured by SHCOH Engineering) attached to the upper side prevents the reflecting mirror from overheating.

Because parallel light can be radiated through fine adjustment of the lighting source position with respect to the reflecting mirror, the temperature can be increased uniformly over the region radiated by the light. Figure 12 shows the exterior and the detailed interior of the radiation heating device developed in this research.

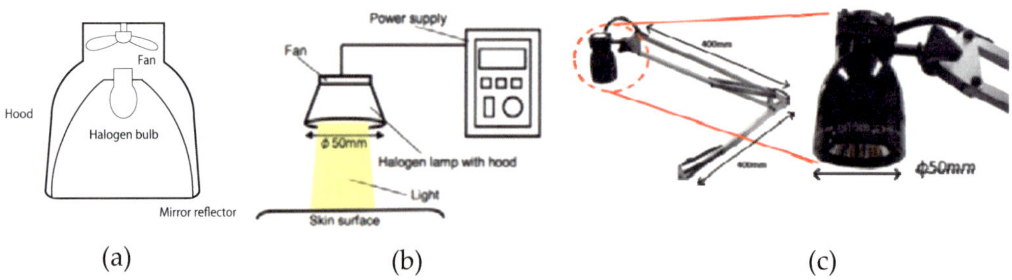


**Figure 12.** a) Detail of components in radiation heater. (b) The configuration drawing of the radiation heater. (c) Photograph of the radiation heater.

### *3.3.3. Performance*

Radiation emission intensity

Figure 13A shows the results from measuring the intensity of the radiation emitted from the radiation heating device for multiple applied voltage values using the Fourier Transform Infrared Spectrophotometer: TTIR (FTIR-8600PC, manufactured by Shimadzu Corporation). The horizontal axis is displayed with the logarithmic axis in the figure. In addition, for comparison, the theoretical value of the ideal black body spectrum at 1,500 K is also stated. The radiation heating device showed a characteristic emission that peaks at about 2 μm, which is within the infrared range. This shows the wavelength range that influences the heating effect from the radiation heating device. Based on this, it is thought that radiation penetrates the skin to a certain degree.

Temperature distribution of the rubber membrane from radiation heating

We evaluated the radiation heating device we developed with the same device used to measure the radiating heat of moxa needle moxibustion and conducted multiple measurements by altering the voltage applied to the radiation heating device (Figure 13B).

Figure 13C shows the temperature distribution at the point where the temperature remains steady (about 10–15 minutes after heating). On the other hand, the temperature caused by the radiation heating device did not increase in an absolutely uniform manner. However, the range indicating the maximum temperature is nearly uniform. Figure 13D shows the temperature distribution of the rubber membrane using infrared thermography. This shows heat application at near uniformity of temperature.

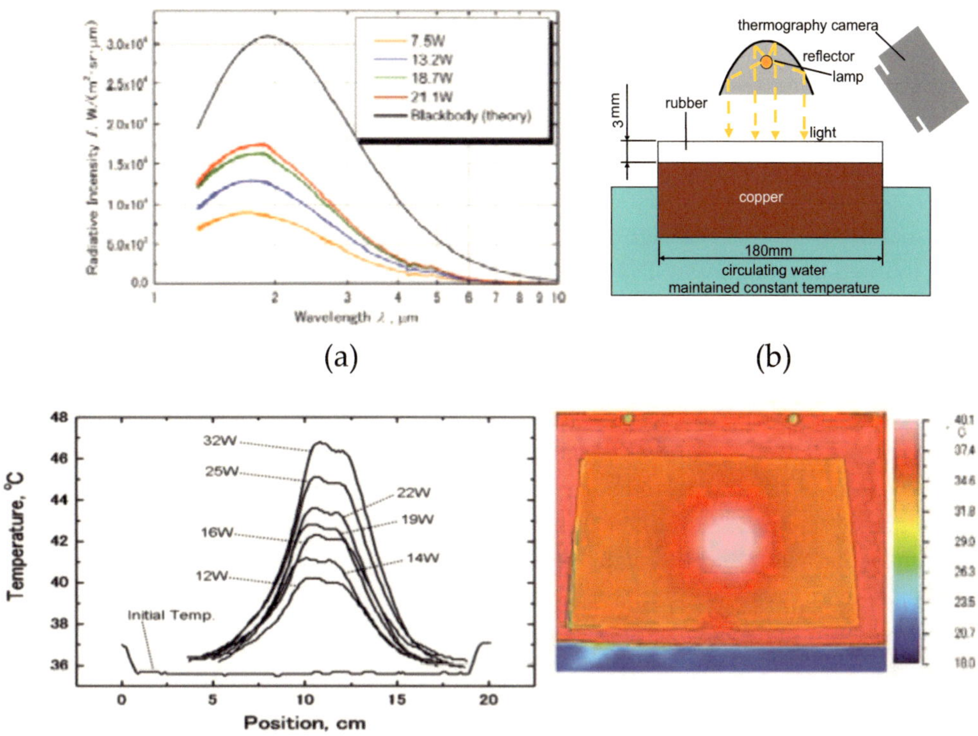


(a) (b) (c) (d)

**Figure 13.** a) Spectral radiative intensity of the radiation heater considering absorption matters. (b) Schematic diagram of the experiment for temperature distribution measurement. (c) Temperature distribution on the surface of the rubber sheet heated by the radiation heater. (d) Thermograph of the rubber sheet heated by the radiation heater.

## Advanced control of heat transfer amount

Figure 14A shows the results calculated for multiple applied voltages of the amount of heat transfer from the radiation heating device. The graph is generally linear except for some minor variability. The amount of heat transfer from the radiation heating device can be calculated by the following formula when the approximate curve is determined by plotting the least squares approximation:

$Q_{heater} = 0.155\ Q_{input}$, wherein

$Q_{input}$ [W] is the applied voltage, and the determination coefficient $R^2$ value is 0.9812.

It is possible to estimate the relationship between the amount of heat transfer and the temperature of the skin at the time of hyperthermia treatment by using this formula.

This finding indicates that it is possible to control the amount of heat transfer by controlling the voltage applied to the radiation heating device. We thus anticipate a precise temperature control within the treated region, which will prevent the risk of burn injury.

Uniform temperature distribution on the skin

Figure 14B shows an image, taken by infrared thermography, of the abdomen of a subject heated by a radiation heater. It was also confirmed that the temperature distribution over the subject's body with the radiation heater was uniform.

The amount of heat transfer and the temperature of the skin

We radiated the subjects with light using the radiation heater and monitored skin temperature using infrared thermography. The abdomen of the subject, lying flat on his back on a bed, was heated by a radiation heater from a distance of 200 mm above. We repeated the experiment multiple times with varied voltages applied to the radiation heater. Further, we conducted the experiments in a temperature-controlled room equipped with air conditioning to maintain the same conditions as much as possible. When applying heat to the human body, it is reported to take approximately 20 minutes for the heat to reach to a stable level (Maruyama et al., 2011; Okajima et al., 2009; Incropera, et al., 2007). In this experiment, we used infrared thermography to monitor the temperature on the surface of the skin and continued the experiment until we observed a stable state with almost no changes in temperature. Hereafter, we deemed temperatures found in this stable state to be post-experiment skin temperature. The temperature indicates the peak value from the temperature distribution. The subjects included five healthy men in their 20s (mean (SD); age: 23 (2) years old; height: 171.4 (2.6) cm; weight: 64.2 (5.1) kg).

Figure 14C is a graph showing the correlation between the heat transfer rate and the subject's skin temperature. As indicated, even after heat has been applied through an identical quantity of heat transfer, the increase in skin temperature varies among different individuals. This suggests that the amount of bioheat varies among individuals. The increase in skin temperature varies between individuals if the body is heated with an equal amount of heat transfer. For example, the difference in the skin temperature among individuals with a heat transfer amount of 1.1 W from the radiation heater varies approximately between 40°C and 43°C.

### 3.4. Clinical studies

#### *3.4.1. Basic research*

##### *3.4.1.1. Variability of temporal and spatial comfort temperature at the time of treatment with a disc-shape heater*

Figure 15 shows the relationship between the optimal heating temperature and number of treatments for one subject. Focusing on the distribution of optimal heating temperature, we detected different values each time for each treatment. This finding appears to depend on the subject's surrounding environment, health condition, and mood at the time treatment is received. This particular patient showed a maximum difference of 5°C, which indicates a significant influence.

http://dx.doi.org/10.5772/53802

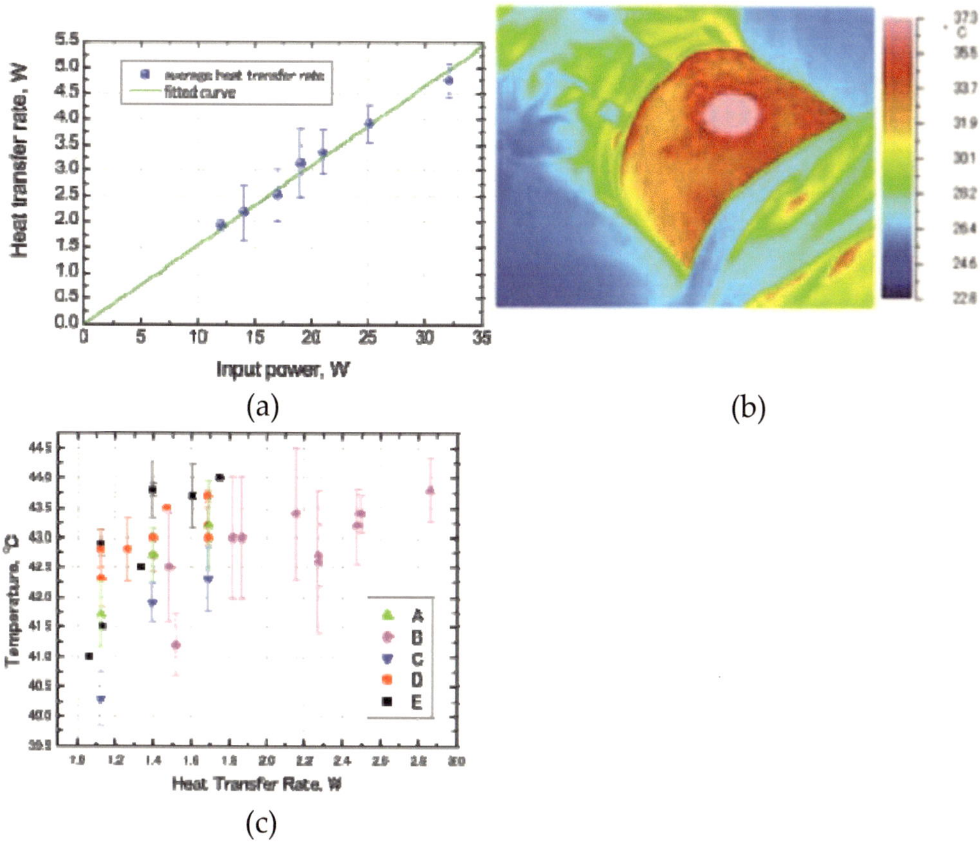


**Figure 14.** a) Correlation between the radiative heat conduction rate emitted by the radiation heater and input electric power. (b) Thermography snapshot of a subject's skin heated by the radiation heater. (c) Correlation between skin surface temperature and radiative heat transfer rate.

#### *3.4.1.2. Individual difference in comfortable temperature at time of treatment with disc-shape heater*

This device, which is able to precisely control the temperature, enabled us to detect the temperature at which a patient feels comfortable, as shown in Figure 16. Each individual has a different level of comfortable temperature that can even vary for the same subject. Figure 16 shows the results from an experiment conducted on 13 subjects.

#### *3.4.1.3. The relationship between patient age and optimal heating temperature with the disc-shaped device*

We measured the most comfortable temperature by applying the disc on the umbilical region of 39 healthy subjects. Figure 17 shows the ages of the subjects and the distribution of the temperature, at which they felt most comfortable. We applied the least squares method for evaluation. This graph indicates that elderly people felt most comfortable at higher tempera-

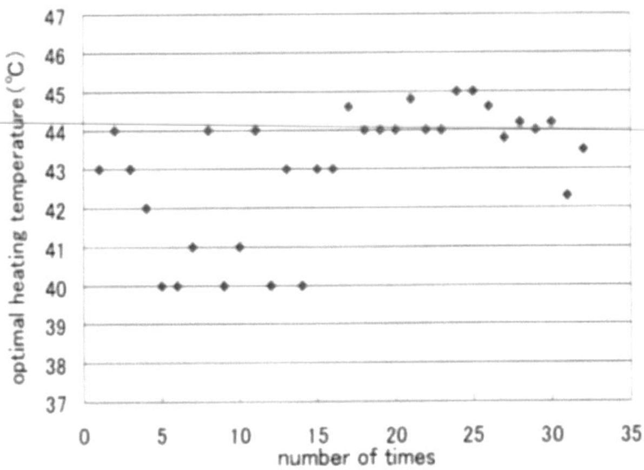


**Figure 15.** Statistical results of optimal heating temperature of one patient.

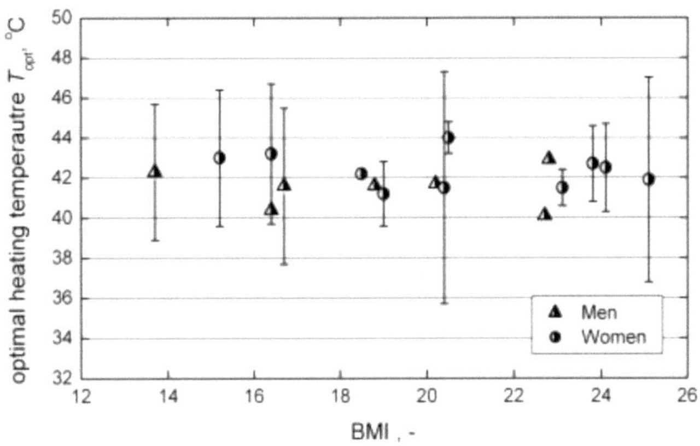


**Figure 16.** Body mass index (BMI) and the optimal heating temperature

tures. It is possible that an elderly person's sense of temperature is blunted, suggesting that they have a higher risk of incurring burn injury at the time of moxibustion treatment.

### *3.4.2. Case reports*

#### *3.4.2.1. Case of a patient who was unable to eat due to long-term vomiting after cord blood stem cell transplantation for treatment of adult T-cell leukaemia: A disc-shaped heat transfer device was used effectively as treatment*

A 49-year-old Japanese woman (height of 150 cm and weight of 54 kg) was referred to our clinic because of difficulty eating. She could not eat any food because she would vomit as she ate, and she felt nauseous just looking at food. She had cacogeusia (bad taste not related to

http://dx.doi.org/10.5772/53802

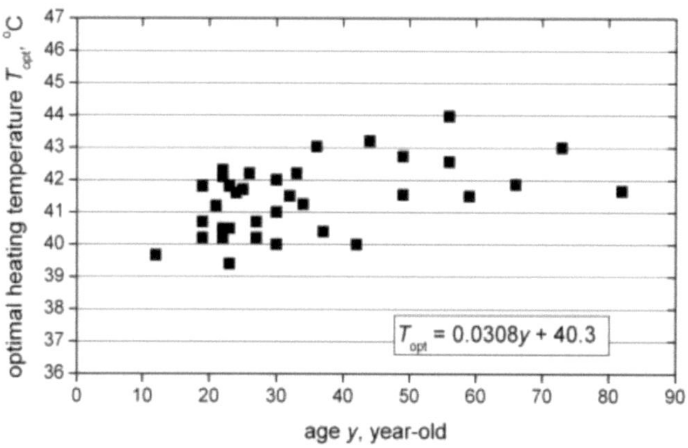


**Figure 17.** Correlation between subjects' age and comfortable temperature.

ingestion of various substances) and reported symptoms of fatigue, insomnia, finger tremor, and algia at the lower extremities. Medical history: She had an automobile accident 5 years ago. Family history: Father had stomach cancer; her mother had lumbar spondylolisthesis. Social history: She had worked at a supermarket; currently, she is a stay-at-home wife.

Clinical history: The patient received a cord blood stem cell transplant with a pre-treatment of total body irradiation, cytosine arabinoside, and cyclophosphamide on Day -157, due to chemotherapy resistance against adult T-cell leukaemia onset two years ago but had a rejection response. She received a second cord blood stem cell transplant with pre-treatment of fludarabine and melphalan on Day -115. Her state was regarded as remission and she was referred to our clinic from the Department of Hematology and Immunology, Tohoku University Hospital, because complications such as nausea and lack of appetite, which are common after transplantation, did not improve easily.

Internal medicine: The patient was treated with one tablet of tacrolimus hydrate 2.0 mg twice daily, one tablet of omeprazole 20 mg once daily, two tablets of Baktar® (sulfamethoxazole 400 mg, trimethoprim 80 mg) twice daily, Scopolamine butylbromide, Ethyl loflazepate, and Flunitrazepam. Medication adherence: None. Drug allergy: None. Findings of physical examination: left-sided upper abdominal tenderness and a cold lower abdomen. (In Kampo medicine, great attention is paid to the findings of the abdominal examination when determining treatment. If the patient had a cold problem, we would choose a heating treatment such herbal medicine and moxibustion.)

Course of treatment: We started the treatment by heating the umbilicus with the disc-shaped heat transfer treatment device on Day 1. At the time the patient started treatment, she was not able to take anything orally. On Day 8, she was able to eat 30% of the food provided by our hospital. She could eat 50% of the food 24 days after the start of treatment, and she could eat more than 80% of the food on the 29th day. After that, she could maintain eating 50–70% of the food.

Conclusion: The patient underwent heating treatment delivered by the disc-shaped heat transfer treatment device to her navel to treat her eating difficulty after cord blood stem cell transplantation. The patient's prolonged eating difficulty was improved.

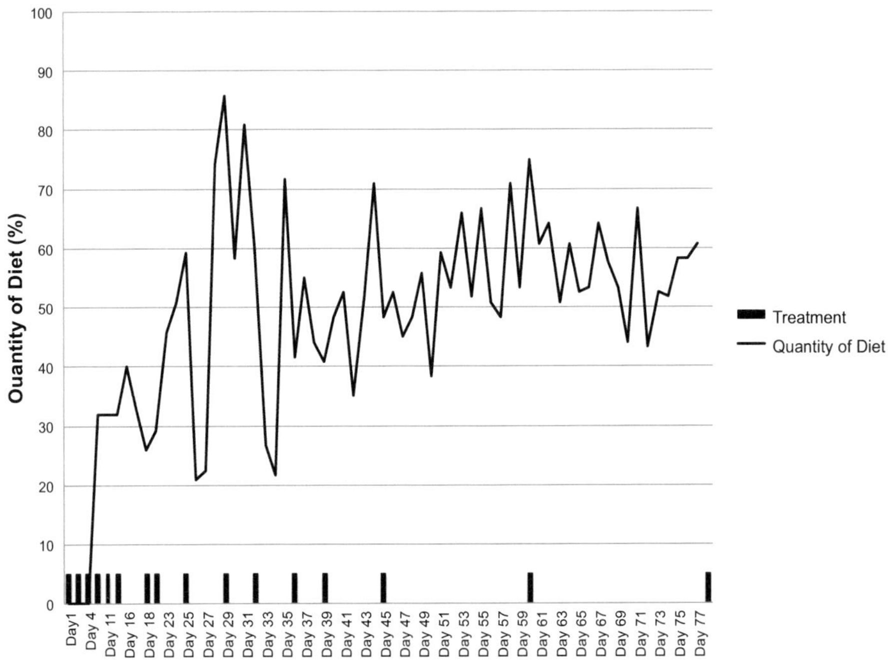


**Figure 18.** Course of treatment. Percent change of quantity of diet.

*3.4.2.2. Case of a patient with refractory melosalgia following an allogeneic bone marrow transplant after extirpation of a granulocytic sarcoma of the lumbosacral spinal cord*

A 27-year-old Japanese woman (height of 161 cm, weight of 54 kg) who had been bedridden for some time, started experiencing pain in her right hip through the lower thigh after starting to walk again. She was referred to our clinic due to the intractable nature of her condition. The pain was relieved when heated and worsened before it rained. Also, she contracted a rash on her face when she was physically fatigued or psychologically stressed. Medical history: She underwent surgery for strabismus at the age of 5 and surgery for appendicitis at Sendai Medical Centre when she was in sixth grade. She became easily tired after giving birth to a child three years ago. Family history: unremarkable. Social history: She was previously employed as a corporate worker.

Clinical history: Two years ago, she had been tired because she had to take her child to various hospitals for a cold. She used massaging tools because she felt numbness in her leg, but she had extreme pain on her left sacrum. She received a nerve block at an orthopaedic clinic, but later she experienced problems with menstrual bleeding that was difficult to stop. Last year,

http://dx.doi.org/10.5772/53802

magnetic resonance imaging showed a tumour and the patient underwent a tumourectomy at Konan Hospital. Granulocytic sarcoma and acute myeloid leukaemia were diagnosed based on a biopsy for vertebral canal tumor. The patient had a partial response after a course of remission induction and nearly a complete response after receiving a high dose of Cytarabine. However, her prognosis was poor, which led to a bone marrow transplant from her sister with matching HLA. Pre-treatment included 12 Gy total body irradiation and 120 mg/kg Cyclophosphamide hydrate. She showed good progress after the transplant, maintained symptom relief, and completed treatment with immune suppressive medication without developing chronic graft-versus-host disease. However, she incurred prolonged pain in the back and buttocks as well as pain and numbness in the back of the thigh after the tumourectomy that interfered with her daily life if she did not take medication for pain relief. She used nonsteroidal anti-inflammatory drugs (NSAIDs) as analgesics. She was not diagnosed with sciatica, and her symptoms were assumed to be associated with the surgery on the lumbosacral spine. At the time, she was 27 years old and too young to be treated with NSAIDs on a long-term basis. Thus, she was referred to our clinic.

Internal medicine: Baktar® (Day -1), Etodolac 3–1 times/day, Loxoprofen sodium hydrate, Sodium azulenesulfonate. External medication: Hot compress (Nippo Pharmaceutical Industries Ltd.; phellodendron bark, red pepper, menthol, camphor, methyl salicylic acid). Medication adherence: None. Drug allergy: None. Dietary history: She likes fruit. Findings on physical examination: MRI scan did not reveal the cause of the pain.

Course of treatment: We initiated heat transfer treatment using the disc-shaped device on Day 1 (first visit). The treatment was conducted by maintaining the temperature of the device between 43°C and 44°C and applied the heat on her right gluteal area and acupoint GV4 (vital point on the back) for 25–40 minutes each time. We evaluated the intensity of the pain by the dose of Etodolac (oral medication) and using a verbal numeric rating scale (NRS) of 0–10 (Farrar et al., 2008). The pain was relieved after the treatment. However, one hour later, there was a gradual recurrence of the pain. On Day 15 (second visit), the dose of Etodolac 200 mg was decreased from 3 tablets/day on the first visit to 2 tablets/day, and we thereafter detected an alleviation of pain. After Day 16, only one tablet was administered each day; moreover, the frequency of the administration was reduced from every day to less than once every 2 days from the $10^{th}$ day to the $23^{rd}$ day. The NRS showed a gradual decrease in pain to 3/10 or 0/10 on Day 39 (10th visit).

Conclusion: We applied heat transfer treatment using the disc-shaped device primarily on the site of pain to treat intractable pain after surgery, which resulted in improvement of the symptom of prolonged pain.

#### *3.4.2.3. A case of patient with intractable stomach pain due to ulceration of the colon caused by Behcet's disease: the portable disc-shaped heat transfer treatment device was used effectively for treatment*

A 39-year-old Japanese woman (height of 158 cm, weight of 43 kg) was referred to our clinic because of a stomach ache. She constantly experienced stomach pain, which became most intense during the night. Her symptoms included nausea, fatigue, poor circulation in her leg, stiff shoulder, headache, eye pain, and frequent throat pain. Medical history: Unremarkable.

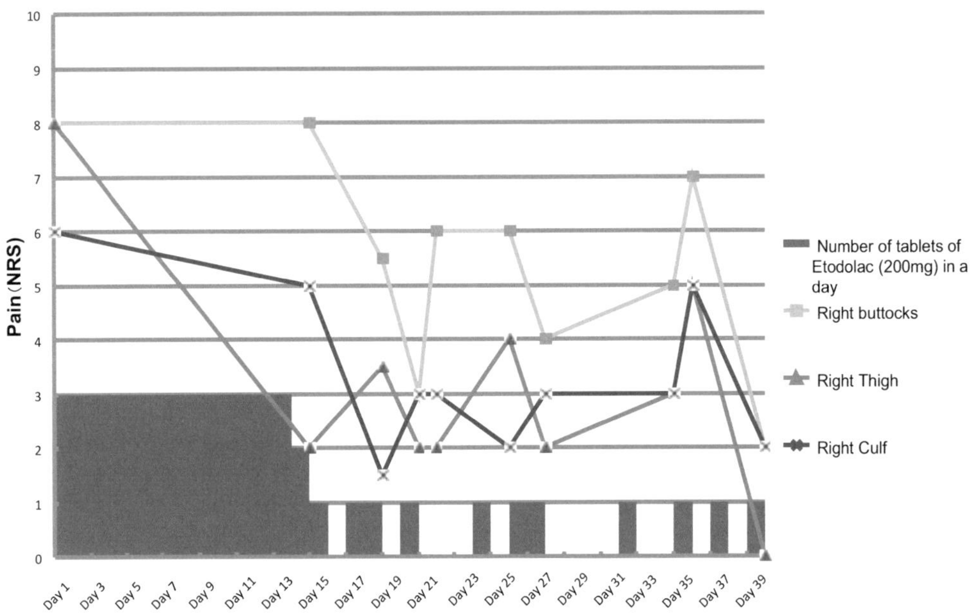


**Figure 19.** Course of treatment. Change of pain and dose of Etodolac.

Family history: Mother had chronic pancreatitis. Social history: She worked in an office between the ages of 30 and 35, and then became a housewife.

Clinical history: She had stomatitis since she was a child and started having it frequently around the age of 30 years. She was hospitalized due to suspected appendicitis two years ago. She was diagnosed with ulcerative colitis caused by Behcet's disease last year.

Administered medication: Rebamipide 100mg, Miya-BM fine granules 1 g, Mesalazine 250mg, Corticosteroid 9 mg/day since five months ago, and Imuran 50 since ten months ago. Medication adherence: None. Drug allergy: She had a history of an allergic reaction to an analgesic medication at the age of 23 years, when her upper lip became itchy and swollen (except when taking Bufferin®). Dietary history: She likes sweets. Findings on physical examination: Pressure pain in the lower stomach.

Course of treatment: This patient was referred to our clinic. Because her pain became more intense on Day 1, we started treatment by affixing portable disc-shaped heater to the patient's lower abdomen with a corset 1–3 times per day for 30 minutes each time. The pain was reduced after 13 days of treatment, showing that the treatment was effective, and the treatment was discontinued.

Conclusion: This patient's prolonged pain was alleviated by treatment using the portable disc-shaped heat transfer device on the lower abdomen for intractable pain due to ulceration of the colon.

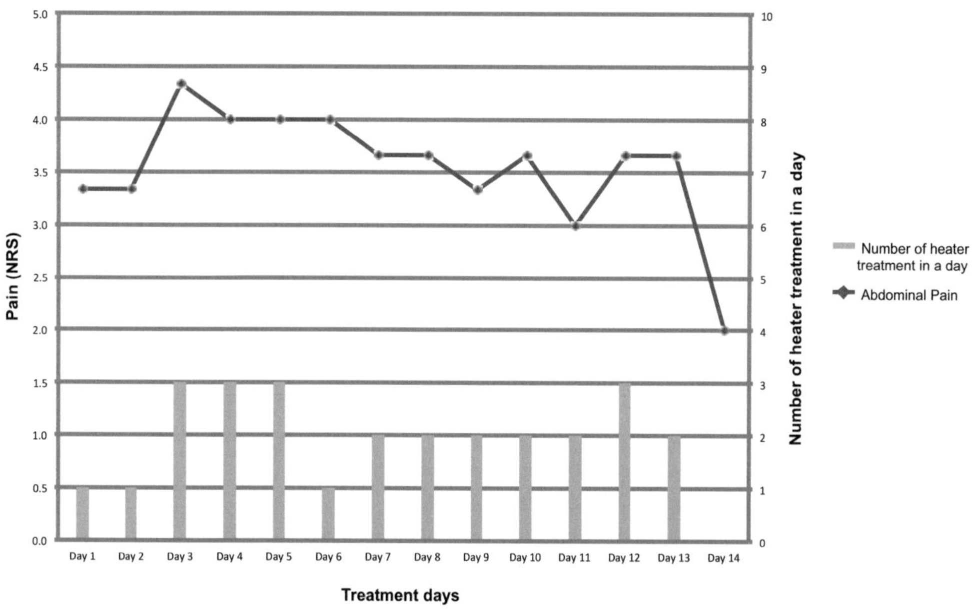


**Figure 20.** Course of treatment. Change of pain and the number of heater treatment in a day.

*3.4.2.4. A case of a patient with cervical and occipital pain after surgery for an extradural cyst tumour in the thoracic vertebra region: Use of the pencil-shaped heater was an effective form of treatment.*

A 57-year-old Japanese woman (height of 156 cm, weight of 56 kg) was referred to our clinic because of pain in her right shoulder blade and heaviness in the neck. Her symptoms included headache, shoulder stiffness, dizziness, and weight loss from loss of appetite and tongue soreness. Medical history: Whiplash injury three times in a year eleven years ago. Family history: Her husband is diabetic. Social history: She had been working as a university staff member since she was 18 years old.

Internal medication: Betahistine mesilate, Zolpidem tartrate (prescribed for difficulty sleeping due to pain in the interior shoulder blade), Neurotropin® (An extract from cutaneous tissue of rabbit inoculated with vaccinia virus), Famotidine, Eperisone hydrochloride, Diclofenac sodium capsules 37.5 mg and Bifidobacterium. External medication: Diclofenac sodium suppositories. Health food: She also consumed Barley Young Leaves Green Juice. Medication adherence: None. Drug allergy: None. Dietary history: Unremarkable. Findings on physical examination: Postoperative cicatrix inside the left shoulder blade and on the right shoulder blade.

Clinical history: Postoperative cicatrix of the right shoulder blade, which was exacerbated by coldness after surgery four months ago. From two months ago, the patient experienced heaviness of the neck, headache, shoulder stiffness, and dizziness. And she visited our clinic.

Course of treatment: The pain during the first visit was rated as 8-10 on the numeric rating scale (NRS), and the patient started general acupuncture and moxibustion treatment. She started treatment using the pencil-shaped device on the algesic region, and the pain appeared to be alleviated (Day 1). The pain (NRS) was 8-6 before heater treatment on Day 35. Pain reduction was detected after every treatments. On Day 48, she received treatment with the pencil-shaped device, which helped to alleviate the pain to a rating of 1-6.

Conclusion: The patient received treatment using a pencil-shaped heat transfer device on the algesic region for postoperative intractable pain, and her protracted pain was alleviated.

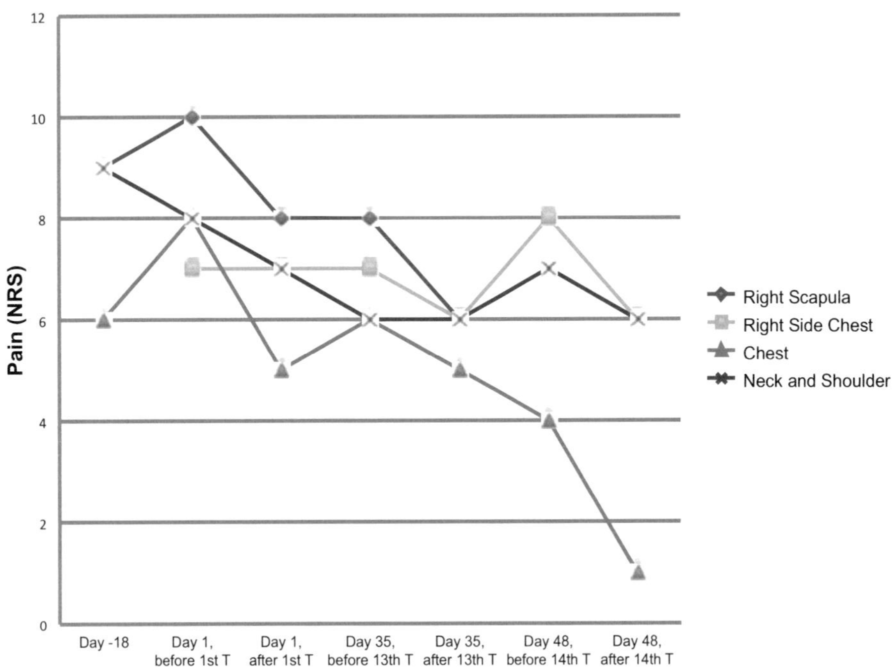


**Figure 21.** Course of treatment. Change of pain. T: heater treatment.

### 3.4.3. *Adverse events*

No adverse events were confirmed in any of the research or medical cases.

## 4. Discussion

### 4.1. The merits of the device

There were many comments by patients that the disc-shaped device in particular was very comfortable (data not shown). The heat transfer treatment device has certain features that

http://dx.doi.org/10.5772/53802

distinguishes it from other medical devices, including patient comfort level, the capability of heating a certain area at a certain temperature, and a precise temperature controller. This device does not emit any fumes and prevents the risk of burn injury.

The portable disc-shaped device possesses the same merits as the stationary disc-shaped device; further, attaching the device with a belt enables it to heat the femoral region, buttocks, and dorsal region even when it is not in a horizontal position, which enables the patient to receive treatment without interfering in his or her daily life. It heats the local area easily and is safe and easy for general users to handle. A smaller-sized version is now in development.

The pencil-shaped device is capable of heating a specific small area using precise temperature control. It can safely heat any part of the body as long as the heater can reach it. Moreover, it can be immediately moved so as to make contact with the skin or can be removed from contact with the skin so that a stimulus similar to direct moxibustion can be achieved. Having a small area of contact with the skin enables application of different temperature stimuli to each region based on the condition of the stimulus region (sensitivity to temperature, intensity of pain). It is also capable of changing the temperature of the contact condition and making instantaneous contact with the skin under certain temperature conditions. Because it is unnecessary to use moxa or ignite it, this makes it possible to stimulate many affected areas (such acupuncture points) consecutively. As a result, it is possible to not only shorten the time for treatment but also alleviate the burden for both patients and practitioners.

The radiation heating treatment device can heat at certain temperatures without making any contact, which keeps the risk of burn injury at a minimum. This device was developed for the purpose of radiation-based treatment of the body without direct contact with or heating of the skin. Because this device is capable of treating the patient without making contact with the skin, the device can be applied to other regions of the body that are difficult to reach during and immediately after surgery.

### 4.2. Study limitations

This research involved only a limited number of subjects.

### 4.3. Future studies

We have shown that there are individual differences in the relationship between the amount of heat transfer of the radiation heating device and the temperature on the surface of the skin. Due consideration must be given to fluctuations of time in different individuals and individual differences of tissue heat. As a result, it is necessary to clarify in greater detail the mechanism of heat phenomena in tissue, such as metabolic response to tissue organization of heat transfer and heat stimulation of blood circulation within tissue. However, such individual differences are possible ground-breaking indicators capable of measuring individual health conditions, which makes it necessary to advance research related to the condition of the human body. Although the difference in temperature (as sensed by a patient) between the acupuncture point and the meridian is said to be tied to the diagnosis, it is possible to quantitatively measure this with the pencil-shaped device.

In the future, we will take steps to increase the number of subjects and conduct comparative experiments.

We are in midst of further studies to identify ways to further reduce the size and weight of the portable disc-shaped version of the contact-type heating controller.

## 5. Conclusion

### 5.1. Safety and sanitariness

The temperature distribution in moxibustion therapy is high in the centre regions. Accordingly, if no appropriate measures are taken, burn injury is a clear likelihood. We have developed a therapeutic device capable of replacing moxibustion therapy that produces no fumes, is non-invasive, is safe, and avoids burn injuries.

### 5.2. Effectiveness and indication

The device has proven to be effective for the treatment of protracted pain and digestive system symptoms in some cases, and it has demonstrated identical effectiveness to older techniques.

We have developed heat conduction treatment devices and radiation heating device capable of controlling temperature with a high degree of precision. Such a device makes it possible to achieve a level of effectiveness on par with moxibustion treatment as currently practiced and is capable of evaluating hyperthermia therapy quantitatively. They make it possible to undertake a scientific study of moxibustion.

### 5.3. Convenience

The device does not require trained skill to use, which means that many more patients can be treated because it is easier to administer than moxibustion treatment.

### 5.4. Characteristics of the devices

These devices make it possible to set the optimal temperature of acupuncture points for each individual patient, which promises to maximally improve the effectiveness of moxibustion without incident of burn injury.

It also optimizes stimulation of each acupoint or area for each individual by allowing precise control of the amount of stimulation possible, which results in the possibility of greater treatment efficacy.

Furthermore, this device advances scientific research of moxibustion therapy, thanks to the ability to quantify the amount of stimulation.

Because this device is capable of temperature regulation, we were able to obtain clear evidence for the first time. At the present time, we are taking steps to commercialize these devices.

## Acknowledgements

Our research owes a great debt to the research of Mr. Hiroshi Mashimo, Mr. Noya Ogasawara and Mr. Shigeru Takashima, who graduated in fluids research. We would like to show our gratitude to the research subjects and patients for their unstinting cooperation.

## Author details

Takashi Seki, Junnosuke Okajima, Akiko Kikuchi, Shin Takayama, Masashi Watanabe, Hiroko Kusuyama, Ayane Matsuda, Soichiro Kaneko, Tetsuharu Kamiya, Atsuki Komiya, Minami Fujiwara, Nobuo Yaegasi, Tomoyuki Yambe and Shigenao Maruyama

Tohoku University, Sendai Medical Center, Japan

## References

[1] Editorial office(2008). Location of whole country massage, shiatzu, acupuncture and moxibustion practitioner training institution, In: Ido no nippon March, 2008), Ido-no nippon sha. Inc., Tokyo., 67(3)

[2] Farrar, J. T, Troxel, A. B, Stott, C, Duncombe, P, & Jensen, M. P. (2008). Validity, reliability, and clinical importance of change in a 0-10 numeric rating scale measure of spasticity: a post hoc analysis of a randomized, double-blind, placebo-controlled trial. *Clinical therapeutics,* , 30(5), 974-985.

[3] Freire, A. O, Sugai, G. C, Blanco, M. M, Tabosa, A, Yamamura, Y, & Mello, L. E. (2005). Effect of moxibustion at acupoints Ren-12 (Zhongwan), St-25 (Tianshu), and St-36 (Zuzanli) in the prevention of gastric lesions induced by indomethacin in Wistar rats. *Digestive diseases and sciences,* , 50(2), 366-374.

[4] Frequently Used Moxibustion Techniques(2012). Beijing Digital Museum of TCM. 1 Sep 2012, Available from: http://en.tcm-china.info/acupuncture/moxibustion/75587.shtml

[5] Incropera, F. P, Dewitt, D. P, Bergman, T. L, & Lavine, A. S. (2007). *Fundamentals of Heat and Mass Transfer* (sixth edition), John Wiley & Sons, Inc.

[6] Jiang, S. C, Ma, N, Li, H. J, & Zhang, X. X. (2002). Effects of thermal properties and geometrical dimensions on skin burn injuries, *Burns,* , 28(8), 713-717.

[7] Kim, S. Y, Chae, Y, Lee, S. M, Lee, H, & Park, H. J. (2011). The effectiveness of moxibustion: an overview during 10 years. *Evidence-based complementary and alternative medicine*: 306515.

[8] Maruyama, S, Ogasawara, N, Okajima, J, Komiya, A, & Seki, T. . (2012). Radiative heat transfer and heating effect of radiation heater forthermal therapy, *The Memoirs of the Institute of Fluid Science Tohoku University*, Vol. 23, pp. 13-19.

[9] Maruyama, S, Takashima, S, Okajima, J, Komiya, A, Seki, T, & Yambe, T. (2011). Thermal therapy and evaluation by a precise temperature control device. *Heat Transfer-Asian Research,* , 40(2), 114-124.

[10] Ministry of EducationCulture, Sports, Science and Technology-Japan, ((2006). Basic research of school 2006, Available from: http://www.mext.go.jp/b_menu/toukei/001/06121219/001/001/005.htm

[11] Ministry of HealthLabour and Welfare-Japan. ((2009). The number of the moxibustion practitioner. *Health administration duties report 2008 (health administration reported case).*

[12] Okajima, J, Maruyama, S, Takeda, H, & Komiya, A. (2009). Dimensionless solutions and general characteristics of bioheat transfer during thermal therapy, *J Therm Biol,* , 34(8), 377-384.

[13] Seki, T, Watanabe, M, & Takayama, S. (2011). Blood Flow Volume as an Indicator of the Effectiveness of Traditional Medicine, In: *Acupuncture- Concepts and Physiology*, Saad, M., InTech, 978-9-53307-410-8Vienna, Austria, 101-124.

[14] SennenqSeptember (2012). Available from: http://www.sennenqshop.net/shop/

[15] Shen, X, Ding, G, Wei, J, Zhao, L, Zhou, Y, Deng, H, & Lao, L. (2006). An infrared radiation study of the biophysical characteristics of traditional moxibustion, *Compl Ther Med,*, 14(3), 213-219.

[16] Tabosa, A, Yamamura, Y, Forno, E. R, & Mello, L. E. A. M. (2004). A Comparative Study of the Effects of Electroacupuncture and Moxibustion in the Gastrointestinal Motility of the Rat, *Dig Dis Sci,* , 49(4), 602-610.

[17] Takayama, S, Seki, T, Watanabe, M, Takashima, S, Sugita, N, Konno, S, Iwasaki, K, Yambe, T, Yoshizawa, M, Nitta, S, Maruyama, S, & Yaegashi, N. (2010). The effect of warming of the abdomen and of herbal medicine on superior mesenteric artery blood flow- a pilot study. *Forsch Komplementmed,* , 17(4), 195-201.

[18] Takayama, S, Seki, T, Watanabe, M, Takashima, S, Sugita, N, Konno, S, Takeda, T, Arai, H, Yambe, T, Yaegashi, N, Yoshizawa, M, Maruyama, S, & Nitta, S. (2011). Changes of blood flow volume in the superior mesenteric artery and brachial artery with abdominal thermal stimulation. *Evidence-based complementary and alternative medicine*: 214089.

[19] Yamaoka, D. (2001). Health promotion by moxibustion. *Zennihon sinkyuu gakkai zasshi,* , 51(1), 38-43.

Chapter 7

# New Development in Sham Acupuncture Needle

Sungchul Kim

Additional information is available at the end of the chapter

http://dx.doi.org/10.5772/55113

## 1. Introduction

Since the inception of clinical research into acupuncture, the dilemma of how to create an appropriate placebo for acupuncture research has hindered the progress. There has been no good method of managing all confounding variables, particularly the implementation of double-blind method into experiments.

Due to the lack of an appropriate placebo, the general scientific society has questioned studies on the effects of acupuncture. The double-blind, placebo-controlled clinical trial is said to be the gold standard for showing that a treatment has a specific effect over placebo. But acupuncture treatments undoubtedly involve placebo effects. In order to support the study of acupuncture's effects and to give more credibility to acupuncture studies in the era of the EBM(Evidence Based Medicine), a thoroughly tested double-blind placebo for acupuncture needs to be developed.

## 2. The need for developing a successful sham acupuncture

Experimental studies of acupuncture have been actively conducted to discover new evidence for acupuncture treatment. To facilitate acupuncture research, the Standards for Reporting Interventions in Clinical Trials for Acupuncture (STRICTA) were published in 2010 as a revision of the 2002 version[1]. Blind study designs are the most important method for diminishing the placebo effect and bias. Due to the lack of an appropriate placebo method, few studies have been conducted in compliance with the standard guidelines for placebo-controlled clinical trials. So far by having appropriate placebo models, research on medical drugs has been advancing strongly while the research on the effects of acupuncture have remained using either single-blind or without any blinding in the study at all. A sham acupuncture needs to be developed for the purpose of double-blind, placebo control research. Acupuncture treatment holds a unique position in the medical research community in that most believe that it cannot be administered in a way both acupuncturist and patient do not know whether the patient is receiving real or sham treatment.

The patient receiving the placebo treatment should believe that they are receiving the real treatment, which entails giving the treatment without actually performing any sort of legitimate operation but still being impossible to distinguish from real treatment.

## 3. Previous studies in Sham acupuncture

Presently there are several sham acupuncture needles that have been invented. Some methods used the Placebo which is pricking[2-3] and superficially stabbing without manipulation at inappropriate acupoints which is not traditional acupuncture point located in the meridian[4]. However, these minimal acupunctures are inadequate Placebos because they can have physiological effects such as DNIC (Diffuse Noxious Inhibitory Controls) on the patient[5-6].

Sham TENS[7-8], sham tablets[9] and un-operative laser acupuncture[10] have been used as control groups, however their effects cannot be appropriately identified as truly having a placebo effect[11] as the participants were comparing their treatment to the real acupuncture group afterwards and finding differences which will cause non-placebo psychological effects. Several other placebo methods include: simply poke the subject with the fingernail[12], without breaking the skin;. stimulating with the acupuncture pipe[13] on the skin and lightly pricking with a real needles on the superficial skin[14];using placebo acupuncture needle with flat tip and only let the acupuncture needle enter to the plastic stopple at the edge of the acupuncture pipe[15] and not puncture the skin but only pressed it[16].

In addition, Streitberger and Kleinhenz, Park et al. developed sham acupuncture devices.

Streitberg's method was designed to use a blunted needle inserted into a prop to give the appearance that acupuncture was being administered through the skin when it was not[17]. By using this method as a placebo in an experiment on the clinical treatment of rotator cuff tendonitis in sportsmen, the results acquired favored real acupuncture over sham acupuncture[18] (Figure 1).

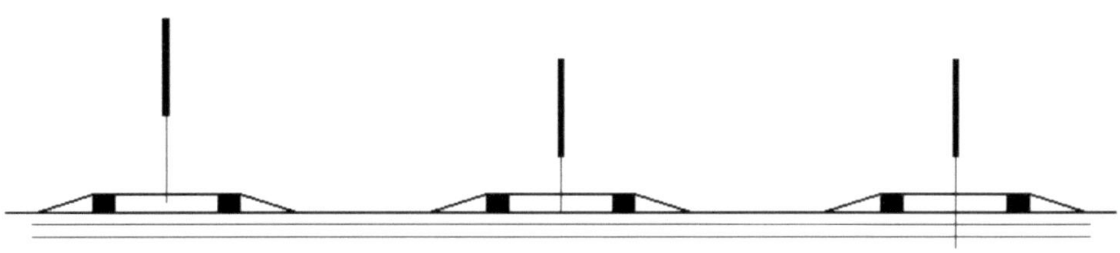

**Figure 1.** Streitberger and Kleinhenz sham and real needle

Park's sham needle[19] was invented independently from Streitberger and Kleinhenz. The apparatus consists of a blunted needle, the shaft of which telescopes into the handle when tapped, so that, while the needle appears to have been inserted, it does not actually pierce the skin. And this consists of an oversize guide tube with a silicon flange at one end which adheres to the skin with double-sided tape. This needle diameter is 0.35mm and its length is 70mm including handle. Real needling can be performed to a depth of up to 15mm. In the published validation study, 22% of volunteers could feel a dull sensation with the sham needle, compared to 57% with a real needle. This needle has not been correctly validated in terms of *deqi* (specific needling sensation) (Figure 2).

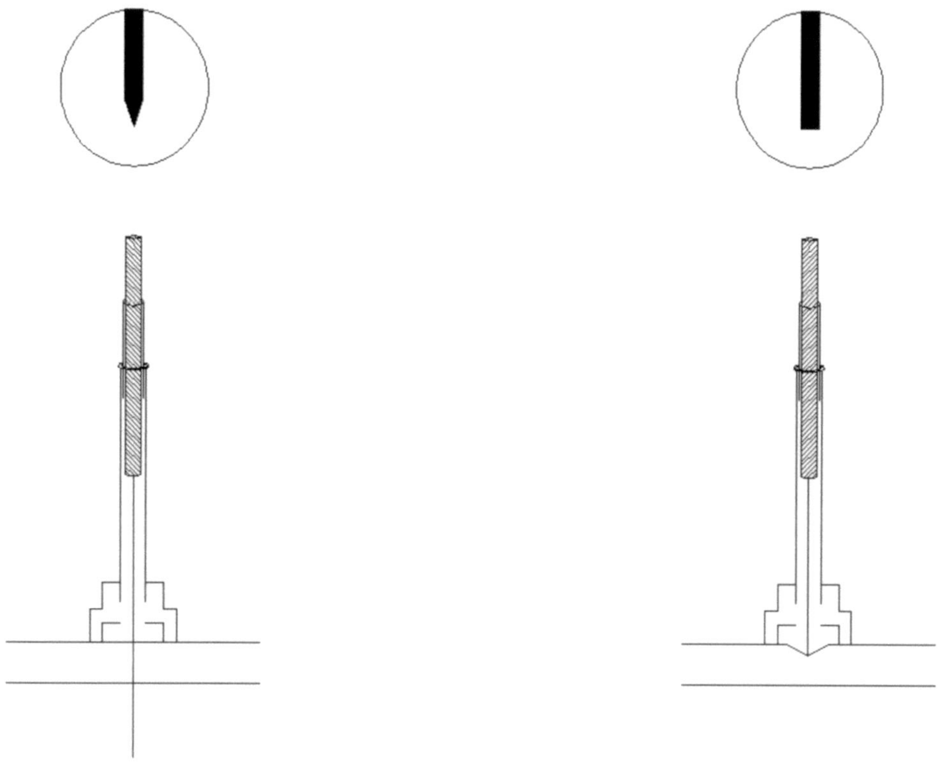

**Figure 2.** Park's real and sham needle

Miyazaki et al.[20] conducted a double-blind clinical trial to compare a press needle to a placebo lacking the needle element. Because of the characteristics of these devices, the ability to blind subjects was limited and double-blind studies are difficult to administer. Therefore, few studies have been conducted in compliance with the standard guidelines for placebo-controlled clinical trials to address this problem. Fregni et al.[21] claimed that an important challenge in using a placebo is the development of a sham device that has a similar appearance and induces a feeling similar to that induced by the real device.

Despite all of this difficulties, Kim[22] came to believe that one could create a type of sham acupuncture needle that would be identical to a real acupuncture needle in structure, color, and form but not break the skin because its edge, while appearing virtually identical to the real needle, is in fact blunt.

## 4. What is Kim's Sham needle?

Kim's sham acupuncture needles was invented as an intradermal T-shaped needle (thickness 0.2 mm, length 1.5 mm, diameter 2 mm).

The sham needles use the exact same manufacturing machines as the real type T. The structure, color, and shape of the sham needle (pre-produced by Dongbang Acupuncture Company, South Korea) were the same as that of the real needle with the exception of the blunt tip. This blunt tip makes it impossible to insert the needle into the skin, and the tactile sensation is similar to that of the real T-shaped intradermal needle. The patch consists of 3 layers, with the first and second film layer securing the needle to the patch and the third layer possessing the adhesive that attaches the needle to the patient's skin. The needle is still 1.5mm long and is secured to the patch to make vertical 90° contact with a skin (Figure 3 and Figure 4).

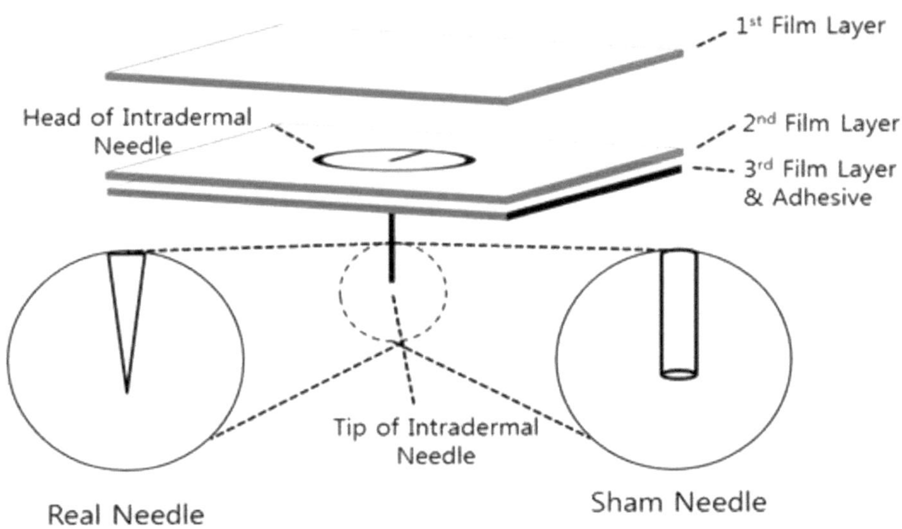


**Figure 3. Differences between real needle and sham needle shape** - The structure, color, and shape of the sham needle were the same as that of the real needle with the exception of the blunt tip.

http://dx.doi.org/10.5772/55113

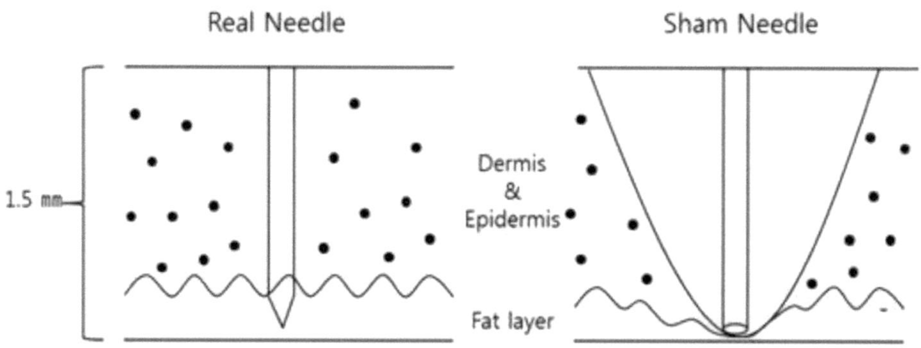


**Figure 4. Difference between real needle and sham needle stimulation** – While the real needle tip is inserted into the epidermis invasively, the sham needles tip simply presses the skin surface non-invasively.

In the packaging process, damage can occur to the tip of the intradermal needle, so suitable holder's development can overcome this problem. This holder was made using a transparent material to see whether or not the needle tips were damaged (Figure 5 and Figure 6).

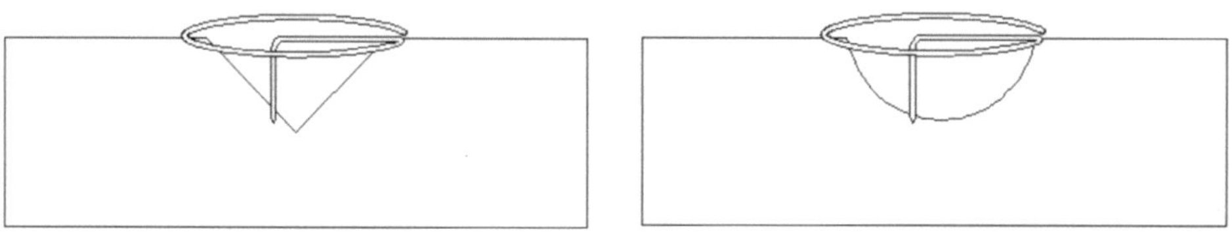

**Figure 5.** Ineffective sham acupuncture needle holders designs

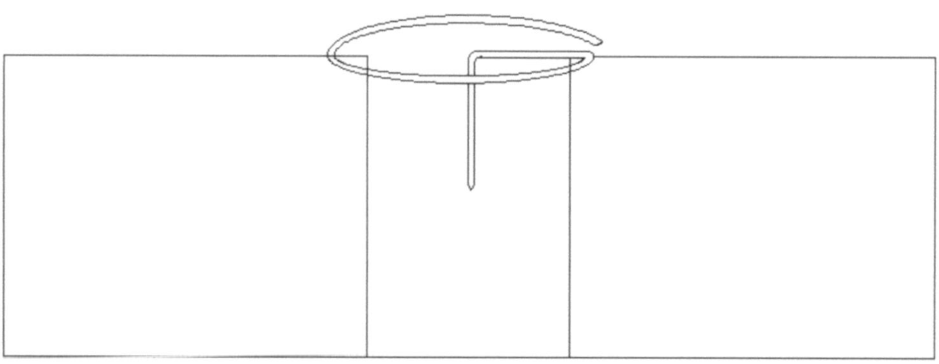

**Figure 6.** Manufactured Kim's sham acupuncture needle holder design

In the 2003 edition of Lee's paper[23], the placebo needles were manufactured type T needles that Lee cut down to 1mm with scissors. This method however caused problems with irregularly shaped needles, some of which that may have actually punctured the skin like a real needle. Kim's sham acupuncture avoids this by using standardized mechanical manufacturing methods that create needles with the same length as real needles and that have edges that will not puncture the skin. In 2004, Menjo tried to test the possibility of a double blind for a sham 0.6mm dermal acupuncture needle at the 1st J-K Workshop meeting in Chiba, Japan. This acupuncture needle is shorter than the mean depth (1.5mm) of the adult dermis. It is very difficult to really prove the effects of acupuncture because the same real needle can't successfully stimulate the skin. Kim's sham acupuncture avoids this problem by using 1.5mm long needles. These experiments were also not successfully implemented in a double-blind manner. Kim's sham acupuncture has the result of using an iron needle to perform subcutaneous stimulation and maintained acupuncture fixed to the skin with a form evolved from classical slight acupuncture to modern short acupuncture. Generally, during normal acupuncture, the acupoint is selected for its corresponding internal organ or for being a tender point, Posterior Referred Point, Limb Referred Point, or Ear Point chosen by meridian theory. The adaptation range is largely applied to chronic internal organ diseases and chronic multiple pains. Kim's sham acupuncture gains several advantages from imitating endermic acupuncture. The simplicity of the puncturing method, the length of treatment (needles remain in for 2 to 3 days), and the uniformity of hand techniques results in standardization of the procedures. This makes Kim's sham acupuncture ideal for the research of endermic acupuncture's effect on pain.

## 5. Validation study of Kim's Sham needle

In order to investigate the possibility of sham acupuncture's application, we examined how well subjects who are accustomed to acupuncture treatment could distinguish between real acupuncture and sham acupuncture.

### 5.1. Determination of real from sham acupuncture by apperance or sensation

Prior to participating in the study, a consent form "Will you please participate in research comparing the appearance and feeling between real acupuncture and sham acupuncture." was obtained from the subjects. The selection criteria were similar with receiving acupuncture treatment. The study targeted 537 people who agreed to participate in the study. Amongst the those 537 people targeted, 120 of them were acupuncturists, 417 of them were from the general public, of which 150 were Korean and 57 were non-Korean.

Group A consisted of 60 Koreans drawn from the public, 40 acupuncturists and the 57 Non-Koreans drawn. These participants were trying to distinguish the real or sham acupuncture needles and all subjects were randomly selected and allocated to the trials by computer (Table 1). Prior to participating in the study, subjects were given a consent form "Will you please participate in research comparing the appearance and feeling between real acupuncture and sham acupuncture." Subjects had been selected for being familiar with receiving acupuncture treatment such as hospital patients, acupuncture assistants and acupuncturists working at the hospital of Korean medicine at Won Kwang University in South Korea and U.S. citizens.

Group B consisted of 60 Koreans drawn from the public, 40 acupuncturists and the 57 Non-Koreans from the public. In this study participants received real or sham acupuncture treatment in the LI4 acupoint and were then asked to distinguish whether the treatment was real or sham (Table 1).

Group C consisted of the remaining 30 Koreans drawn from the public, 40 acupuncturists and the 57 Non-Koreans drawn from the public. In this study participants were shown real and sham acupuncture using the double-blind method in their left and right hands in varying orders as well as being given acupuncture in the LI4 acupoint. After receiving treatment in both hands, the subjects were asked to identify which hand received the real acupuncture. Whether the needle was placed on the right or the left was randomized to eliminate potential bias. Those who could not distinguish between the two needles after treatment were recorded as "wrong answers" (Table 1).

(C-1) left -real- right - real

(C-2) left -sham- right - sham

(C-3) left-real-right-sham

(C-4) left-sham-right-real

| **Subjects** | | *Public (120 Korean)* | | *Acupuncturists(40)* | | *Public(57Non-Korean)* | |
|---|---|---|---|---|---|---|---|
| **Methods** | | **Correct** | **Incorrect** | **Correct** | **Incorrect** | **Correct** | **Incorrect** |
| A | From appearnce | N=67(56%) | N=53(44%) | N=18(45%) | N=22(55%) | N=31(54.4%) | N=26(45.6%) |
| | | P=.201 | | P=.527 | | P=.508 | |
| B | From sensation | N=68(57%) | N=52(43%) | N=22(55%) | N=18(45%) | N=27(47.4%) | N=30(52.6%) |
| | | P=.144 | | P=.527 | | P=.691 | |
| C | From appearnace and sensation | N=59(49%) | N=61(51%) | N=14(35%) | N=26(65%) | N=16(28.1%) | N=41(71.9%) |
| | | P=.855 | | P=.058 | | P=.001** | |

**Table 1. Results from the public and acupuncturists in correctly distinguishing real and sham acupuncture treatment.** The analysis of the statistics were done with a chi-square test which produced a statistically significant result at the $p<0.05$ * and $p<0.01$**level.

Regardless of whether the subject is an acupuncturist or a regular acupuncture patient; the order in which real and sham acupuncture are performed; or the exposure to the needle's appearance, the subjects ability to discriminate real endermic (intradermal) acupuncture from Kim's sham acupuncture was between 28.1% and 57%.

Examining the results of this experiment, the acupuncturists were unable to distinguish between real and sham acupuncture treatment by either appearance or sensation. It also may be inferred that the general public cannot distinguish by sensation whether it was real or sham acupuncture treatment and that this may indicate that Kim's sham acupuncture could be applied to other double-blind acupuncture clinical studies.

### 5.2. Validation study of Kim's Sham needle by measuring facial temperature[24]

Physiological stimulation of Kim's sham needle is different from that of a real needle. This study tested the feasibility of using Kim's sham needle in a double-blind clinical trial on the efficacy of acupuncture to reverse smoking-induced decreases in facial temperature.

This was conducted in N-of-1 randomized controlled trial with a double-blinded evaluation process, and the results were based using a statistical analysis. N-of 1 trials can be used in medical practice to determine the optimum treatment for an individual patient.

Seven healthy male smokers who met the following inclusion criteria were enrolled in this clinical trial.

The inclusion criteria was as follows : (1) a submission of the written informed consent, (2) a lack of exercise within the previous 24 hours, (3) a lack of intake of tobacco, alcohol, green tea and coffee within eight hours and (4) more than one hour elapsing after a meal before participating.

The exclusion criteria were as follows: (1) subjects with cardiovascular diseases,including hypertension, arrhythmia, and ischemic heart disease, (2) those with endocrine diseases, including diabetes mellitus and thyroid diseases, (3) those with kidney diseases, including chronic renal failure, (4) those with a past history of surgery for diseases, such as gastric cancer, (5) those with febrile diseases, such as epileptic seizure, and (6) other cases (e.g., dysautonomia, cancer or alcoholism).

| | A | B | C | D | E | F | G |
|---|---|---|---|---|---|---|---|
| 1 | Sham | Verum | Verum | Sham | Sham | Sham | Sham |
| | Verum | Sham | Sham | Verum | Verum | Verum | Verum |
| 2 | Verum | Sham | Verum | Verum | Verum | Sham | Verum |
| | Sham | Verum | Sham | Sham | Sham | Verum | Sham |
| 3 | Verum | Verum | Sham | Sham | Sham | Verum | Sham |
| | Sham | Sham | Verum | Verum | Verum | Sham | Verum |
| 4 | Sham | Sham | Verum | Sham | Verum | Sham | Sham |
| | Verum | Verum | Sham | Verum | Sham | Verum | Verum |
| 5 | Sham | Verum | Sham | Verum | Sham | Verum | Verum |
| | Verum | Sham | Verum | Sham | Verum | Sham | Sham |
| 6 | Verum | Sham | Verum | Sham | Verum | Sham | Sham |
| | Sham | Verum | Sham | Verum | Sham | Verum | Verum |

**Table 2.** Allocation of stimulation

The subjects were randomized and one set of needles was chosen randomly for use in one session of the trial(Table 2). The set was composed of two types of needles: a real needle and a sham needle. The experimental sequence of the needle types was set randomly by a third

http://dx.doi.org/10.5772/55113

party. Both the physicians and subjects were blinded using a masking test. One session was composed of two stimulations separated by a two hour washout period.

Following traditional Korean medicine literature, 'Saam Five Element Acupuncture', HT8 and KI2 acupoint on both sides were selected to stimulate the blood circulation. All the operations were performed by the acupuncturist according to the WHO(World Health Organization) criterion[25]for standard acupuncture point locations (Figure 7).

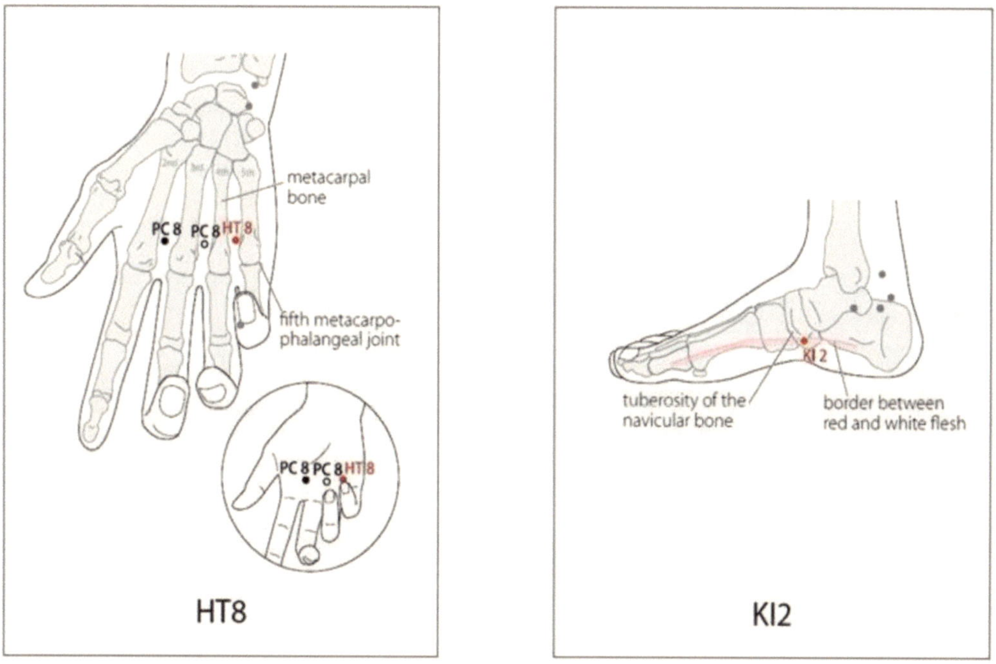


**Figure 7. Location of selected acupuncture points for tonification of heart fire** – HT8 is used to generate warmth by tonification of the heart fire and KI2 is used to generate warmth by tonification of the kidney fire. The selection of acupuncture points located were based on the publication of WHO standard acupuncture point locations.

The experimental procedures were as follows:

i. Following a thirty minutes stabilization period, the subjects were encouraged to smoke 1 cigarete during 3minutes (DunHill Light, Korea).

ii. After five minutes (once smoking was finished), with the use of DITI(digital infrared thermographic imaging, Dorex, DTI-16UTI, U.S.A.) photography, the facial temperature was photographed.

iii. Either an invasive needle or noninvasive needle was randomly applied to the subjects.

iv. After retaining a needle for fifteen minutes, DITI photographs were taken again.

v. Following a two hour rest period, the subjects were encouraged to smoke 1 cigarete during 3minutes.

**vi.** After five minutes (once smoking had finished), DITI photographs were taken again.

**vii.** Subjects were received the remaining needles.

**viii.** After retaining a needle for fifteen minutes, DITI photographs were taken again.

The above procedure was considered one pair. 1 pair of procedure was carried out six days with each subject (Figure 8.).

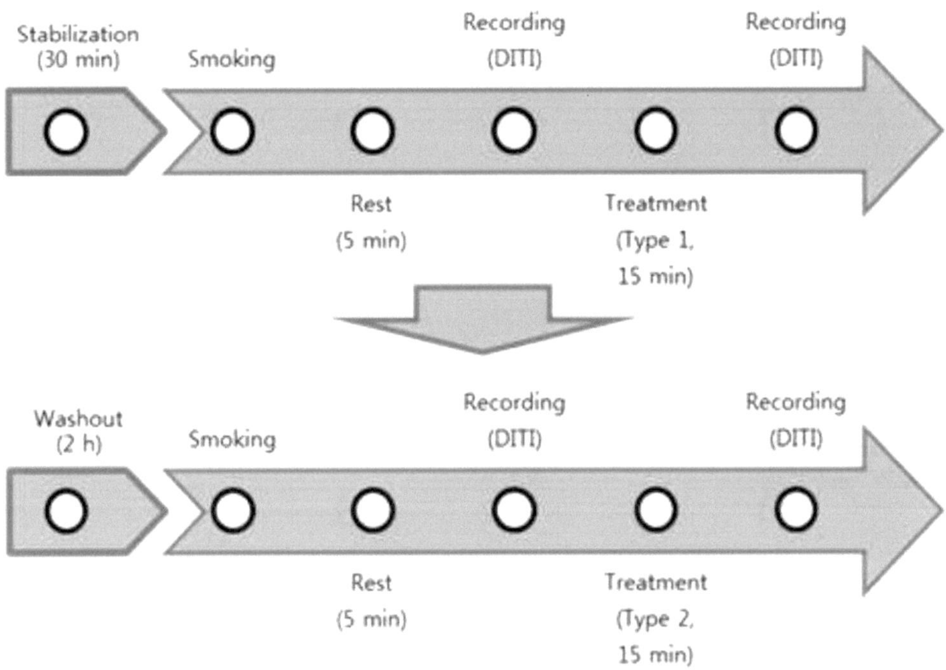


**Figure 8. Flow of participants through the trial -** The top panel represents the first treatment (either sham or real) that the subject underwent. This was followed by a 2 hr. washout period followed by the alternate treatment (either real or sham), as shown in the bottom panel.

DITI (digital infrared thermographic imaging, Dorex, DTI-16UTI, U.S.A.) was used to measure facial temperature, it is a method of measuring body temperature the apparatus for which is

http://dx.doi.org/10.5772/55113

installed in a photographic laboratory (DITI studio). The mean temperature was measured by drawing a circle with a diameter that extended from a 1 cm above the median point between the eyebrows to 1 cm below the midpoint of the philtrum midline.

In subjects who were treated with a sham needle following smoking, DITI showed a marked decrease in facial temperature (Figure 9). In subjects who were treated with a real needle following smoking, however, DITI showed a marked increase in the facial temperature (Figure 10).

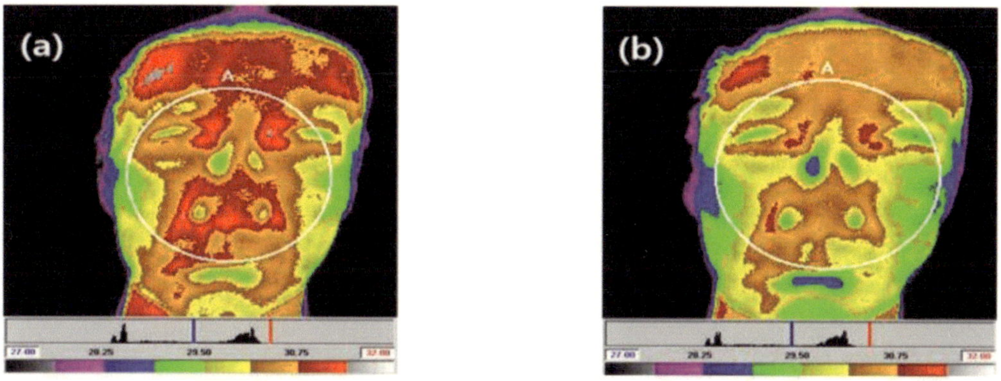


**Figure 9.** Facial temperature before and after treatment with a sham needle - The changes in facial temperature after smoking (a) and after being treated by sham needle (b). After treatment with sham needle, the average facial temperature shows an overall decrease. On the color bar below the photos, lower temperatures are located on the left.

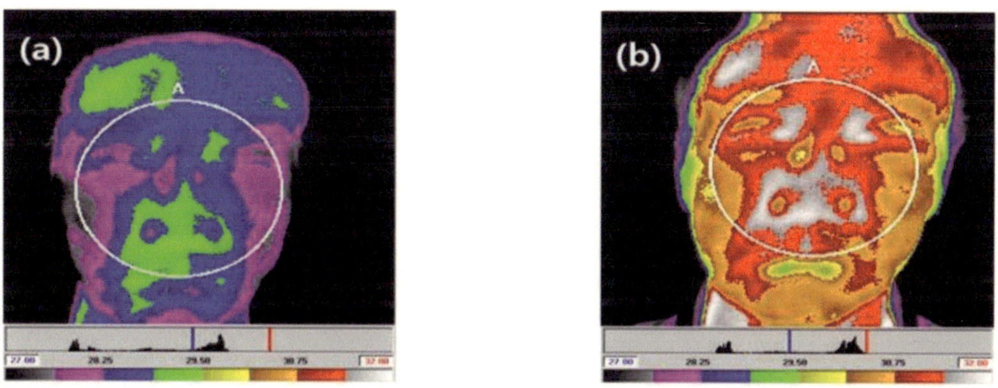


**Figure 10.** Facial temperature before and after treatment with a real needle -The changes in facial temperature after smoking (a) and after being treated by real needle (b). After treatment with a real needle, the average facial temperature shows an overall increase. On the color bar below the photos, higher temperatures are located on the right.

Considering the mean values of the differences in facial temperature, all subjects demonstrated decreased facial temperatures after treatment with sham needles, while 5 of the 7 subjects showed increased facial temperatures after treatment with real needles. Where as for 6 of the 7 subjects, a paired-sample T-test showed a significant difference ($p < 0.05$) in the facial temperature between the treatments with real and sham needles (Table 3 and Figure 11).

| Subject | Needle | After smoking(°C) | After needling(°C) | Temperature difference(°C) | * P value < 0.05<br>** P value < 0.01<br>(paired t-test) |
|---|---|---|---|---|---|
| A | Real | 30.01±0.99 | 30.89±1.03 | 0.87±1.60 | 0.0270* |
| | Sham | 30.71±0.96 | 29.89±1.20 | -0.81±0.35 | |
| B | Real | 31.72±0.62 | 31.78±0.53 | 0.06±0.20 | 0.0072** |
| | Sham | 32.04±1.32 | 31.65±1.41 | -0.38±0.33 | |
| C | Real | 32.05±0.94 | 32.01±0.72 | -0.03±0.26 | 0.0138* |
| | Sham | 31.66±0.42 | 31.23±0.33 | -0.43±0.26 | |
| D | Real | 31.16±0.92 | 31.50±0.73 | 0.20±0.39 | 0.0164* |
| | Sham | 31.57±0.71 | 30.90±1.01 | -0.67±0.92 | |
| E | Real | 31.86±1.10 | 32.17±1.01 | 0.31±0.32 | 0.0688 |
| | Sham | 32.49±0.65 | 32.20±0.37 | -0.28±0.67 | |
| F | Real | 32.60±0.76 | 32.36±0.68 | -0.24±0.21 | 0.0450* |
| | Sham | 33.24±0.79 | 32.42±0.74 | -0.81±0.39 | |
| G | Real | 32.32±1.03 | 32.67±0.78 | 0.34±0.34 | 0.0431* |
| | Sham | 32.97±0.51 | 32.47±0.45 | -0.50±0.57 | |

**Table 3.** Temperature changes after smoking and treatment with real or sham needle.

In conclusion, an N-of-1 trial was performed to validate Kim's sham by measuring facial temperature. Real needle treatment after smoking caused a significant increase in the facial temperature in 6 of 7 subjects compared to Kim's sham needle. This result indicates that Kim's sham needle has a different physical effect on skin temperature. After acupuncture treatment

http://dx.doi.org/10.5772/55113

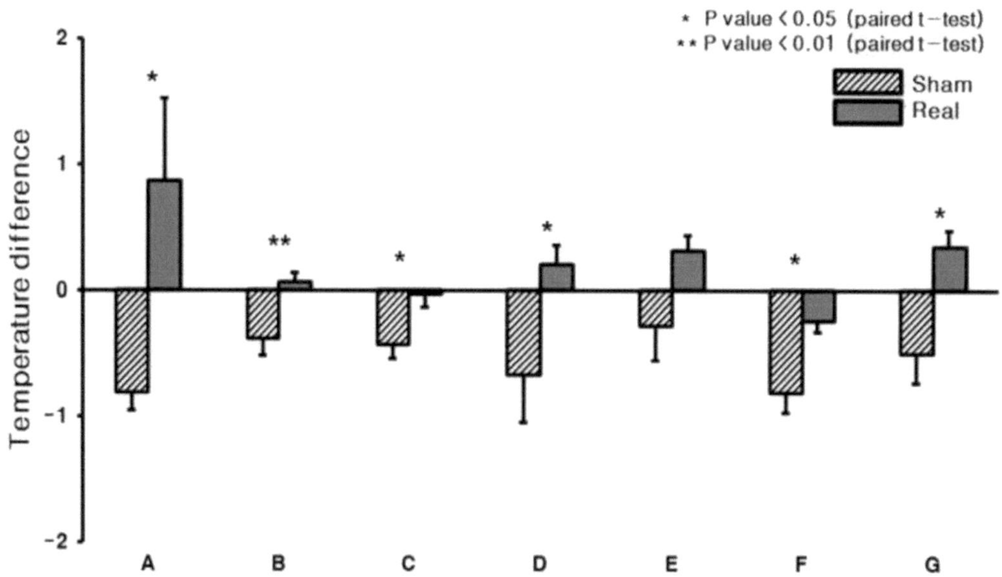


**Figure 11. Temperature change before and after treatment with real or sham needle:** Seven male smokers (A–G) were treated with either a sham needle or a real needle 5 mins after smoking and their facial temperature was monitored by DITI. The results show that treatment with a sham needle resulted in an overall decrease in facial temperature, while treatment with a real needle resulted in an overall significant increase in facial temperature in 6 subjects. Values on the graph represent the mean (SD) of 6 independent treatments with 2 hr intervals.. **For six out of the seven subjects,a paired sample T-test showed a significant difference ($p<0.05$) in facial temperature between treatments with verum and sham needle.**

with the sham needle, facial temperature decreased in all subjects. However, in real needle group, facial temperature increased in five subjects and decrease in two subjects. An analysis of seven subjects was performed using a paired T-test, and the results showed that all subjects but one had a significant difference in facial temperature. These results indicate that the real needle was more effective than the sham needle in raising the temperature, which was initially lowered because of smoking. However, Kim's sham needle was a realistic enough simulation to raise peripheral skin temperature.The results showed that real and sham acupuncture were significantly different in six of seven subjects. Further studies using this sham needle might provide more evidence and improve the scientific quality of clinical trials on acupuncture.

## 6. Conclusion

In conclusion the study on Real versus Sham needle the results show that the acupuncturists, Koreans and Non-Koreans were all unable to distinguish between Real and Sham needles. Also in the study for validation the effectiveness of the real needle, the results showed that the real needle caused a significant increase in the facial temperature of smokers, compared with the Sham needle. Indicatory that the Sham needle has a different physical effect on the skin. As these studies were carried out as a double blind trial. The results would infer that Kim's Sham needle could be applied to the double blind study of acupuncture. Further research regarding acupuncture and non-acupuncture point treatments with real and sham needles may help garner sufficient scientific evidence to validate Kim's sham needle and increase scientific precision and accuracy in clinical trials on acupuncture.

## Index

## Acknowledgements

The author wishes to thank Dr. Sanghun Lee for help in obtaining good information on Kim's sham needle holder design and also thanks Dr. Sunmi Choi at the Korea Institute of Oriental Medicine and Sungha Kim at the Wonkwang ALS clinical center in South Korea.

## Author details

Sungchul Kim[1,2,3*]

Address all correspondence to: kscndl@hanmail.net

1 Wonkwang University in Iksan, South Korea

2 Wonkwang University Oriental Medicine Hospital in Gwangju, South Korea

3 Won ALS Clinical Center, South Korea

## References

[1] Mac, H. . Hammerschlag, et al. Revised STandards for Reporting Interventions in Clinical Trials of Acupuncture (STRICTA): extending the CONSORT statement. Journal of Evidence-Based Medicine 2010; 3(3):140-155,

[2] Gaw, A. C, Chang, L. W, & Shaw, L. C. Efficacy of acupuncture on osteoarthritic pain. N Engl J Med (1975).

[3] Godfrey, C. M, & Morgan, P. A controlled trial of the theory of acupuncture in musculoskeletal pain. J Rheumatol (1978).

[4] Vincent, C. A. A controlled trial of the treatment of migraine by acupuncture. the clinical Journal of Pain (1989).

[5] Le Bars DDickenson AH, Besson JM. Diffuse noxious inhibitory controls (DNIC). I. Effects on dorsal horn convergent neurones in the rat. Pain (1979).

[6] Lewith, G, & Vincent, C. The evalution of the clinical effects of acupuncture. Pain Forum (1995).

[7] Macdonald AJRMacrae KD, Master BR, Rubin AP. Superficial acupuncture in the relief of chronic low back pain. Ann R Coll Surg Engl (1983).

[8] Dowson, D. I, Lewith, G, & Machin, D. The effects of acupuncture versus placebo in the treatment of headache. Pain (1985).

[9] Thomas, M, Eriksson, S. V, & Lundeberg, T. A comparative study of diazepam and acupuncture in patients with osteoarthritis pain. Am J Chin Med (1991).

[10] Irnich, D, Behrens, N, Molzen, H, Konig, A, Gleditsch, J, Krauss, M, et al. Randomised trial of acupuncture compared with conventional massage and sham laser acupuncture for treatment of chronic neck pain. BMJ (2001).

[11] Kaptchuk, T. J, Goldman, P, Stone, D. A, & Stason, W. B. Do medical devices have enhanced placebo effects? J ClinEpidemiol (2000).

[12] Junnila SYTAcupuncture therapy for chronic pain. Am J Acupunct (1982).

[13] Lao, L, Bergman, S, Langenberg, P, Wong, R. H, & Berman, B. Efficacy of Chinese acupuncture on postoperative oral surgery pain. Oral Surg Oral Med Oral Pathol Oral RadiolEndod (1995).

[14] Marks, N. J, Emery, P, & Onisiphorou, C. A controlled trial of acupuncture in tinnitus. J Laryngol Otol (1984).

[15] Taub, H. A, Mitchell, J. N, Stuber, F. E, Eisenberg, L, Beard, M. C, & Mccormack, R. K. Analgesia for operative dentistry: a comparison of acupuncture and placebo. Oral Surg Oral Med Oral Pathol (1979).

[16] Hesse, J, Mogelvang, B, & Simonsen, H. Acupuncture versus metoprolol in migraine prophylaxis: a randomized trial of trigger point inactivation. J Intern Med (1994).

[17] Streitberger, K, & Kleinhenz, J. Introducing a placebo needle into acupuncture research. Lancet (1998).

[18] Kleinhenz, J, Streitberger, K, Windeler, J, Gussbacher, A, Mavridis, G, & Martin, E. Randomised clinical trial comparing the effects of acupuncture and a newly designed placebo needle in rotator cuff tendinitis. Pain (1999).

[19] Jongbae ParkAdrian White, Hyejung Lee, Edzard Ernst. Development of a New Sham Needle. Acupuncture in Medicine (1999). , 17(2), 110-2.

[20] Miyazaki, S, Hagihara, A, Kanda, R, Mukaino, Y, & Nobutomo, K. Applicability of press needles to a double-blind trial: a randomized, double-blind, placebo-controlled trial, Clinical Journal of Pain (2009). , 25(5), 438-444.

[21] Felipe, F, Marta, I, Husin, F. C, Henry, L. L, Paulo, B, Ted, J. K, Marcelo, R, Wu, T. H, Linamara, R. B, & Andrea, F. Challenges and Recommendations for Placebo Controls in Randomized Trials in Physical and Rehabilitation Medicine, Am J Phys Med Rehabil (2010). , 89(2), 160-172.

[22] Kim, S. Creating an instrument for a successful double-blind acupuncture placebo, Journal of Acupuncture and Meridian Studies (2008). , 1(1), 36-41.

[23] Lee, K. M, Lee, S. Y, Kim, S. W, Ha, I. H, Cho, G. H, Park, H. J, et al. Is it possible to apply placebo auricular acupuncture to Korean? The effects of placebo auricular acupuncture through single blind method and randomized controlled trial. J Korean Acupuncture & Moxibustion Soc (2003). In Korean]

[24] Lee, S, Lim, N, Choi, S, & Kim, S. Validation study of Kim's sham needle by measuring facial temperature, Evidence-Based Complementary and Alternative Medicine (2011). , 2012, 7-14.

[25] Western Pacific Region Officeeditors. WHO Standard Acupuncture Point Locations in the Western Pacific Region. WHO: 1st edition; June (2008).

Chapter 8

# Fu's Subcutaneous Needling, a Modern Style of Ancient Acupuncture?

Zhonghua Fu and Ryan Shepherd

Additional information is available at the end of the chapter

http://dx.doi.org/10.5772/53970

## 1. Introduction

Fu's Subcutaneous Needling (FSN), originated from Chinese traditional acupuncture, is a therapeutic approach for localized diseases, especially for musculoskeletal painful disorders. This procedure is performed by inserting a special trocar needle into the subcutaneous layer around the afflicted spot (Fig. 1) or nearby limbs (Fig. 2) to achieve the desired effect. In some cases, FSN could provide immediate and significant relief of the pain in trigger points (TrPs) more effectively than anesthesia.

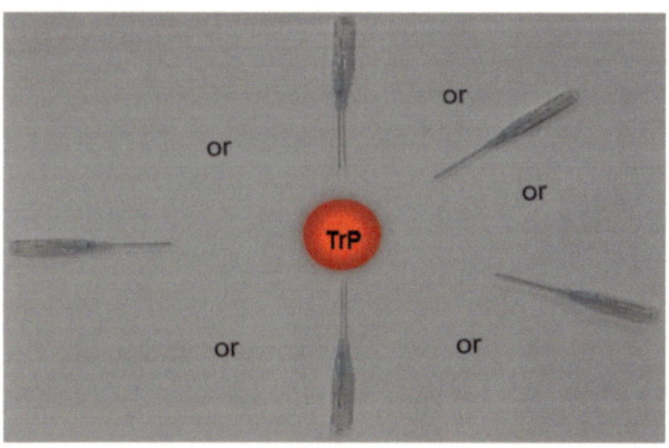


**Figure 1.** The situation of FSN needles with TrP

FSN, Chinese pronunciation of which is "*Fu Zhen*" (浮, in simplified Chinese; 浮針, in Traditional Chinese), has double implications: Fu is the surname of the inventor (also the first author of this chapter); in Chinese, "Fu, 浮" also means floating or superficial. "Zhen" means acupuncture or needling. Therefore, in some English-language papers, FSN was also called Floating Acupuncture[1], Fu's Acupuncture [2], Fu Needling [3] and Floating Needling [4]. However, neither *floating* nor *superficial* is a precise translation, and it has been decided that the word *subcutaneous* is a better substitute in terms of demonstrating where the effects of FSN are acting upon, and where the FSN needle is being manipulated..

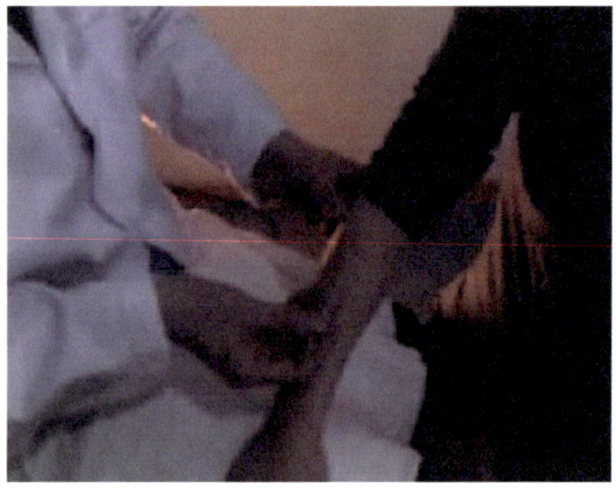

**Figure 2.** For neck pain, ipsilateral arm is the one chosen to be inserted in

Although it originated from classic acupuncture, FSN's manipulation and theory have little to do with the concepts of acupuncture, such as meridians, acupoints, Yin-Yang, and *Qi*. Therefore, it is not a kind of acupuncture and hence should no longer be called acupuncture, but rather FSN should be classified as its own separate identity..

The specific name, *Fu's Subcutaneous Needling*, was first mentioned in the article by Fu and Xu in the *Pain Clinic* to describe the treatment method [5]. Since then, a series of research papers have adopted the use of the name [6, 7].

FSN should be clearly distinguished from the narrow sense of dry needling, which is well known in the Western medical world. Since the 1940s, dry Needling [8-14], which refers to the insertion of a fine, single-use sterile needle, into a TrP [15-18] for myofascial pain [19-26] based on Western anatomical and neuro-physiological principles, has been increasingly utilized in the Western world, especially in the United States, United Kingdom, Australia, Germany, Brazil and Spain [27]. Unlike traditional acupuncture, dry needling ignores ancient Chinese philosophy and traditional ideas. Therefore, the manipulation method used in classic acupuncture differs from that used in dry needling because each one follows different theoretical instructions.

FSN stemmed from some ideas of traditional acupuncture, but its essential features are different from those of traditional acupuncture: 1. they are based on different theories; 2. their manipulation is different; and, 3. they use different kinds of needles. The theory of traditional acupuncture is a mystifying concept, even to Chinese doctors. FSN makes the job much easier by ignoring the traditional theories and placing more emphasis on the anatomical model. This makes FSN a modern form of acupuncture to some extent.

Compared with the current practice of common dry needling, FSN also has unique features. There are at least two differences between FSN and dry needling: 1, FSN inserts needles into non-diseased areas, but dry needling inserts the needles into TrPs; 2, FSN is confined to the subcutaneous layer, whereas dry needling goes deep into the muscles.

FSN is also considered as one type of dry needling in its "broad sense" because: 1, they both share the same theory surrounding modern scientific neurophysiology and anatomy; 2, In clinical practice, the end goal for both dry needling and FSN is to manage myofascial pain.

## 2. Features of Fu's Subcutaneous Needling (FSN)

FSN is differentiated from traditional acupuncture and other alternatives in terms of manipulation and effects.

### 2.1. Manipulation features

The manipulation of FSN is mainly devised of the following features:

*The selection of FSN insertion areas are based on the nature of TrPs or focal disorders*

FSN abandoned traditional acupuncture theories, such as meridians, acupoints, and the reinforcing-reducing method, and the selection of FSN points mainly depends on the different relevant muscles or situations of the disorders.

*The FSN needle inserts into non-diseased areas*

Different from medicated plasters, dry needling, and cupping, which are located directly on the afflicted or painful area, FSN acts on non-afflicted areas. The tip of the FSN needle usually does not reach the lesion area. The FSN needle stimulates a healthy area to heal the unhealthy area or organ. If the area is unhealthy, FSN needles are usually not inserted. For example, if the surrounding area of the painful spot is swollen or inflamed, the FSN needle should not be inserted into the swollen part.

*The insertion of the FSN needle stops at the subcutaneous tissue*

The needle used in dry needling goes through the skin, passes through the subcutaneous layer, and then enters deep into muscles, whereas the FSN needle stops at the subcutaneous layer (Fig. 3).

*Deqi is not required during an FSN treatment*

In traditional acupuncture, *Deqi* is considered an omen of its curative effect [28-30], which is why most acupuncturists try to induce *Deqi*. However, FSN aims for the patient not to have sensations of soreness, swelling, or numbness, and for the acupuncturist not to feel any mild resistance or "needle grasp".

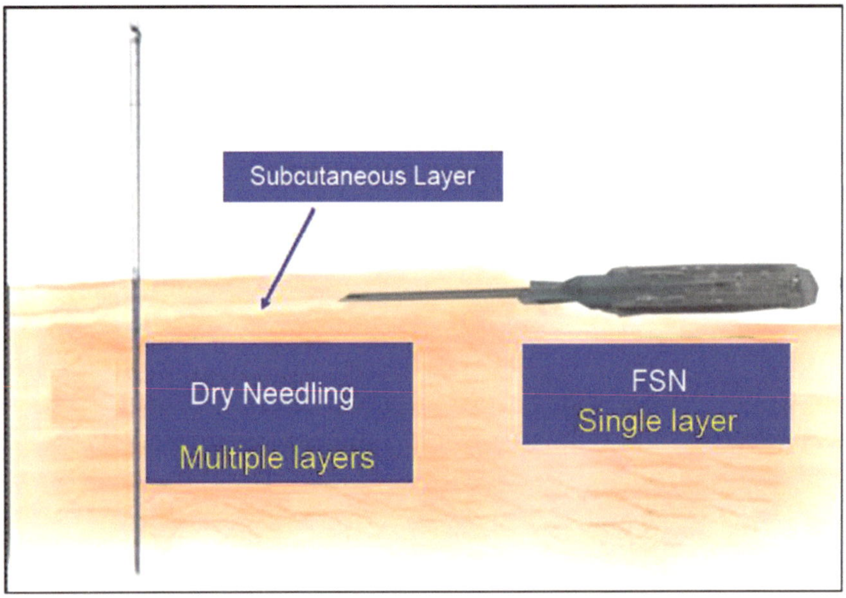


**Figure 3.** The different relevant layers of FSN and dry needling

*The FSN needle is retained in the subcutaneous tissues for a long duration*

The retention of the needles was seldom mentioned in ancient acupuncture. In modern acupuncture, however, retention is widely used, and the retention often lasts for 15 or 20 minutes. FSN needs a longer retention time, often lasting more than one hour. The patient should be allowed to move or exercising in a mild way with the FSN needles retained in the subcutaneous layer.

*The tip of the FSN needle directs to the painful region*

The acupuncture needle is often inserted perpendicularly or obliquely, whereas the tip of the FSN needle is inserted horizontally and is directed toward the TrP or localized disorder.

*The FSN needle has to be swayed from side to side*

The FSN applies a special technique, which is the swaying movement. The swaying movement is essential to FSN treatment and provides a curative effect, especially when dealing with chronic disorders. In most circumstances, FSN does not work well without the swaying movement.

*The involved muscles and joints can move easily during FSN treatment*

Moving afflicted joints and relevant muscles can effectively speed up the recovery from musculoskeletal injury. This kind of movement in an FSN clinic is called the reperfusion approach, which will be introduced in detail afterwards in this chapter. As mentioned above, the FSN needle is manipulated above the muscular layer, which makes it easy for the medi-

http://dx.doi.org/10.5772/53970

cal staff or the patients themselves to extend/contract the afflicted muscles even during FSN's swaying movement.

### 2.2. Characteristics of effectiveness

After clinical observations for about 16 years, FSN was found to have the following characteristics:

a. FSN focuses on treating painful problems, although FSN can also have positive effects on some non-painful disorders, such as numbness, chronic cough without sputum, and acute onset of asthma.

b. FSN can provide relief under most conditions. After the swaying movement, the pain completely goes away or is reduced to some extent.

c. Retention of the FSN needle is usually necessary in order to aviod symptoms from recurring frequently, although they can be easily suppressed after therapy.

d. FSN has adverse effects, such as minor hemorrhage, dizziness, and fainting. However, FSN is safer than acupuncture because its needles do not go deeply and do not touch focal diseases.

e. FSN has short-term and long-term effectiveness in the treatment of a majority of soft tissue non-traumatic lesions if the relevant muscles can have enough rest. However, for painful problems caused by malignant tumors, trigeminal neuralgia, and post-herpetic neuralgia, FSN often only have short-term effects.

f. The treatment room of an FSN clinic can be better utilized than that of an acupuncture clinic because patients can keep retention of the casing pipe, a soft part of the FSN needle, and go home after the treatment.

g. FSN treatment is inexpensive for patients because FSN can achieve the same effect with fewer treatments compared with acupuncture. In addition, FSN is much cheaper than surgery because it can often relieve painful problems, such as lower back pain with sciatica, without an invasive surgical procedure.

h. The effects of FSN can be seen immediately to confirm the accuracy of the diagnosis and technique. The doctor can then modify the diagnosis and treatment accordingly. FSN could provide feedback much quicker than acupuncture and medication could.

Although FSN is superior to traditional approaches in many respects, it also has its disadvantages: for example, doctors spend more time and energy on each subject, and FSN can be easily misunderstood by patients and other doctors because the FSN rationale seems too unconventional for the general public to understand. Chinese physicians doubt the results and effects of FSN because it does not obey the rules of traditional Chinese medicine. Furthermore, Chinese patients who have never previously been exposed to FSN often think that their physicians have discreetly injected them with an anaesthetic and/or steroid. Nevertheless, future studies confirming these clinical assumptions are imperative to further determine the effectiveness of FSN versus classic acupuncture.

## 3. Origin of Fu's Subcutaneous Needling (FSN)

The following three sources led to FSN's evolution from traditional acupuncture.

### 3.1. Contemplation of *De-Qi*

*De-Qi* [31], is an acupuncture phenomenon that occurs during needle manipulation. During needle manipulation, when the patient feels sensation, e.g. soreness, aching, numbness, and "needle grasp," and/or the acupuncturist feels a pulling sensation, it suggests that *De-Qi* is achieved [30, 32, 33 ]..

Traditionally, *De-Qi* must be achieved in the process of acupuncture regardless of the manipulation used; otherwise, the therapeutic results are poor [31]. In every textbook on acupuncture in Chinese, the importance of *De-Qi is* always emphasized and reiterated. Acupuncturists also repeatedly emphasize *De-Qi*. As a result, most Chinese patients believe in the adage, "no *De-Qi*, no effect." Sometimes, patients will be disappointed in the acupuncturist if they fail to acquire *De-Qi*, which causes discomfort to the patient.

Acupuncturists and patients are not the only ones who consider *De-Qi* to be essential, as some scientists also believe that *De-Q*i plays an important role in acupuncture analgesia [28, 34]. Acupuncture needling could activate the afferent fibers of peripheral nerves to elicit *De-Qi*, which ascends to the brain, activates the antinociceptive system, including certain brain nuclei, modulators (opioid peptides) and neurotransmitters, and through the descending inhibitory pathway, results in analgesia [34].

However, acupuncture could work without *De-Qi* every now and then, and could fail even when the patients achieve strong *De-Qi*. Furthermore, many acupuncture substitutes, such as cupping, moxibustion, trans-cutaneous electrical nerve stimulation (TENS), and so on, do not elicit *De-Qi*, but they appear to be effective [35].

Therefore, it is supposed that *De-Q*i might be not as pivotal as traditional comments suggest. To prove the insignificance of *De-Qi*, the best method is to stimulate the tissue with less nerve endings and then observe what will happen. The elicitation of *De-Qi* is related to the needling depth[32]. There are few free nerve endings and proprioceptive receptors in the subcutaneous layer, whereas free nerve endings are abundant in the epidermis and dermis, and proprioceptive receptors exist in the muscular layer [36]. Therefore, there should be no occurrence of *De-Qi* even if the subcutaneous layer is stimulated. Under such a condition, does the needling effect still exist? For an acupuncturist, it is simple to verify the existence of the needling effect, and this simple trial was one of the factors resulting in the development of FSN.

### 3.2. Clinical application of wrist-ankle acupuncture

Wrist-ankle acupuncture (WAA) [37] is also called wrist-ankle needling [38]. Dr. Xinshu Zhang, a neurologist who has worked at the Second Military Medical University in Shanghai, developed WAA in 1972. WAA divides the whole body into 12 longitudinal districts, 6 for each half of the body, 3 for each side of the central line.

http://dx.doi.org/10.5772/53970

There are 6 points 2 *cun* (about 50 mm) above the wrist joint corresponding to the 6 districts above the diaphragm, and there are 6 points 3 *cun* (about 75 mm) above the ankle joint corresponding to the other 6 districts. If a disorder occurs in one of the districts, the corresponding point should be chosen.

Unlike conventional acupuncture, WAA inserts an acupuncture needle only superficially in the subcutaneous layer; some authors claim that WAA is effective in the treatment of pain with various origins [39]. Needling superficially in WAA wrist or ankle point to treat distant disorders often has good effect [38], leading to the idea that needling close to the afflicted area could be at least as effective as needling in an area remote from that which is afflicted, and that needling closer maybe better. These thoughts motivated the author to seek answers through clinical trials.

### 3.3. Ancient techniques

*The Medical Classic of the Yellow Emperor* (also known as *The Yellow Emperor's Canon on Internal Medicine* or *Yellow Emperor's Inner Classic*), written thousands of years ago, is a fundamental book of traditional Chinese medicine. The book says needling superficially and needling nearby are two characteristics of the ancient techniques for the treatment of painful problems. The author of the chapter learned from, and were inspired by, these techniques in the process of FSN initiation. In *The Medical Classic of the Yellow Emperor*, there is a chapter entitled "*Guanzhen,*" which records 26 special techniques. The 26 techniques are classified into three groups: 9-technique group, 12-technique group, and 5-technique group.

The characters of superficial needling refers to quite a few techniques, such as *MAO Ci* in the 9-technique group, *Zhizhen Ci* and *Fu Ci* in the 12-technique group, and *Ban Ci* in the 5-technique group. Among them, *Zhizhen Ci* significantly resembles FSN: Hold up the skin with the thumb and index finger of the left hand; insert the filliform needle into the skin; and then go forward toward the painful spot obliquely. *Zhizhen Ci* of thousands of years ago can be said to be FSN without the use of FSN needle and its swaying movement.

Needling nearby is often seen in the 26 techniques, such as *Fen Ci* in the 9-technique group, *Hui Ci, Qi Ci, Yang Ci, Duan Ci,* and *Pangzhen Ci* in the 12-technique group, and *Baowen Ci, Guan Ci,* and *Hegu Ci* in the 5-technique group.

Aside from the practicable techniques mentioned above, *The Medical Classic of the Yellow Emperor* also describes many systemic theories, such as meridians, acupoints, and Yin–Yang. Nevertheless, from then on, the most ancient acupuncture texts took meridians, acupoints, and other theories instead of practicable techniques as their main interests. The long-term neglect of practicable techniques resulted in today's acupuncturists having little knowledge about this valuable ancient technique, which is a wise shortcut to FSN.

Based on the above ideas and thoughts, Fu, the first author of the chapter, devoted himself to seeking a new and effective treatment strategy and finally invented FSN in 1996, while the author worked at the First Military Medical University in Guangzhou, China. The university ran a TCM Clinic in Zengcheng, a city near Guangzhou. In the clinic, the patients who were in great pain were more numerous than the author could deal with, which encouraged him to find ways to more quickly relieve the painful problems.

The author, Fu, made an attempt and received a positive response when he treated a patient with tennis elbow (lateral epicondylitis) by needling near the painful spot; this was the first successful case of FSN. From then on, a series of clinical trials were made and positive results were achieved. FSN then came into being. In the same year, Fu wrote a brief introduction to FSN, and it was published in a Chinese health newspaper. Fu also published his first research paper in Chinese in the *Journal of Clinical Acupuncture and Moxibustion* the following year.

## 4. Development of Fu's Subcutaneous Needling (FSN)

Fu continued using FSN in his clinics and in accumulating evidence to improve FSN. The development took place in two main aspects: the innovation of the FSN needle and the increase of FSN's indications.

### 4.1. Innovation of the FSN needle

In physics, scientific theories always come out first, followed by technologies. However, in traditional medicine, these phenomena often occur the other way around: technologies or therapies come first, followed by theories. Without past experience to draw from or previous theories to follow, the author had to develop FSN by trial and error. During FSN's early months, the author used a filiform acupuncture needle, but the following factors made him change his mind:

- When the lesion range is large or deep, FSN did not work well with the filiform needles despite the simultaneous usage of many needles.
- FSN needs a long period of retention, and the patients could not stay in any settled position for extended periods of time. The patients should be able to move their bodies and limbs during needle retention. If the stainless-steel filiform needle is in use, patients are easily hurt.
- FSN requires the needle to sway from side to side. The filiform needle is too elastic to allow for the swaying movement.

Fu knew that some changes to the FSN needle must be made. However, the problem was determining the kind of needle that could go through the skin quickly and stay beneath the skin safely.

- Initially, a physical method was developed: a needle was invented using a new material. The material is solid at low temperature, and becomes soft at high temperature. When not in use, the needle is stored in a refrigerator. When FSN is being done, the needle is taken out and inserted into the patient's body, and the needle then becomes soft due to body temperature. It is a fine idea except that both the material used for the needle and the refrigerators are too expensive for most acupuncturists to afford.

- A chemical method was also considered. The author tried to produce a biological hard needle made of a high-polymer material, such as absorbable catguts, which is subsequently dissolved by the tissue fluids. A large amount of time and energy were devoted to finding such a material, but none was found.
- Finally, the author was inspired by the i.v. catheter and then invented a trocar needle of the compound structure used at present. Since 1997, the FSN needle has mainly consisted of two parts: a solid stainless-steel needle and its soft casing pipe. The former is hard enough to break through the skin quickly and to ensure that the FSN needle can be easily controlled; the latter is soft enough to remain beneath the skin without pricking.

An application for the patent of the FSN needle was made in December 1997, and the Chinese invention patent was granted in August 2002.

### 4.2. Increase of FSN indications

When the author mentioned that a certain disorder is one of FSN's indications, the following criterion was applied: an immediate effect can come into play when FSN is used to treat the disorder or release the symptoms. This criterion is called the *gold criterion*. Disorders or symptoms for which FSN is unable to get immediate results are not incorporated into the indications for FSN.

After the first successful case, the tennis elbow case previously mentioned, the author unceasingly searched for FSN indications. The search procedure could roughly be divided into four stages.

*Stage 1: FSN was mainly used to treat soft tissue injuries in the four limbs.*

In the early months after the formation of FSN, the diseases treated with FSN were all painful problems in the four extremities, such as tennis elbow, stenosing tenosynovitis of the styloid process of the radius, snapping finger, osteoarthritis of the knee, sprain and strain of ankle, and so on. Due to the limited experience with FSN in its early days, the success rate of the treatment of painful problems of the extremities was only about 40%. Therefore, FSN was not useful for the treatment of complex diseases of the trunk of the body.

*Stage 2: FSN was utilized to treat non-visceral diseases in the trunk.*

One day in the autumn of 1998, the author and a friend met on the university campus. The friend was seeking advice for her father-in-law, who was suffering from severe neck pain and who had been treated in the university hospital for nearly one month but did not respond to the treatment. The friend inquired if Fu can do something her father-in-law before leaving in a couple of days. The author had no better choice of treatment than FSN. Surprisingly, the neck pain was immediately relieved after the FSN trial. From then on, the author started using FSN to treat non-visceral painful diseases in the trunk, such as lower back pain with or without sciatica, cervical syndrome, and slight ankylosing spondylitis.

*Stage 3: FSN treats visceral benign painful problems.*

FSN is performed superficially; hence, superficial illnesses such as soft tissue injuries were regarded as FSN indications. FSN was never expected to treat visceral diseases until an 80-year-old acupuncturist, who worked in Luzhou, Southwest China, wrote to Fu that he treated a patient with appendicitis using FSN. Although FSN may not be suitable for the treatment of appendicitis for safety reasons, the letter implied that FSN may possibly treat visceral diseases. From then on, FSN was used to treat acute/chronic gastritis, cholecystitis, pain due to urinary calculus, painful menstruation, and so on.

*Stage 4: FSN was used to handle painful problems in the head and face and non-painful diseases.*

After the successful treatments of visceral diseases, more confidence in FSN was gained. The author moved on to treat head pain and face problems. These experiences convincingly showed that FSN is effective in relieving localized headaches and in painful problems of the face caused by temporomandibular and accessory sinusitis. FSN was mainly used to deal with painful problems where an immediate response could always be achieved. A query was raised regarding FSN's capacity for effectively managing non-painful diseases. After long-term practice, it was found that FSN could also deal with non-painful problems. At present, the following non-painful indications have been determined: chronic cough without sputum, onset of chronic asthma, localized numbness, chronic cold, chronic constipation, long-term diarrhoea and so on.

## 5. Fu's Subcutaneous Needling (FSN) manipulations

Although FSN originated from traditional acupuncture, its manipulation is quite different.

### 5.1. Structure of the FSN needle

FSN needles, individually packaged and pre-sterilized with ethylene oxide gas, are designed for single use. The FSN needle is made up of three parts (Fig. 4): a solid steel needle core (bottom), a soft casing pipe (middle), and a protecting sheath (top).

The needle core consists of a steel needle stick and the needle-core handle. The former is made of stainless steel, with a beveled tip. When the needle pricks the skin, the bevel of the tip should face upward. The latter is made of plastic and is square-shaped; one of the four sides has 10 protuberances. The protuberances are on the same side as the bevel of the tip. If the protuberances face upward, the bevel will also face upward. The needle core allows the FSN needle to have sufficient rigidity to quickly go through the skin, go forward along the subcutaneous layer, and smoothly sway from side to side. A soft casing pipe encases the FSN needle.

The soft casing pipe consists of two parts: the pipe body of fluoroplastic and the pipe neilsbed of common plastic. A metal wedge connects the two parts to one another. The tip of the casing pipe is about 3 mm behind the tip of the needle core when the needle core is embedded inside the casing pipe. The casing pipe has two functions: 1, it could cover the tip of needle stick until the needle stick is pulled back by 3 mm; thus, the tip of needle stick will not hurt the surrounding organs during the swaying movement; and, 2, substituting the steel needle core with the casing pipe beneath the skin can ease the patient's pain during retention.

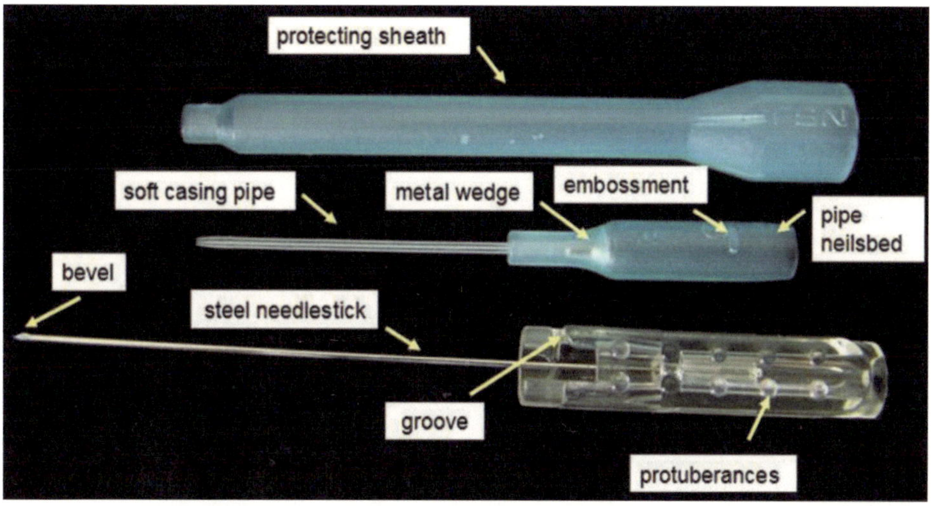


**Figure 4.** Three parts of FSN needle

The protective sheath is an affiliated structure and is made of common plastic. The protective sheath shields the needle core and the casing pipe from collision with something else, and it also keeps the FSN needle sterile.

## 5.2. Preparation prior to treatment

### *5.2.1. Select a treatment posture*

The FSN needle is thicker than acupuncture filiform needles, and FSN manipulation lasts longer; hence, selecting a suitable posture is crucial for FSN manipulation compared with acupuncture and dry needling. The following are the common postures used when FSN is used:

**Sitting position:** Appropriate for manipulating locations in the head, face, neck, shoulders, upper back and upper extremities.

**Supine position:** A fine choice when manipulating in the abdomen.

**Prone or lateral decubitus position:** An appropriate posture when treating diseases of the back and the rear of lower extremities.

The demonstrations in the above figures are only several of the common examples used in an FSN clinic. In fact, the postures can be modified depending on the patient's condition.

To be more precise, we should often change the positioning of the patient under the following two conditions: 1, when there is no immediate effect after several minutes of the FSN swaying movement, another posture should be considered. For example, the sitting posture is the first choice for the treatment of neck and upper back pain. However, if the sitting position does not work, letting the patient lie down may be a better choice; 2, when a patient is sensitive to a certain position or the painful problem becomes extraordinarily uncomfortable when a patient assumes a certain position, this special posture may be the best choice for the particular patient. For example, if the back pain is felt only when the patient stands, the FSN needle could be inserted while the patient is in a prone position, and then the patient could be asked to stand up before doing the swaying movement (Fig.5 ).

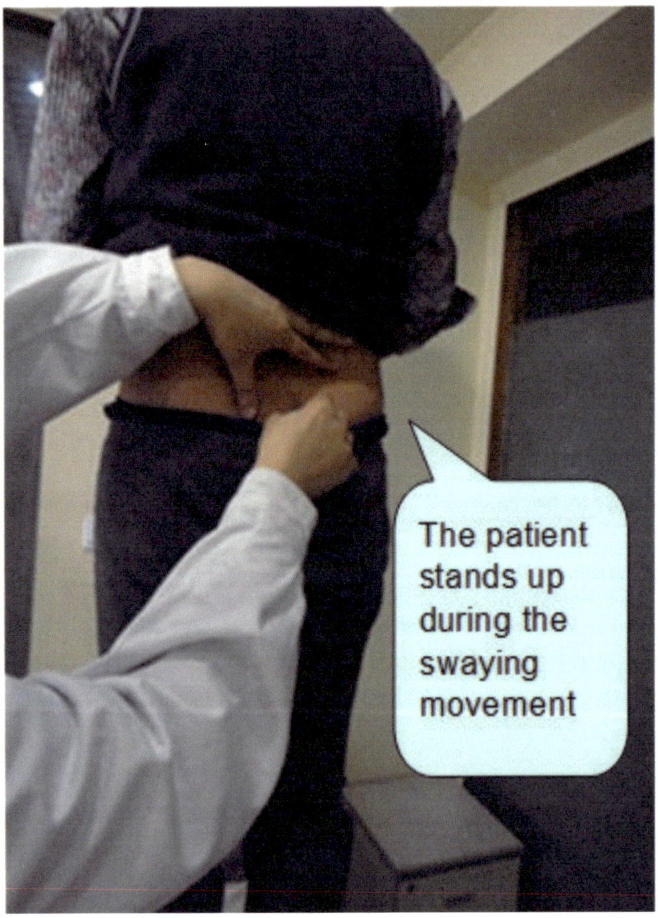


**Figure 5.** The needling technique when low back pain is worse while the patient is bending forward

### *5.2.2. Palpate the Trigger Point (TrP)*

In most cases, TrPs are the cause of painful musculoskeletal problems and are also the main targets of the FSN needle. In the following introduction to the treatment details of common diseases, the locations of relevant common TrPs are mentioned. Readers are referred to some current books for TrP dry needling.

### *5.2.3. Locate the insertion area*

Unlike traditional acupuncture, FSN does not require the insertion of the needles into acupoints or Ah-shi points. The needles are inserted into the area surrounding the TrPs or in the nearby limbs. After ascertaining the TrP, the needles can be inserted anywhere within the district around the TrP or in the adjacent limb. How is the area chosen? Here are some principles:

**Principle A:** For a single small-sized TrP, the insertion area should be close to this TrP. For a large-sized TrP or for TrPs clustered in one area, the insertion points should be in the nearby limbs. For example, the insertion points should be close to the TrP in the case of tennis elbow, whereas they should be far away from the TrP cluster in the case of upper back pain. The reason being is that when the distance between the TrP and the FSN needle tip is farther, the level of FSN effectiveness may be reduced, but its coverage area may be considerably enlarged. This phenomenon is called the *flashlight* \

**Principle B:** Between the insertion points and TrP, there should not be scars or hollow or prominent, especially there should not be the olecranon of ulna, patella, styloid processes of the radius and ulna, malleolus lateralis, or malleolus medialis.

**Principle C:** For different types of diseases, the FSN needle insertion site should follow the guidelines listed in **Table 1** if the needle insertion area should be far from the lesion site.

**Principle D:** To reduce pain during needle insertion, the needling points should be kept away from surface blood vessels, most of which are veins.

| Diseased Region | Insertion Area |
|---|---|
| Head, face, upper back | Thumb side of the forearm, outside of the upper arm |
| Chest, epigastric zone | Inner side of the forearm and upper arm |
| Hypogastrium | Middle part of the inner side of the leg, anteromedial part of thigh |
| Low back | Rear or outside part of the leg, outside of the thigh |
| Genitals, anus | Middle part of the inner side of the lower limb |

**Table 1.** Insertion areas corresponding to the diseased region

#### *5.2.4. Sterilize*

Sterilization is necessary and essential before FNS insertion. Both the surface of the insertion point and the practitioner's fingers should be sterilized.

### 5.3. Needling method

The needling procedure for FSN, including needle insertion, needle swaying, needle direction, needle retention, etc., is described below.

#### *5.3.1. Needle insertion*

The posture of the patient should be adjusted to ensure that the skin on the inserting point is neither tight nor loose. If the skin is too tight, relevant blood vessels dilate, and the FSN needle is more prone to inducing pricking; on the other hand, if the skin is too loose, it is harder to penetrate. During the whole process, the needle tip should always be directed toward the TrP.

First, the protective sheath of FSN needle is gently taken off, and then Fix the FSN needle into fixing groove of a kind of inserting device (Fig.6 ), which was specially designed for FSN Needle inserting, and then pull the fixing groove back to the locked position..

Hold the device as shown in Fig. 7.

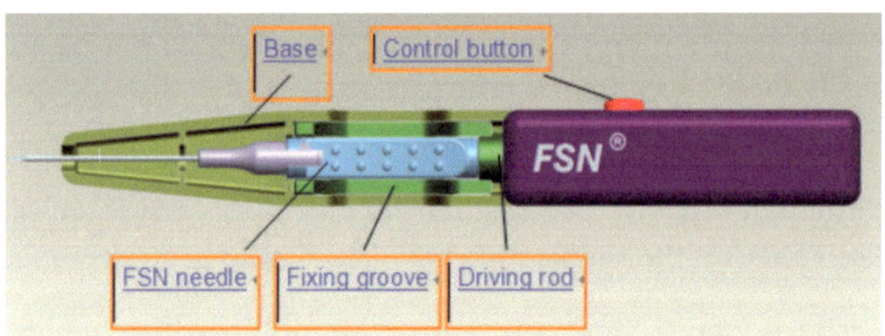


**Figure 6.** A FSN inserting device with a FSN needle in

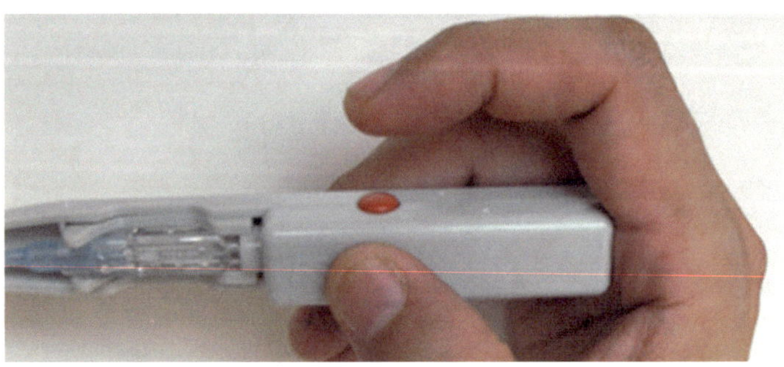

**Figure 7.** The way of holding the inserting device

Push and press the device to the area of intended insertion to form an indentation (Fig.8).

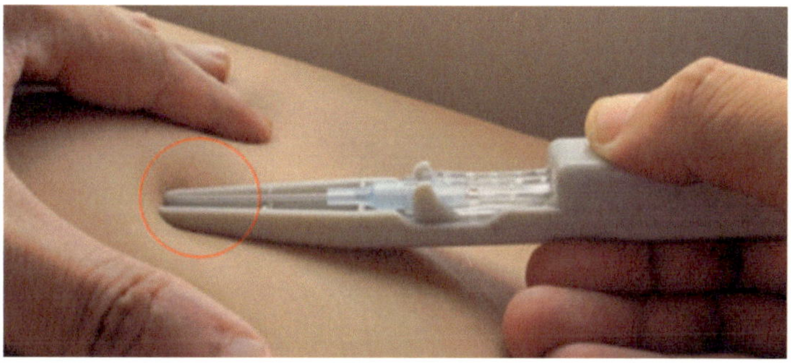

**Figure 8.** Before ejecting, the device should be pushed in

Press the control button with your right index finger, and then the FSN needle will immediately eject and penetrate the surface of the skin.

Use your left hand to take the FSN needle out from the fixing groove, and remove the device with your right hand (Fig.9).

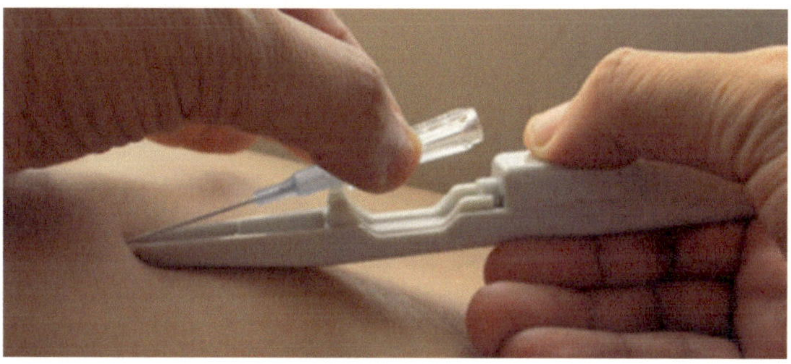

**Figure 9.** After insertion of the needle tip into the skin, the method to separate the device from the needle

Afterward, the needle should be laid flat and then carefully pushed in until the needle has been fully inserted. While being pushed forward, the needle tip should be slightly elevated in order to observe if the skin hunch is moving along with the needle tip. At this point, the therapist's right hand should feel loose with no resistance; while the patient feels something moving under the skin, but there is no feeling of *De-Qi*.

After the casing pipe is totally embedded beneath the skin, the needle-core handle should be withdrawn by about 3 mm and turned 90º to the left; this way, an embossment in the pipe neilsbed goes into a groove in the needle-core handle. The swaying movement can be done. Once the swaying movement is finished, the needle-core handle is turned right by 90º out of the groove, and then the steel needle core is withdrawn. The steel needle core is placed into the protective sheath so as not to hurt the medical staff and the garbage collector.

The casing pipe is then embedded beneath the skin using an adhesive tape. After 1-2 hours of retention, the adhesive tape is removed and the casing pipe is pulled out. At the same time, the insertion point should be pressed using a sterilized cotton ball for at least one minute to prevent bleeding.

### *5.3.2. Swaying movement*

The swaying movement, a key procedure for FSN, is a smooth, soft, fan-style waggle using the thumb as its fulcrum. The index finger, middle finger, and ring finger stay in a line. The middle finger and thumb affix the needle in a face-to-face way, while the index finger and ring finger alternately move back and forth (Fig. 10).

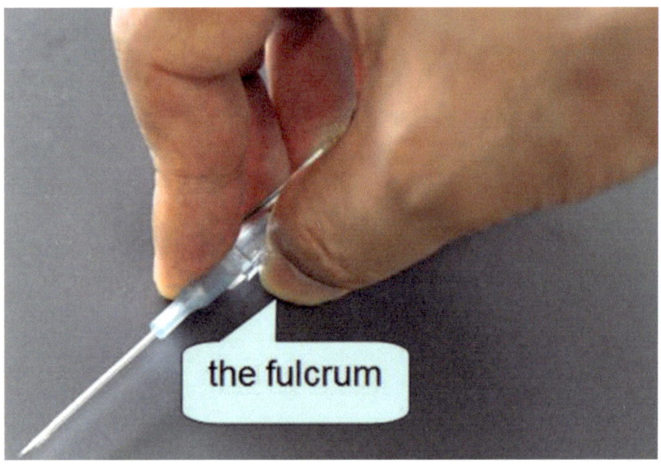


**Figure 10.** The way of hold the needle while the swaying movement.

The frequency of the swaying movement is about 100 times a minute. The duration of the swaying movement for one insertion point is often within 2 minutes. After 50 repetitions of the swaying movement (about half a minute), you can palpate the TrP or ask the patient about the condition of his/her problems. If the TrP has been deactivated or the patient says the problem is gone, the swaying movement should be stopped; otherwise, it should be continued. If the problem persists, the entire needle should be pulled out and the insertion point should be adjusted.

At the same time of swaying movement, the clinicians should move or ask the patient himself to move the relevant muscles or joints. Fig. 11 shows consecutive photos taken while manipulating the needle in upper extremity pain. The lifting of the sleeve by the practitioner's left hand and the movement of the left thigh should be noted. The rocking of the relevant muscles or joints is one of methods called the *reperfusion technique*.

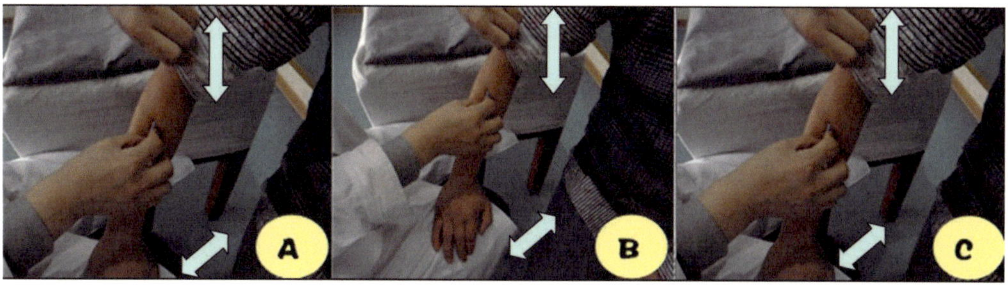


**Figure 11.** The consecutive photos of needle manipulation for upper extremity pain.

*5.3.3. Reperfusion technique*

Chinese acupuncturists often make use of a kind of technique for the treatment of acute painful problems. This technique is often conducted by the patients' themselves: the patients exercise their afflicted body part while acupuncturists insert the needles in an area other than the afflicted region. For example, when a Chinese acupuncturist treats pain associated with a sudden sprain in the lower back, he will ask the patient to stand up and rock his back during needling at the acupoint *Renzhong* (DU26). Although widely used, this practical rocking technique has seldom been introduced in textbooks. At present, this technique has no regular name; sometimes, it is called *Yundong needling* (kinetic needling) [40], other times, *Dong-qi* (meaning moving the energy) therapy and movement therapy [41]. In the Western world, there are also some similar techniques, such as exercise [42] or ischemic compression [43.44].

Inspired by these techniques, Fu tried to apply them in conjunction with FSN. To his surprise and delight, these techniques immediately enhanced FSN in many patients, especially for stubborn pain. To say that FSN is a much better fit for these conditions than acupuncture is no exaggeration. The reason is that the insertion point of acupuncture should be far from the afflicted area if these techniques are applied; there is no such restriction in FSN because FSN needles are not inserted deep into the muscles. Thus, these techniques could be done easily during FSN manipulation, regardless of whether your FSN insertion point is far from or near the afflicted area.

Fu once wondered about the mechanism of these techniques, and then searched for relevant studies. To his disappointment, there are only a few studies on these techniques both in Chinese and English papers. The limited number of studies could probably be blamed on the shortage of appropriate techniques, such as ischemic compressions, that could be done while exercising. These techniques are known to increase the effectiveness of FSN. Why do they work this way?

In the energy crisis theory [17,25], the contraction of a muscle segment creates a demand for energy and cuts off local circulation. Thus, improving local circulation is crucial. FSN can relieve muscle contraction from TrPs and then improve the local circulation, but this consumes both time and the practitioner's energy. FSN can be better utilized with the help of other methods that can help to impove circulation. Can these reperfusion techniques help in improving circulation? The answer can be illustrated using the change in the hand's skin color when the fist is clenched and loosened alternately (Fig. 12)

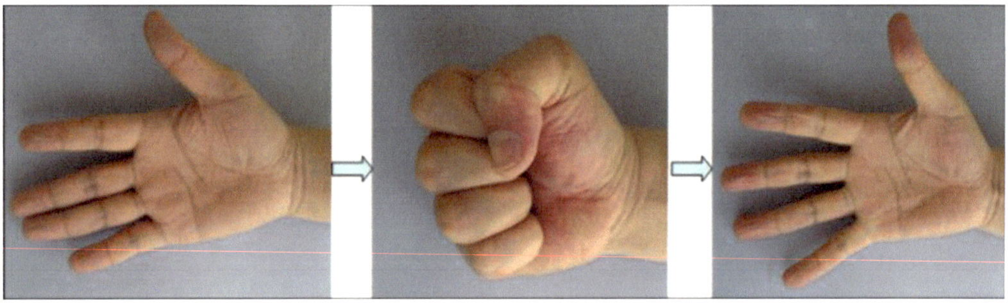

**Figure 12.** The changes of the skin color when the fist clenches and unclenches,

Fu named the course of techniques the *reperfusion approach (RA)*. RA here refers to the mechanical methods that extent/contract repetitively the relevant muscles to improve the local circulation in non-inflamed ischemic tissues, especially in musculoskeletal injured tissues.

*Reperfusion* is a word often found in the phrase *reperfusion injury*, which refers to tissue damage caused when blood supply returns to the tissue after a period of ischemia. Reperfusion injury is often involved in stroke and brain trauma, and sometimes, also in muscular trauma.

Could RA lead to reperfusion injury in ischemic tissues? This possibility should not exist because: (1) the ischemic state is a chronic one; and (2) the approach calls for the actions to be performed in a sequential and repetitive way; each action can only slightly improve the circulation.

There are two kinds of RA: active RA and passive RA. Active RA means that the actions are carried out by the patient's afflicted joints or some afflicted organs. Passive RA means that the actions are implemented by the practitioner or the patient's healthy limbs. The application range of active RA is larger than that of passive RA. Active RA can be used in most conditions. Passive RA is more applicable in the following conditions: (1) the patient does not know how to perform the RA; (2) the patient does not know how to control the amplitude and frequency; and (3) the TrP is located in a body part that the patient finds hard to move, such as in the scalp.

Active RA and passive RA could be used alternatively. Passive RA in small joints can often be implemented by the practitioner, whereas passive RA in large joints could be carried out by either the practitioner or the patient. For different muscles afflicted with musculoskeletal disease, practitioners should use different methods of RA during FSN.

With RA, the range of extension or contraction should be as large as possible under the safe condition. The transition between extension and contraction had better be slow.

*5.3.4. Retention*

After the swaying movement and RA, the solid steel needle core should be taken out (Fig. 13), and then go to retention. Retention is the process of retaining the casing pipe beneath the skin after the needle core is pulled out. The goal of retention is to maintain the immediate effects of the treatment. Therefore, if the treatment has no immediate effect, retention is meaningless. If the treatment has an immediate effect, then retention is necessary. The pain that just disappeared might recur without retention.

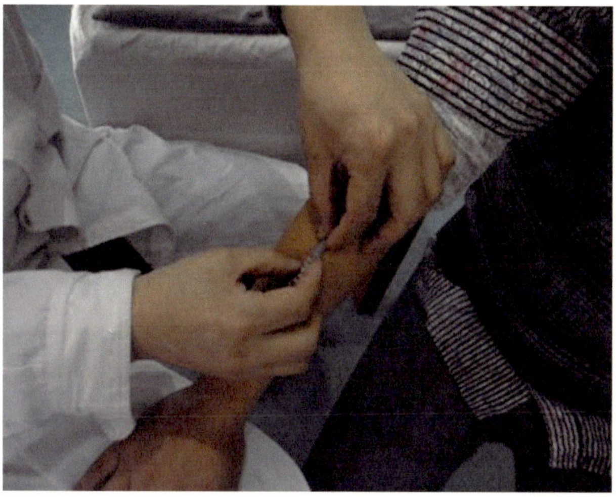

**Figure 13.** The method of separating the needle core from the tube.

The rubberized fabric that is used for retention should be big enough to cover the pipe neils-bed and insertion point (Fig. 14). Sometimes, rubberized fabrics can cause local itching and swelling due to allergy. In this case, the rubberized fabric should be changed.

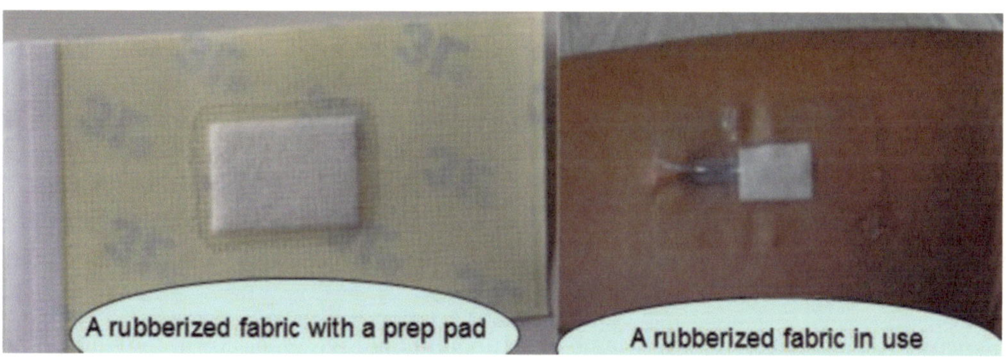
A rubberized fabric with a prep pad
A rubberized fabric in use

**Figure 14.** Fixing the soft tube by an adhesive tape.

For the sake of safety, retention time should last for 1 hour. According to our experience, the patients had better to stay in your clinic and to feel the condition. After 1 hour, if the pain is still present, do another swaying movement or insert other FSN needle. If the pain goes away or there is no change at all, take the whole FSN needle out without retention and let the patient go home.

## 6. Precautions, contraindications, and management of side effects

During traditional acupuncture, many people feel a brief stinging sensation, like a pinprick, when the needles are inserted. Others experience a dull ache around the needle after it goes in. A handful of patients have been injured because the needle was pushed into a vital organ, such as a lung. Nevertheless, acupuncturists have an extremely good safety record.

Given that an FSN needle does not go deep and does not elicit *De-Qi*, it is also a safe form of therapy, even safer than traditional acupuncture. However, no form of therapy is absolutely safe. When using FSN, close attention should be given to the following to gain satisfactory effects and to avoid causing patients discomfort:

**a.** FSN treatment should be delayed for those patients who are famished or who have overeaten, and also those who are intoxicated, over fatigued, or very weak.

**b.** The insertion of an FSN needle into the lower abdomen of pregnant women is contraindicated.

c. During needling, the blood vessels should be avoided to prevent bleeding, especially in the region of the superficial temporal artery, posterior auricular artery, and radial artery. When a patient suffers from spontaneous hemorrhage, do not give FSN treatment..

When performed correctly, FSN is free from any adverse effects. However, there are some potential yet temporary side effects that the practitioner should be aware of.

**Bruise:** A bruise appears where small blood vessels have broken, leaking blood under the skin. Bleeding under the skin results in a red or purple mark, which fades to yellow or green over time? Bruises often feel tender or swollen in the first few days. There are many small blood vessels, mostly veins, in the subcutaneous layer. During FSN manipulation, care should be taken to avoid the veins. However, some conditions make it impossible to avoid all blood vessels; hence, bruising under skin sometimes occurs. If the bruise under skin is not severe, there is no need to manage it. What needs to be done is to tell the patient not to worry, and ask him/her to relax. If the congestion is severe and causes pain or affects local function, the casing pipe should be pulled out immediately, and then cold, soft materials, for example, cold and wet towels, should be applied to compress the local area and stop or reduce the bleeding.

**Syncope:** People occasionally feel faint while undergoing FSN, especially at the start of the first treatment. When the patient is faint, he/she feels tired, dizzy, and nauseous, and his/her face turns pale. Sometimes, the patient also exhibits profuse sweating, flushing, and cold-

http://dx.doi.org/10.5772/53970

ness of the extremities, or even goes into a coma or falls to the ground. The prevention of fainting is more important than its treatment. When a patient undergoes FSN treatment for the first time and feels nervous or is in a weak condition, you should explain the FSN procedure and help the patient relax by selecting the suitable posture. During manipulation, the patient's expression should be observed; if any aura of faintness is seen, stop the FSN and let the patient lie down on a bed. In most cases, the patient will recover with the help of drinking water within 3-5 minutes.

## 7. Factors that influence Fu's subcutaneous needling effects

Many factors influence the effects of FSN, but some of them, for example, smoking, have not been proven. However, some of the factors have already been clinically proven in some cases.

### 7.1. Main factors that influence short-term effects

*Edema:* Stopping FSN treatment is advisable if the patient is suffering from general edema, such as when patient with lupus or rheumatoid arthritis received steroid treatment. Moreover, even if the patient has a concurrent painful problem, using FSN will have no effect.

*Fever:* Regardless of the cause of fever, the effects of FSN would not be as good as when a patient is in a normal healthy state. FSN should be stopped and the fever should be managed

*Other previous treatments:* Some previous treatments, such as local steroid injections, heavy cupping, plaster medicine, local ointment medicine, and local application of the coupling medium for an ultrasound check, will obviously influence the effects of FSN.

*Bad manipulation:* Any type of manipulation has an impact on the effect. If one step has not been performed well, the short-term effect will be influenced.

*Wrong diagnosis:* FSN is good for soft tissue non-traumatic lesions, but not for traumatic lesions, such as acute ankle sprain or pain caused by a hairline fracture

### 7.2. Factors that influence long-term effects

*Short-term effectiveness:* If there is a good short-term effect, there is likely to be a good long-term effect. If the short-term effect is not easily achieved, the long-term effect will probably not be good.

*Chronicity of the lesion:* If the soft tissue non-traumatic lesion has been present for a long time, the long-term effect will not be as good as if the lesion has only been present for a short time.

*Completeness of FSN treatment for TrPs:* Beginners of FSN can easily deactivate active TrPs, but ignore the palpation and the treatment of latent TrPs, which are also the engines of soft tissue lesions.

*Personal Habits:* Some routine habits or customs aggravate FSN's long-term effects. These routine habits include watching TV in the bedroom, playing poker or mahjong for extended periods of time, using an electric fan while sleeping, indulging in online gaming, walking or standing for long time, and not having enough sleep.

*Health Condition:* If the patient also suffers from other diseases such as immunologic diseases, chronic infection, hypothyroidism, diabetes, hyperuricemia or malignant change, the therapeutic effects may be poor.

## Author details

Zhonghua Fu[1] and Ryan Shepherd[2]

1 Fu´s Subcutaneous Needling, Nanjing University of Chinese Medicine, Nanjing, China

2 Optimum Health Centre, Toronto, ON, Canada

## References

[1] Huang Y, Fu ZH, Xia DB, Wu RK. 1998. Introduction to floating acupuncture: Clinical study on the treatment of lateral epicondylitis. Am J Acupuncture 26: 27-31.

[2] Zhang C. 2004. An investigation on fu's acupuncture treating lumbago. J Clin Acupuncture Moxibustion 20: 2.

[3] Xia DB, Huang Y. 2004. Combination of Fu needling with electric acupuncture for tennis elbow. Di Yi Jun Yi Da Xue Xue Bao 24: 1328-1329.

[4] Fu Z, Huang Y. 1999. Floating Needling. Int J Clin Acupuncture 10: 51-52.

[5] Fu Z, Xu J. 2005. A brief introduction to Fu's subcutaneous needling. Pain Clinic 17: 343-348.

[6] Fu ZH, Chen XY, Lu LJ, Lin J, Xu J. 2006. Immediate effect of Fu's subcutaneous needling for low back pain. Chin Med J 119: 953-6.

[7] Fu ZH, Wang JH, Sun JH, Chen XY, Xu JG. 2007. Fu's subcutaneous needling: possible clinical evidence of the subcutaneous connective tissue in acupuncture. J Altern Complement Med 13: 47-51.

[8] Baldry P. 1995. Superficial dry needling at myofascial trigger point sites. J Musculoskel Pain 3 (3): 117-126.

[9] Chu J. 1995. Dry needling (intramuscular stimulation) in myofascial pain related to lumbosacral radiculopathy. Eur J Phys Med Rehabil 5: 106-121.

[10] Baldry P. 2000. Superficial dry needling. In: Chaitow L (Editor). Fibromyalgia syndrome: a practitioner's guide to treatment. Edinburgh: Churchill Livingston.

[11] Cummings T, White A. 2001. Needling therapies in the management of myofascial trigger point pain: a systemic review. Arch Phys Med Rehabil 82: 986-992.

[12] Baldry P 2002. Superficial versus deep dry needling. Acupuncture Med 20: 78-81.

[13] Ga H, Choi JH, Park CH, Yoon HJ. 2007. Dry needling of trigger points with and without paraspinal needling in myofascial pain syndromes in elderly patients. J Altern Complement Med 13: 617-623.

[14] Hsieh YL, Kao MJ, Kuan TS et al. 2007. Dry needling to a key myofascial trigger point may reduce the irritability of satellite MTrPs. Am J Phys Med Rehabil 86: 397-403.

[15] Fischer AA. 1988. Documentation of myofascial trigger points. Arch Phys Med Rehabil 69: 286-291.

[16] Hong CZ. 1996. Pathophysiology of myofascial trigger point. J Formosan Medical Ass (Taiwan yi zhi) 95: 93-104.

[17] Hong CZ, Simons DG. 1998. Pathophysiologic and electrophysiologic mechanisms of myofascial trigger points. Arch Phys Med Rehabil 79: 863-872.

[18] Hong CZ. 2000. Myofascial trigger points: Pathophysiology and correlation with acupuncture points. Acupuncture Med 18: 41-47.

[19] Travell JG, Simons DG. 1983. Myofascial pain and dysfunction: The trigger point manual. Vol. 1. Baltimore: Williams & Wilkins.

[20] Simons DG. 1988. Myofascial pain syndrome due to trigger points. In: Goodgold J, editor. Rehabilitation Medicine. St Louis: CV Mosby Co.

[21] Travell JG, Simons DG. 1992. Myofascial pain and dysfunction: The trigger point manual. Vol. 2. Baltimore: Williams & Wilkins.

[22] Simons DG. 1999. Diagnostic criteria of myofascial pain caused by trigger points. J Musculoskeletal Pain 7 (1-2): 111-120.

[23] Hong CZ. 2004. Myofascial pain therapy. J Musculoskeletal Pain 12 (3-4): 37-43.

[24] Simons DG. 2004. New aspects of myofascial trigger points: etiological and clinical. J Musculoskeletal Pain 12 (3/4): 15-21.

[25] Hong CZ. 2006. Treatment of myofascial pain syndrome. Current Pain Headache Reports 10: 345-349.

[26] Simons DG. 2008. New views of myofascial trigger points: Etiology and diagnosis. Arch Phys Med Rehabil 89: 157-159.

[27] Lewit K. 1979. The needle effect in the relief of myofascial pain. Pain 6: 83-90.

[28] Park J, Park H, Lee H et al. 2005. Deqi sensation between the acupuncture- experienced and the naive: a Korean study II. Am J Chin Med 33: 329-37.

[29] Hui KK, Nixon EE, Vangel MG et al. 2007. Characterization of the deqi response in acupuncture. BMC Complement Altern Med 7: 33.

[30] White P, Bishop F, Hardy H et al. 2008. Southampton needle sensation questionnaire: development and validation of a measure to gauge acupuncture needle sensation. J Altern Complement Med 14: 373-9.

[31] Cheng X. 1987. Chinese Acupuncture and Moxibustion, Beijing: Foreign languages press.

[32] Lin JG. 1997. Studies of needling depth in acupuncture treatment. Chin Med J 110: 154-6.

[33] Langevin HM, Bouffard NA, Badger GJ, Churchill DL, Howe AK. 2006. Subcutaneous tissue fibroblast cytoskeletal remodeling induced by acupuncture: evidence for a mechanotransduction-based mechanism. J Cell Physiol 207: 767-74.

[34] Cao X. 2002. Scientific bases of acupuncture analgesia. Acupunct Electrother Res 27: 1-14.

[35] Chen CJ, Yu HS. 2003. Acupuncture, electro-stimulation, and reflex therapy in dermatology. Dermatol Ther 16: 87-92.

[36] Tortora GJ. 1989. Principles of Human Anatomy, Fifth Edition.

[37] Jiang H, Shi K, Xuemei L et al. 2006. Clinical study on the wrist-ankle acupuncture treatment for 30 cases of diabetic peripheral neuritis. J Tradit Chin Med 26: 8-12.

[38] Song BZ, Wang XY. 1985. Short-term effect in 135 cases of enuresis treated by wrist-ankle needling. J Tradit Chin Med 5: 27-8.

[39] Zhu Z, Wang X. 1998. Clinical observation on the therapeutic effects of wrist-ankle acupuncture in treatment of pain of various origins. J Tradit Chin Med 18: 192-4.

[40] Liu WA, Wu QM, Lei F et al. 2010. Effect of kinetic needling combined with blood-letting puncturing and cupping on functions of upper limbs of patients with shoulder-hand syndrome after apoplexy. World J Acupuncture-Moxibustion 1: 24-27.

[41] Luo BH, Han JX. 2010. Cervical spondylosis treated by acupuncture at Ligou (LR 5) combined with movement therapy. J Tradit Chin Med 30: 113-7.

[42] Carneiro KA, Rittenberg JD. 2010. The role of exercise and alternative treatments for low back pain. Phys Med Rehabil Clin N Am 21: 777-792.

[43] Vernon H, Schneider M. 2009. Chiropractic management of myofascial trigger points and myofascial pain syndrome: a systematic review of the literature. J Manipul Physiol Ther 32: 14-24.

[44] Montanez-Aguilera FJ, Valtuena-Gimeno N, Pecos-Martin D et al. 2010. Changes in a patient with neck pain after application of ischemic compression as a trigger point therapy. J Back Musculoskelet Rehabil 23: 101-4.

Chapter 9

# Explore Laser Acupuncture's Role

Wen-Long Hu, Yu-Chiang Hung and I-Ling Hung

Additional information is available at the end of the chapter

http://dx.doi.org/10.5772/55092

## 1. Introduction

Acupuncture has been widely used in the treatment of many diseases for over 2000 years. It is traditionally performed by inserting thin needles into acupuncture points in human body; this is known to affect the functions of various organs. According to the theory of traditional Chinese medicine, energy (or Qi) flows through the body along specific paths known as meridians. Any disturbance in this Qi results in an energy imbalance in the body; this imbalance may in turn result in disease. Acupuncture attempts to regulate and restore energy balance by stimulating specific acupoints along the meridians and thereby treat the underlying disease. In 1979, the World Health Organization (WHO) identified 43 conditions that might benefit from acupuncture. In 1996, WHO confirmed 64 indications for acupuncture treatment.

Recently, laser acupuncture (LA) has been used as a complementary and alternative therapy in addition to traditional acupuncture. It was first introduced clinically in the 1970s [1, 2]. LA is defined as the stimulation of traditional acupuncture points with low-intensity, non-thermal laser irradiation [3]. A laser beam is an electromagnetic wave and can stimulate the acupuncture points in the human body by depositing energy without heating. In doing so, the beam excites the channels and properties, regulates the function of organs, and promotes metabolism. It can function as both acupuncture and moxibustion via different frequencies, e.g., the information of the needle type (steel, gold/silver, left/right turn etc.). According to the research of Manfred Reininger et al, frequencies (Reininger frequencies: LU= 824 Hz, LI= 553 Hz, ST= 471 Hz, SP= 702 Hz, HT= 497 Hz, SI= 791 Hz, BL= 667 Hz, PC= 530 Hz, TE= 732 Hz, GB= 583, LR= 442 Hz; Bahr frequencies: B1= 599.5 Hz, B2= 1199 Hz, B3= 2388 Hz, B4= 4776 Hz, B5= 9552 Hz, B6= 19104 Hz, B7= 38208 Hz; Nogier frequencies: A′= 292 Hz, B′= 584 Hz, C′= 1168 Hz, D′= 2336 Hz, E′= 4672 Hz, F′= 9344 Hz, G′= 18688 Hz) can be applied to acupuncture points to improve the meridian energy. In this chapter, we explore laser acupuncture's role in modern medicine with a focus on how it strengthens and promotes the current methods of treatment.

## 2. Laser acupuncture vs. acupuncture

Instead of using a metal acupuncture needle, LA uses red or near-infrared light with a wavelength between 600 and 1000 nm and power between 5 and 500 mW. It is also referred to as low level laser therapy (LLLT), with 0.1–0.5 J/cm$^2$ being deposited per acupoint, or 1–4 J/cm$^2$ per Ashi point. Because of the low absorption of laser light by human skin in the given wavelength range, it has been hypothesized that laser light can penetrate deeply into the tissue, where it may have a photobiostimulation effect [4].

LA combines the advantages of traditional Chinese acupuncture and modern laser medicine. However, in some ways, laser energy may be more suitable than the traditional needle for stimulating the oscillating energy field of the meridian system. The correct frequency modulation of the monochromatic laser beam energizes the meridian and acupuncture point and thereby improves the oscillation of the meridian's own frequency. In addition, some patients may avoid acupuncture because of fear of pain and LA may be less invasive, less painful, and safer than traditional acupuncture. It may also be an improvement over traditional moxibustion, because it uses similar energy levels but avoids harmful effects related to smoke and heat (Table 1).

## 3. Review of the clinical literature

### 3.1. Pain

Assessment of the methods and findings of clinical trials on LA is confounded by the lack of detail in some studies in the literature. It is also noteworthy that all studies reporting negative results (no significant benefit of LA compared with control or sham conditions) lacked details regarding treatment parameters, such as laser power or dose [5].

| Treatment | Instrument | Invasiveness | Sensations | Pain |
|---|---|---|---|---|
| Traditional acupuncture | Needle | Invasive | Soreness, numbness, expansion, or pain | Painful |
| Laser acupuncture | Low-level laser | Non-invasive | None or slight warmth (if > 10 J/cm$^2$) | Painless |

**Table 1.** Comparison of traditional and laser acupuncture

*3.1.1. Low back pain*

Glazov used multiple regression analysis to identify which baseline characteristics predicted pain changes in the immediate, short, and intermediate terms. They found that higher pain scores at baseline predicted greater pain relief after LA for chronic non-specific low back pain. Adjusted analysis suggested a clinically significant effect on pain with LA compared to sham treatment ($P < 0.05$), at short term follow-up only [6]. Later, Glazov et al. performed a randomized controlled trial comparing the effects of laser acupuncture (LA) and sham laser treatment in reducing pain and disability in adults with chronic non-specific low back pain. Their results showed no effect of LA in reducing pain using infrared light at 0.2 J/point [7]. A possible reason for this result is dose dependency issue [8].

On the other hand, Fiore et al. [9] examined the short-term effects of high-intensity laser therapy versus ultrasound therapy for the treatment of low back pain in a randomized controlled trial without placebo control group. At the end of a 3-week intervention period with 5 treatments per week, participants in the laser therapy group showed a significantly greater decrease in pain and an improvement in related disability compared with the ultrasound group. This study suggests that laser therapy is a promising treatment option for the rehabilitation of low back pain.

*3.1.2. Myofascial pain*

LA has been used to treat myofascial pain in the masticatory musculature and trapezius muscles. Some trials focusing on the ability of LA to relieve myofascial pain found negative or contradictory results, which may reflect the poor methodologies used before 2001 [10]. In recent years, randomized controlled trials revealed significant decreases in pain during both rest and activity, and an increase in pain threshold in patients treated with LA compared to those treated with needle-acupuncture and placebo, respectively. Although no definite conclusions can be drawn due to the low number of participants ($n = 11$), LA may be a good treatment option for patients wanting a noninvasive, complementary therapy [11]. LA appears to be an effective form of acupuncture for the management of these conditions [12].

*3.1.3. Temporomandibular dysfunction*

The effectiveness of LLLT for the control of pain in patients with temporomandibular disorder (TMD) has been evaluated in studies with various research designs. In one study, LA was applied to acupuncture points in TMD patients, and the results showed significant pain reduction and improvement in the electromyographic behavior of masseter muscles in maximal habitual occlusion after treatment, but no significant improvement was observed in mandibular movement. This shows that LA may have an effect for controlling pain in TMD patients [13, 14].

#### *3.1.4. Lateral epicondylitis*

LLLT is a conservative treatment for lateral epicondylitis (LE). A recent systemic review evaluated therapeutic effects of LLLT in treating LE in terms of pain, grip strength, range of motion (ROM), and weight tests. The results revealed that applying LLLT on myofascial trigger points is an effective means for pain reduction and also led to increases in grip force, ROM, and weight test [15]. However, most of the reviewed studies, which were all several decades old, showed no significant differences between the laser treatment and the placebo groups [16]. This may be related to dose or wavelength effects. LLLT at optimal doses of 0.5–7.2 J at 904 nm and possibly 632 nm administered directly to the lateral elbow tendon insertions, has been shown to offer short-term pain relief and reduce LE disability. No serious side effects were reported in that study. This finding contradicts the conclusions of the previously mentioned review [16], which failed to assess treatment procedure, wavelength, or optimal dose [17].

#### *3.1.5. Knee osteoarthritis*

Laser acupuncture has been widely used in treating knee osteoarthritis. A study by the Western Ontario and McMaster Universities (WOMAC) found a significant decrease in pain score in knee osteoarthritis patients treated with LA compared sham treatment [18]. Yurtkuran et al. used a range of pain indices to investigate the effects and minimum effective dose of LA in treating this condition. Although they found some pain reduction in the placebo group, statistically significant reduction in knee circumference was observed only in the laser group. They concluded that LA was effective in reducing periarticular swelling. They also noticed different effects for different knee joint acupoints. The most common acupoints they used were Dubi (ST35) and Neixiyan (EX-LE 4) [19].

#### *3.1.6. Headache*

Several randomized controlled trials have found LA to be an effective treatment for headache, especially in children, including both migraine and chronic tension-type headaches [20, 21]. LA was shown to decrease headache intensity, duration of attacks, as well as number of headache days per month.

### 3.2. Other conditions

#### *3.2.1. Obesity*

LA has been reported to be effective in weight control. Wozniak (2003) compared the efficacy of a low-calorie diet with and without concurrent LA in reducing visceral obesity in postmenopausal women. They observed a significantly greater drop in body weight, body mass index, and waist-to-hip ratio with the combined treatment [22]. More recently, Hu et al. evaluated the therapeutic effects of LA in subjects with simple obesity using a non-restrictive diet protocol. Significant reductions in body weight and body mass index were seen after 4 weeks of LA treatment. Moreover, patient compliance was high, since this is a comfortable and non-restrictive diet protocol [23].

#### 3.2.2. Carpal tunnel syndrome

In patients with carpal tunnel syndrome (CTS), lower-level-laser therapy plus microamperes transcutaneous electric nerve stimulation (TENS) applied to acupuncture points has been shown to significantly reduce pain. In this study, both subjective (McGill Pain Questionnaire scores) and objective (sensory and motor latencies and Phalen and Tinel signs) measurements revealed that this combined approach was effective in treating CTS [24]. Branco examined the effects of various conservative treatments on CTS patients, including LA, TENS, needle acupuncture, and Chinese herbal medicine formulas, pain reductions were significantly greater with the LA compared to the other treatments, including some patients failed to have symptom relief after surgical release. Suggested mechanisms of pain reduction they proposed included increased adenosine triphosphate (ATP) at the cellular level, decreased inflammation, and temporarily increased serotonin level [25].

#### 3.2.3. Postoperative vomiting

Postoperative nausea and vomiting (PONV) are frequent side effects of general anesthesia in children. In 1998, LA was shown to reduce PONV in children after strabismus surgery. In this study, laser stimulation of PC6 occurred 15 min before administration anesthesia and again 15 min after arriving in the recovery room. In the laser stimulation group, the incidence of vomiting was significantly lower (25%) than that in the placebo group (85%) [26]. In another study, Butkovic et al. compared the effectiveness of LA to that of metoclopramide in preventing PONV in children after sevoflurane anesthesia. There were no statistically significant differences between the LA and metoclopramide groups in occurrence or timing of vomiting ($P < 0.001$). They concluded that LA is equally as effective as metoclopramide in preventing PONV in children [27].

#### 3.2.4. Smoking cessation

A prospective observational 2 year study showed that the Smokex-Pro method (Table 2) is an effective aid in smoking cessation. The treatment was well tolerated and showed only mild and temporary side effects. Additional advantages included lower cost and shorter treatment duration compared to other smoking cessation programs. However, controlled clinical trials are still needed to confirm the results of this study and to refine the treatment for maximum efficacy [28].

#### 3.2.5. Alcohol addiction

Auricular acupuncture has been used in the treatment of alcohol addiction for many years. Zalewska-Kaszubska et al. performed a study aimed at intensifying this method by adding laser biostimulation for treatment of patients with alcohol dependence syndrome. The patients received a single helium-neon laser neck biostimulation and 10 auricular acupuncture treatments with an argon laser. After 2 months of treatment, improvements in Beck Depression Inventory-Fast Screen (BDI-FS) scores and increases in beta-endorphin level were observed. These results suggest that laser therapy can be useful as an adjunct treatment for alcoholism [29].

#### *3.2.6. Asthmatic children*

It has been shown that LA significantly decreases mean weekly PFV as a measurement of bronchial hyper reactivity in asthmatic children. In this study there were no significant effects on FEV1, quality of life, or additional medication [30]. Another randomized control trial concluded that a single LA treatment offers no protection against exercise induced bronchoconstriction in pediatric and adolescent patients [31].

#### *3.2.7. Neurogenic pruritus*

Stellon described successful LA treatment in a 6-year-old girl with neurogenic pruritus of the abdomen, which was the first case report on LA treatment for this condition. The main advantage of using low energy laser light to stimulate points, as opposed to using acupuncture needles, was that it causes little or no sensation during the treatment which is particularly useful in pediatric population [32].

#### *3.2.8. Depression*

Depression is a major public health problem, and there is some evidence supporting the effectiveness of needle acupuncture in its treatment. Quah-Smith et al. investigated the effects of LA in treating depression patients and found that Depression Inventory scores decrease from baseline by 16.1 points in the intervention group and by only 6.8 points in the sham control group ($P < 0.001$). However, the beneficial effect was short-lived. The LA was well tolerated, with transient fatigue being the most common adverse effect [33]. Additional controlled clinical trials are needed to confirm the results of this study and to refine the treatment for maximum efficacy.

#### *3.2.9. Nocturnal enuresis*

LA therapy has been shown to be significantly more effective in reducing bed-wetting in primary monosymptomatic nocturnal enuresis patients compared to placebo treatment. In this study, they found no significant effects on maximal voided volume (first morning void excluded), maximal morning voided volume, voiding frequency, enuresis frequency before and after treatment, or nocturnal urine production after LA treatment. However, they did find significant increases in average daytime voided volume compared to the placebo group. They concluded LA was a safe but inefficient treatment for these patients [34]. However, a different study showed subtle effects on bladder reservoir function after LA treatment [35]. In comparison with pharmacological therapy using desmopressin, another study showed no statistically significant differences in success rates between desmopressin therapy and LA. LA is an alternative, noninvasive, painless, cost-effective, and short-term therapy for children with primary nocturnal enuresis, normal bladder function, and high nighttime urine production [36].

### 3.2.10. *Autonomic nervous activity of night shift workers*

Many studies have demonstrated high levels of affective disorders in night-shift workers. Wu et al. examined the impact of LA on autonomic nervous system (ANS) and heart-rate variability (HRV) of such workers. Compared with a placebo group, the treatment group had a statistically significant improvement in high-frequency (HF) HRV, low-frequency (LF) HRV, and LF:HF HRV ratio. This suggests LA may increase vagal activity and suppression of cardiac sympathetic nerves and could be used to help patients who have circadian rhythm disorders [37].

### 3.2.11. *Whiplash injuries*

Following introduction of compulsory seat belt use in cars, whiplash injuries of the cervical spine have become commonplace. Current treatment approaches resolve symptoms within a short time in most cases, but a small proportion of patients still develop persistent health problems. Aigner et al. combined LA with cervical collar treatment and medication (paracetamol and chlormezanone) to treat whiplash patients. They did not observe significantly greater improvements in any outcome measure at any time for LA compared to the other treatment protocols [38].

### 3.2.12. *Postural instability*

It is well known that the risk of falling is high among elderly people. Bergamaschi compared the effectiveness of auriculopuncture, ultralow-power LA, and placebo treatment in improving postural control in an elderly population. Balance performance was measured on a force platform before and after treatment. Although the small sample size did not allow reliable statistical analysis, the observed balance improvements were remarkable, and some differences were observed between the two kinds of stimulation. They found that both LA and auriculopuncture reduced nociceptive interference, thus improving postural control [39].

### 3.2.13. *Peripheral artery disease*

Cardiovascular disease is the most common cause of death in humans. The use of acupuncture as a complementary and alternative treatment for cardiovascular disease has been suggested in both humans and animals. Possible advantages of using acupuncture are the low cost of treatment and the low risk of collateral damage when used in combination with other medical treatments. In 2010, a trial was performed to compare the effects of traditional acupuncture and LA on arterial pressure and peripheral circulation of the inferior limbs in patients with circulatory deficiencies. The results showed that only those treated with LA exhibited a significant increase in systolic pressure in their lower limbs, with a resulting improvement in Revascularization Index. This suggests that different stimuli on acupuncture points generate different variations of peripheral resistance in the lower limbs [40].

*3.2.14. Cerebral cortical and subcortical activations*

As recent studies have demonstrated, acupuncture can elicit activity in specific areas of the brain. Siedentopf et al. investigated the cerebral effects of LA at both GB43 acupoints with functional magnetic resonance imaging. Their results showed that LA produced significant, predominantly ipsilateral, brain activation within the thalamus, nucleus subthalamicus, nucleus ruber, the brainstem, and the Brodmann areas 40 and 22. No significant brain activations were observed within the placebo group. The fact that the observed effects were primarily ipsilateral supports the assumption that LA is mediated by meridians, since they do not cross to the other side of the body [41].

## 4. Discussion and conclusions

LA is a non-invasive technique involving the stimulation of traditional acupoints with low-intensity, non-thermal laser irradiation. Its clinical application is widespread even though its mechanisms are not well understood. LLLT can decrease inflammation by reducing the levels of biochemical markers (prostaglandin E2, messenger ribonucleic acid cyclooxygenase-2, IL-1$\beta$, TNF-$\alpha$), neutrophil influx, oxidative stress, edema, and hemorrhaging [42]. Analgesia induced by laser phototherapy is mediated by peripheral opioid receptors [43], however LA has both local and distant analgesic effects that may be mediated by different mechanisms.

LA combines the positive effects of traditional acupuncture with LLLT. Compared with needle-based methods for manipulating Qi, LA has the advantages of being non-invasive and aseptic. Moreover, it is painless and safe because no heat is generated during the procedure, and it is more effective in some medical condition and requires less time than needle-based acupuncture [23]. No side effects or complications resulting from LA have been reported in any study so far.

We have presented evidence supporting the use of LA in the treatment of various types of acute and chronic pain, postoperative nausea and vomiting, nocturnal enuresis, alcohol addiction, smoking cessation, obesity, and cerebral cortical activation (Table 2). Inappropriate selection of points and frequencies, insufficient energy and therapeutic sessions will lead to a failure in laser acupuncture therapy. Further studies are needed to better define optimal treatment parameters, including wavelength, dose, and intensity, and to maximize the physiological benefit and cost effectiveness of treatment (Figure 1). In conclusion, LA integrates traditional acupuncture with LLLT, and is effective in treating many conditions. In the hands of an experienced physician, LA can be an effective alternative treatment method in modern medicine.

| Study | Subjects | Design | Parameters | Acupoints | Intervention | Results |
|---|---|---|---|---|---|---|
| Fiore et al, 2011 [9] | Low back pain n=30 | RCT | 1064 nm, 760 mJ/cm$^2$, pw | Trigger points | 5 times/ week for 3 weeks | Greater decrease in pain and an improvement of related disability |
| Katsoulis et al, 2010 [11] | Myofascial pain n=108 | NR, blind control study | 690 nm, 40 mW, 40–60 J, 15 min | ST6, SI18, SI3, LI4 | Twice a week for 3 weeks | Pain reduction > 50% |
| Hotta et al, 2010 [13] | TMD n=10 | Case series | GaAlAs laser, 780 nm; 70 mW, 35 J/cm$^2$ | LI4, HT3, ST6, ST7 | Once a week for ten sessions | Improve painful symptoms and electromyographic activities of masseter muscles |
| Mazzetto et al, 2010 [14] | TMD n=40 | RCT, double-blind | GaAlAs laser, 830 nm, 40 mW, 5 J/cm$^2$ | Affected condyle lateral pole: superior, anterior, posterior, posterior-inferior | Twice a week for 4 weeks | Immediate decrease of painful symptoms and increased range of mandibular movements |
| Ren et al, 2010 [18] | Knee OA n=41 | RCT | Semiconductor laser, 650 nm, 36 mW; and $CO_2$ laser, 1006 nm, 200mW, 40 Hz; 2 min | ST35 and EX-LE 4 | Thrice a week for 2 weeks, then twice a week for 4weeks | Improve the pain, stiffness and functional limitation of knee |
| Yurtkuran et al, 2007 [19] | Knee OA n=52 | RCT | 904 nm, 10 mW/cm$^2$, 4 mW, 0.48 J, 120 s | SP 9 | 5 times per week for 2 weeks | Reducing periarticular swelling |
| Gottschling et al, 2008 [20] | Headache n=43 | RCT | 30 mW, 830 nm, cw, 3.8 W/cm$^2$, 0.9 J/ point, 30 s | Frontal: LI4, ST36; lateral: TE5, GB34; occipital: SI3, BL60; holocephalic: GV20 | Once a week over 4 weeks | Headache decreased |
| Ebneshahidi et al, 2005 [21] | Tension Headache n=50 | RCT | GaAsAl laser, 830nm, 39 mW/cm$^2$, 1.3 J/ point, 43s | LU7, LI4, GB14, GB20 bilaterally | Thrice a week for 10 sessions | Improvement for headache intensity, median duration of attacks, and median number of days with headache per month |

| Study | Subjects | Design | Parameters | Acupoints | Intervention | Results |
|---|---|---|---|---|---|---|
| Wozniak et al, 2003 [22] | Viseral obesity after menopause n= 74 | RCT | 900 Hz, 24 mW, 0.1 J, 10–15 s/ point, 150 s | CV12, ST36, ST25, LR3, PC6, HT7; auriculotherapy: 55, 87 | Twice a week with low-calorie diet for 6 weeks | Higher efficacy in lowering body weight, body mass index and waist-to-hip-ratio |
| Hu et al, 2010 [23] | Simple obesity n=95 (M/F 22/73) | Case series | GaAlAs laser, 785 nm, 50 mW, 0.25 J/ point | Stomach, Hunger, ST25, ST28, ST40, SP15, CV9 | Thrice a week with non-restrictive diet for 4 weeks | Reduce body weight and body mass index |
| Naeser et al, 2002 [24] | CTS n=11 | RCT | 632.8 nm, cw, 15 mW on shallow acupoints; 904 nm, pulsed, 9.4 W on deeper points | PC7 | 35 to 45 min, thrice a week for 3-4wk | Significant decreases in MPQ score, median nerve sensory latency, and Phalen and Tinel signs |
| Branco et al, 1999 [25] | CTS n=36 | open protocol study | HeNe laser, 670 nm, cw, 5 mW, 1-7 J/point, TENS; 904 nm, pw, 10 W, 1 J/ point and/or needle acupuncture | PC7, 8, 9; LU9, 10, 11; LI1, 4; TE1, 5; SI1 | Thrice a week for 4-5 weeks | 33 of 36 hands (91.6%) no pain, or pain reduced by more than 50% |
| Schlager et al, 1998 [26] | PONV n=91 | RCT | 670 nm, 10 mW, cw, 30 s | PC6 | 15 min before induction of anaesthesia and 15 min after arriving in the recovery room | Lower incidence of PONV (25%) |
| Butkovic et al, 2005 [27] | PONV n=120 | RCT | GaAlAs laser, 780 nm, 20 mW, cw, 1 J/ point, 60 s | PC6 | 15 min before induction of anesthesia | Equally effective as metoclopramide in preventing PONV |
| Breivogel et al, 2011 [28] | Smoking cessation n=156 | prospective observational study | Smokex-Pro method (electric stimulation and laser at 650 nm, 1.5 mW, 10 Hz) | Defined regions in the ear and nose | For 24 months | Long-term abstinence rates were 49.3% (1 year) and 47.95% (2 years) |

| Study | Subjects | Design | Parameters | Acupoints | Intervention | Results |
|---|---|---|---|---|---|---|
| Zalewska - Kaszubska et al, 2004 [29] | Alcohol addiction n=53 | Case series | HeNe laser 632.8 nm, 25 mW (neck); Argon laser, 514 nm, 100 mW, 10 s (ear) | Neck and auricular acupoints: 82, 83, 87, 51, 55 | For 20 days | Improved BDI-FS and increase in beta-endorphin level |
| Stockert et al, 2007 [30] | Asthmatic children n=17 | RCT | 670 nm,10 mW, 20 s/point up to 16 points + probiotics | LU1, 5, 7, 9, 11; LI4, 6, 19, 20; BL13, 17, 18, 20, 21, 23; ST13, 25, 36, 40, 44; SP3, 6, 9, 10; HT3, 5, 7; SI3; KI3, 6, 8, 27; PC6; TE5, 15; GB3, 34, 40, 41; LR2, 3, 8, 13; CV4, 6, 9, 17, 21; GV4, 13 | For 10 weeks | Decreased mean weekly Peak flow variability and days of acute febrile infections |
| Quah-Smith et al, 2005 [33] | Depression n=30 | RCT | 100 mW, 0.5 J, 5 s | LR14, CV15, CV14, HT7, LR8 | Twice weekly for 4 weeks then weekly for a further 4 weeks | BDI scores fell from baseline by 16.1 points in the test group and by 6.8 points in the control group |
| Karaman et al, 2011 [34] | Nocturnal enuresis in childern, n=91 | RCT, single blind | 635~670 nm, < 5 mW, 1 min/ point | CV3, 4, 6, and bilateral SP6, ST36 | Thrice a week for 4 weeks | Decreased the mean number of weekly bed-wetting episodes |
| Radvanska et al, 2011 [35] | Monosymptomatic nocturnal enuresis n=31 | RCT, single-blind | 670 nm, 20 s | GV20, HT7, ST36, SP6, LR3, KI3, CV3, CV4, BL23, GV4 | Thrice a week in the first 2 weeks, then Twice a week in the next 3 weeks | Increase in average daytime voided volume |
| Wu et al, 2009 [37] | Healthy night shift worker n=45 | Case series | 830 nm, 60mW, 9.7 J/cm$^2$, 10 min | PC6 | Single treatment | Increase vagal activity and suppression of cardiac sympathetic nerves |
| Bergamaschi et al, 2011 [39] | Postural instability n= 34 | preliminary report | 0.03 mW, 100Hz, 0.3 mJ/ point | BL60, KI3, Auriculotherapy zones | Single treatment | Reduce nociceptive interference and improve postural control |

| Study | Subjects | Design | Parameters | Acupoints | Intervention | Results |
|---|---|---|---|---|---|---|
| Cunha et al, 2010 [40] | Peripheral artery disease n=40 | RCT | AlGaAs laser, 650 nm, 2.4 J/cm$^2$ | 10 acupoints | Single treatment | Increase in systolic pressure of lower limbs, improvement in Revascularization Index |
| Siedentopf et al, 2005 [41] | Healthy male n=22 | RCT | 10 mW, 670 nm, cw | GB43 | Time series RARARARAR (on: A/off: R) | Significant brain activations within the thalamus, nucleus subthalamicus, nucleus ruber, brainstem, Brodmann areas 40 and 22 |
| Aigner et al, 2006 [38] | Whiplash injury n=45 | RCT | HeNe laser, 632.8 nm, cw, 5 mW, 0.075 J/cm$^2$, 15 s | B10, B40, G20, G34, TE5, SI6, LG14; ear points 29, 37, 41, 55 | Thrice a week for three weeks | No statistically significant advantage in the acute or chronic phase |

**Table 2.** Summary table of clinical researches into laser acupuncture

BDI-FS: Beck Depression Inventory–Fast Screen, CTS: carpal tunnel syndrome, cw: continuous wave, MPQ: McGill Pain Questionnaire, NR: non-randomized, OA: osteoarthritis, PONV: Postoperative nausea and vomiting, pw: pulsed wave, RCT: randomized controlled trial, TMD: temporomandibular disorders.

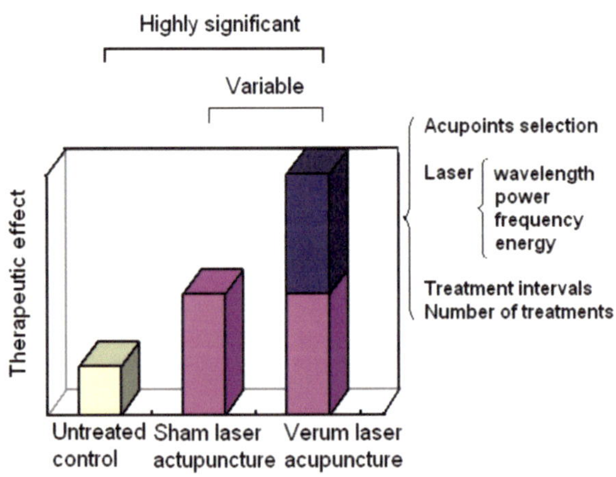


**Figure 1.** Graph of the therapeutic effects of laser acupuncture divided into psychological (pink) and physiological (dark blue) effects. The latter is determined by the shown factors

http://dx.doi.org/10.5772/55092

## Author details

Wen-Long Hu[1,2,3,4], Yu-Chiang Hung[1,2] and I-Ling Hung[1]

1 Department of TCM, Kaohsiung Chang Gung Memorial Hospital, Taiwan

2 Chang Gung University College of Medicine, Taiwan

3 Kaohsiung Medical University College of Medicine, Taiwan

4 Fooyin University College of Nursing, Taiwan

## References

[1] Hill, S. Letter: Acupuncture research in the USSR. American Journal of Chinese Medicine (1976). , 4(2), 204-5.

[2] Miklánek, J, & Kriz, V. st experiences with the utilization of lasers for acupuncture. The Akuplas device. Fysiatrický a reumatologický vestník (1978). , 56(1), 36-40.

[3] Whittaker, P. Laser acupuncture: past, present, and future. Lasers in Medical Science (2004). , 19(2), 69-80.

[4] Cigna Medical Coverage Policy: Low-Level Laser Therapy. (2012). http://www.cigna.com/assets/docs/health-care-professionals/coverage_positions/mm_0115_coveragepositioncriteria_lowlevel_laser_therapy.pdf,.

[5] Baxter, G. D, Bleakley, C, & Mcdonough, S. Clinical effectiveness of laser acupuncture: a systematic review. Journal of Acupuncture and Meridian Studies (2008). , 1(2), 65-82.

[6] Glazov, G. The influence of baseline characteristics on response to a laser acupuncture intervention: an exploratory analysis. Acupuncture in Medicine (2010). , 28(1), 6-11.

[7] Glazov, G, Schattner, P, Lopez, D, & Shandley, K. Laser acupuncture for chronic non-specific low back pain: a controlled clinical trial. Acupuncture in Medicine (2009). , 27(3), 94-100.

[8] Baxter, G. D. Laser acupuncture: effectiveness depends upon dosage. Acupuncture in Medicine (2009).

[9] Fiore, P, Panza, F, Cassatella, G, Russo, A, Frisardi, V, Solfrizzi, V, & Ranieri, M. Di Teo L, Santamato A. Short-term effects of high-intensity laser therapy versus ultrasound therapy in the treatment of low back pain: a randomized controlled trial. European Journal of Physical and Rehabilitation Medicine (2011). , 47(3), 367-373.

[10] Fargas-babjak, A. Acupuncture, transcutaneous electrical nerve stimulation, and laser therapy in chronic pain. The Clinical Journal of Pain (2001)., 17(4), 105-13.

[11] Katsoulis, J, Ausfeld-hafter, B, Windecker-gétaz, I, Katsoulis, K, Blagojevic, N, & Mericske-stern, R. Laser acupuncture for myofascial pain of the masticatory muscles. A controlled pilot study. Schweizer Monatsschrift für Zahnmedizin (2010)., 120(3), 213-25.

[12] Baxter, G. D, Bleakley, C, & Mcdonough, S. Clinical effectiveness of laser acupuncture: a systematic review. Journal of Acupuncture and Meridian Studies (2008)., 1(2), 65-82.

[13] Hotta, P. T, Hotta, T. H, Bataglion, C, & Bataglion, S. A. de Souza Coronatto EA, Siéssere S, Regalo SC. Emg analysis after laser acupuncture in patients with temporomandibular dysfunction (TMD). Implications for practice. Complementary Therapies in Clinical Practice (2010)., 16(3), 158-60.

[14] Mazzetto, M. O, Carrasco, T. G, & Bidinelo, E. F. de Andrade Pizzo RC, Mazzetto RG. Low intensity laser application in temporomandibular disorders: a phase I double-blind study. The Journal of Craniomandibular Practice (2007)., 25(3), 186-92.

[15] Chang, W. D, Wu, J. H, Yang, W. J, & Jiang, J. A. Therapeutic effects of low-level laser on lateral epicondylitis from differential interventions of Chinese-Western medicine: systematic review. Photomedicine and Laser Surgery (2010)., 28(3), 327-36.

[16] Haker, E, & Lundeberg, T. Laser treatment applied to acupuncture points in lateral humeral epicondylalgia. A double-blind study. Pain. (1990)., 43(2), 243-7.

[17] Bjordal, J. M, Lopes-martins, R. A, Joensen, J, Couppe, C, Ljunggren, A. E, Stergioulas, A, & Johnson, M. I. A systematic review with procedural assessments and meta-analysis of low level laser therapy in lateral elbow tendinopathy (tennis elbow). BMC Musculoskeletal Disorders (2008).

[18] Ren, X. M, Wang, M, Shen, X. Y, Wang, L. Z, & Zhao, L. Clinical observation on acupoint irradiation with combined laser or red light on patients with knee osteoarthritis of yang deficiency and cold coagulation type. Zhongguo Zhen Jiu (2010)., 30(12), 977-81.

[19] Yurtkuran, M, Alp, A, Konur, S, Ozçakir, S, & Bingol, U. Laser acupuncture in knee osteoarthritis: a double-blind, randomized controlled study. Photomedicine and Laser Surgery. (2007)., 25(1), 14-20.

[20] Gottschling, S, Meyer, S, Gribova, I, Distler, L, Berrang, J, Gortner, L, Graf, N, & Shamdeen, M. G. Laser acupuncture in children with headache: a double-blind, randomized, bicenter, placebo-controlled trial. Pain. (2008)., 137(2), 405-12.

[21] Ebneshahidi, N. S, Heshmatipour, M, Moghaddami, A, & Eghtesadi-araghi, P. The effects of laser acupuncture on chronic tension headache--a randomized controlled trial. Acupuncture in Medicine (2005)., 23(1), 13-8.

[22] Wozniak, P, Stachowiak, G, Piêta-doliñska, A, & Oszukowski, P. Laser acupuncture and low-calorie diet during visceral obesity therapy after menopause. Acta Obstetricia et Gynecologica Scandinavica (2003). , 82(1), 69-73.

[23] Hu, W. L, Chang, C. H, & Hung, Y. C. Clinical observations on laser acupuncture in simple obesity therapy. The American Journal of Chinese Medicine (2010). , 38(5), 861-7.

[24] Naeser, M. A, Hahn, K. A, Lieberman, B. E, & Branco, K. F. Carpal tunnel syndrome pain treated with low-level laser and microamperes transcutaneous electric nerve stimulation: A controlled study. Archives of Physical Medicine and Rehabilitation (2002). , 83(7), 978-88.

[25] Branco, K, & Naeser, M. A. Carpal tunnel syndrome: clinical outcome after low-level laser acupuncture, microamps transcutaneous electrical nerve stimulation, and other alternative therapies--an open protocol study. The Journal of Alternative and Complementary Medicine. (1999). , 5(1), 5-26.

[26] Schlager, A, Offer, T, & Baldissera, I. Laser stimulation of acupuncture point reduces postoperative vomiting in children undergoing strabismus surgery. British journal of anaesthesia (1998). , 6.

[27] Butkovic, D, Toljan, S, Matolic, M, Kralik, S, & Radesiæ, L. Comparison of laser acupuncture and metoclopramide in PONV prevention in children. Pediatric Anesthesia (2005). , 15(1), 37-40.

[28] Breivogel, B, Vuthaj, B, Krumm, B, Hummel, J, Cornell, D, & Diehl, A. Photoelectric stimulation of defined ear points (Smokex-Pro method) as an aid for smoking cessation: a prospective observational 2-year study with 156 smokers in a primary care setting. European Addiction Research (2011). , 17(6), 292-301.

[29] Zalewska-kaszubska, J, & Obzejta, D. Use of low-energy laser as adjunct treatment of alcohol addiction. Lasers in medical science (2004). , 19(2), 100-4.

[30] Stockert, K, Schneider, B, Porenta, G, Rath, R, Nissel, H, & Eichler, I. Laser acupuncture and probiotics in school age children with asthma: a randomized, placebo-controlled pilot study of therapy guided by principles of Traditional Chinese Medicine. Pediatric Allergy and Immunology (2007). , 18(2), 160-6.

[31] Gruber, W, Eber, E, Malle-scheid, D, Pfleger, A, Weinhandl, E, Dorfer, L, & Zach, M. S. Laser acupuncture in children and adolescents with exercise induced asthma. Thorax. (2002). , 57(3), 222-5.

[32] Stellon, A. The use of laser acupuncture for the treatment of neurogenic pruritus in a child--a case history. Acupuncture in Medicine (2005). , 23(1), 31-3.

[33] Quah-smith, J. I, Tang, W. M, & Russell, J. Laser acupuncture for mild to moderate depression in a primary care setting-a randomized controlled trial. Acupuncture in Medicine (2005). , 23(3), 103-11.

[34] Karaman, M. I, Koca, O, Küçük, E. V, Öztürk, M, Güne, M, & Kaya, C. Laser acupuncture therapy for primary monosymptomatic nocturnal enuresis. The journal of Urology (2011). , 185(5), 1852-6.

[35] Radvanska, E, Kamperis, K, Kleif, A, Kovács, L, & Rittig, S. Effect of laser acupuncture for monosymptomatic nocturnal enuresis on bladder reservoir function and nocturnal urine output. The journal of Urology (2011). , 185(5), 1857-61.

[36] Radmayr, C, Schlager, A, Studen, M, & Bartsch, G. Prospective randomized trial using laser acupuncture versus desmopressin in the treatment of nocturnal enuresis. European Urology (2001). , 40(2), 201-5.

[37] Wu, J. H, Chen, H. Y, Chang, Y. J, Wu, H. C, Chang, W. D, Chu, Y. J, & Jiang, J. A. Study of autonomic nervous activity of night shift workers treated with laser acupuncture. Photomedicine and laser surgery (2009). , 27(2), 273-9.

[38] Aigner, N, Fialka, C, Radda, C, & Vecsei, V. Adjuvant laser acupuncture in the treatment of whiplash injuries: a prospective, randomized placebo-controlled trial. Wiener Klinische Wochenschrift (2006).

[39] Bergamaschi, M, Ferrari, G, Gallamini, M, & Scoppa, F. Laser acupuncture and auriculotherapy in postural instability--a preliminary report. Journal of Acupuncture and Meridian Studies (2011). , 4(1), 69-74.

[40] Cunha, R. G, Rodrigues, K. C, Salvador, M, & Zangaro, R. A. Effectiveness of Laser treatment at acupuncture sites compared to traditional acupuncture in the treatment of peripheral artery disease. Engineering in Medicine and Biology Society (EMBC), 2010 Annual International Conference of the IEEE (2010). , 2010, 1262-5.

[41] Siedentopf, C. M, Koppelstaetter, F, Haala, I. A, Haid, V, Rhomberg, P, Ischebeck, A, Buchberger, W, Felber, S, Schlager, A, & Golaszewski, S. M. Laser acupuncture induced specific cerebral cortical and subcortical activations in humans. Lasers in Medical Sciense (2005). , 20(2), 68-73.

[42] Bjordal, J. M, Johnson, M. I, Iversen, V, Aimbire, F, & Lopes-martins, R. A. Photoradiation in acute pain: a systematic review of possible mechanisms of action and clinical effects in randomized placebo-controlled trials. Photomedicine and Laser Surgery (2006). , 2, 158-68.

[43] Serra, A. P, & Ashmawi, H. A. Influence of Naloxone and Methysergide on the Analgesic Effects of Low-Level Laser in an Experimental Pain Model. Revista Brasileira de Anestesiologia (2010). , 60(3), 302-310.

Chapter 10

# New Technology: Femtosecond Laser May be Used for Future Acupuncture Therapy

Yutaka Takaoka, Mika Ohta, Aki Sugano,
Akihiko Ito and Yoichiroh Hosokawa

Additional information is available at the end of the chapter

http://dx.doi.org/10.5772/54315

## 1. Introduction

Acupuncture therapy is utilized to cure many diseases and to maintain health. We have been studying the molecular mechanism of acupuncture and obtained its molecular evidence [1-4]. The World Health Organization has listed more than 40 indications for acupuncture [5], and the National Institutes of Health (NIH) has accepted the validity of acupuncture treatment [6,7]. One of the popular uses of acupuncture treatment is to treat muscle exhaustion, including stiff shoulders. Major acupuncture techniques involve penetration of the skin by thin, solid metallic needles, which are manipulated manually or are stimulated electrically. The efficacy of such muscle therapy is attributed to the over-proliferation of muscle cells induced by the damage of muscle in response to the needle penetration. We recently reported that myostatin gene expression is suppressed by electroacupuncture (EA) [1].

However, we cannot exclude the possibility of infection for use of acupuncture, and thus a noncontact method without using needles is needed. Furthermore the laser treatment has a potential for high-throughput therapy. When an intense femtosecond laser is focused on biological tissue, laser ablation is induced at the laser focal spot. Since the main component of the tissue is water, the initiation process occurs with the mutual interaction between water molecules and the femtosecond laser pulse. In comparison with picosecond or nanosecond laser irradiation, the excitation energy of water molecules after the femtosecond laser irradiation is effectively converted to energy to generate shock and stress waves [8,9]. This means simultaneously that heat generation at the laser focal spot is suppressed because of effective energy conversion to these kinetic waves [10]. As a result, when the femtosecond laser is focused on the tissue with suitable irradiation conditions, we can expect that the tissue will be stimulated mechanically, rather than thermally, by the photomechanical ablation. In previous studies we realized several single-cell manipulation techniques using shock and stress waves under a microscope, including noncontact detachment of an animal cell from its cultured substrate [11,12], control of cell multiplication [13], and estimation of intercellular adhesion strength [14,15]. These techniques can be utilized not only for single cells but also for tissues and organs of living animal. As one of the promising approach, our attention is directed to acupuncture treatment.

In this study, we focused a femtosecond laser (FL) on the skin of the hind leg muscles of living mice and investigated the clinical influence of the common acupuncture (ACP) on muscle disease via histological examination and expression analysis of the gene encoding myostatin [16]. In the histological examination, we observed damage of the skeletal muscle due to the femtosecond laser irradiation. We then used real-time PCR to estimate the gene expression and western blotting to estimate the protein translation of myostatin in the skeletal muscle after the laser irradiation. Myostatin is a growth repressor in muscle satellite cells [17]. The suppression of myostatin gene expression and protein translation indicates the facilitation of muscle cell proliferation. In comparison with the common acupuncture treatment, we recognized the potential of the femtosecond laser as a tool for the acupuncture.

## 2. Materials and methods

### 2.1. Laser stimili

The experimental setup for the femtosecond laser (FL) is shown in Figure 1. Eight-week-old inbred strain C57BL/6 male mice were purchased from Japan SLC, Inc., Tokyo, Japan. After anesthesia treatment for the mice, hairs of the hind legs were saved and then mounted on an XY motorized stage (Sigma Koki, BIOS-215T). A femtosecond laser pulse train from a regeneratively amplified femtosecond laser system (Spectra Physics, Hurricane, 800 nm, 150 fs) was focused on the top of the hind leg through a quartz convex lens with a focus length of 150 mm. The laser irradiation was controlled by a mechanical shutter positioned in front of the laser system. The three-dimensional position of the laser focal spot was guided by a HeNe laser, with beams divided into two lines introduced on the focal spot from different directions. The laser focal spot was changed on the 1.5-cm-square area on the hind leg point to point with the XY motorized stage. The irradiation area was a little larger than the hind leg. The interval between the focal spots was set to 1 mm, and thus the laser irradiation was performed at 256 (16x16) points on the surface of the hind leg. Although the sample position fluctuated along the optical axis with a precision of a few millimeters, the focal spot size remained almost the same throughout the irradiation because the fluctuation is much smaller than the focus length of the focus lens (150 mm). By this manipulation, the laser irradiated almost the entire area of the hind leg. For each laser focal spot, a single- or 1000-shot laser pulse irradiated the target. For single-shot laser irradiation, a single-shot pulse was extracted from the pulse train at a repetition rate of 20 Hz by the mechanical shutter with a gate time of 50 ms. The 1000-shot laser pulse irradiation was performed by focusing the pulse

http://dx.doi.org/10.5772/54315

train at a rate of 1 kHz for 1 sec. The laser pulse energy was tuned to 300 mJ/pulse by a half-wave plate and polarizer.

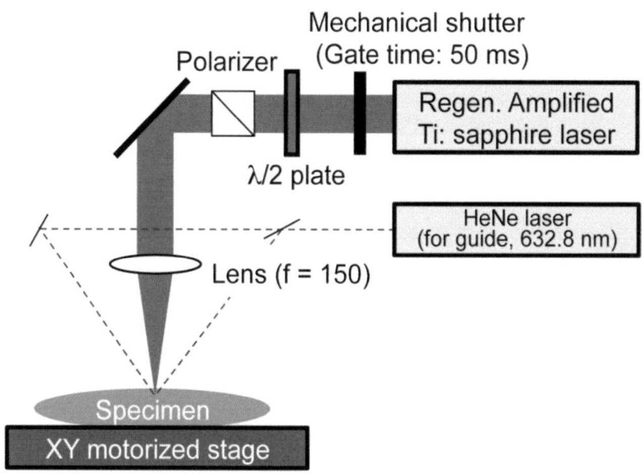


**Figure 1.** Experimental setup for femtosecond laser acupuncture.

After the laser stimulation, mice were treated for biological analyses to describe in the following sections. All mice in this research project were treated according to the Standards Relating to the Care and Management of Experimental Animals (Ministry of the Environment, Tokyo, Japan) [18]. This study was approved by the Committee for Safe Handling of Living Modified Organisms at Nara Institute of Science and Technology (permission number 1132) and Kobe University (permission number 17-21) and was carried out according to the guidelines of the committee.

### 2.2. Histochemical analysis

Tissue samples after the laser irradiation were fixed in 10% neutral buffered formalin and embedded in paraffin. Paraffin sections (3 mm thick) were stained with hematoxylin and eosin (H&E) as described previously [1,19].

### 2.3. Creatine kinase analysis

Blood samples were collected from mice after 3 hours of the laser irradiation. Creatine kinase (CK) assay was measured according to the manufacturer's instructions (L-Type CK kit, Wako Pure Chemical Industries, Japan) [20]. CK activity was determined by using a Hitachi autoanalyzer 7180 (Hitachi, Japan). The number of mice for each group in CK analysis was as follows: 9 for control, 11 for FL, 6 for ACP.

### 2.4. Real-time PCR analysis

To examine myostatin gene expression, total RNA was extracted from triceps surae muscle. Total RNA (5-μg samples) was reverse-transcribed into cDNA by using SuperScript RT (SuperScript First-Strand Synthesis System; Life Technologies, Gaithersburg, MD), according to the company's instructions. Expression levels were compared by using real-time quantitative RT-PCR analysis with gene-specific primers as follows: myostatin: sense: 5'-GACAAAACACGAGGTACTCC-3'; antisense: 5'-GATTCAGCCCATCTTCTCC-3'. Real-time PCR was performed by using Power SYBR Green PCR Master Mix and StepOne (Applied Biosystems, Foster City, CA), according to the manufacturer's instructions. The reaction mixture consisted of 2 ml of SYBR Green, 4 ml of cDNA, and each primer at 5 pmol, plus water to a final volume of 20 ml. The PCR conditions were 95°C for 10 min followed by 50 cycles for 95°C for 15 s, 60°C for 60 s, and then 95°C for 15 s, 60°C for 60 s, and 95°C for 15 s. Internal control gene for this research was glyceraldehyde-3-phosphate dehydrogenase (GAPDH) [21,22]. The values of each group were expressed relative to those obtained for the control. The number of mice for each group in this analysis was as follows: 4 for control, 5 for FL, 6 for ACP.

### 2.5. Western blotting analysis

The triceps surae muscles were homogenized in PhosphoSafe reagent (Novagen, Madison, WI) supplemented with a protease inhibitor cocktail tablet (Roche, Indianapolis, IN). After centrifugation at 12,000 g for 25 min, the supernatant was frozen until use. Protein concentration was determined with Micro BCA Protein Assay Kit (Pierce, Rockford, IL) using bovine serum albumin as standard. For western blotting analysis, protein samples were resolved by SDS-PAGE and blotted on PVDF (*Amersham*, Piscataway, NJ). The primary antibodies used in this study were polyclonal anti myostatin antibody (Millipore, Billerica, MA) and α-tubulin loading control (Abcam, Cambridge, MA) [23]. The secondary antibody was a goat anti-rabbit IgG horseradish peroxidase (HRP) conjugate (Cell Signaling Technology, Danvers, MA). Immunoreactive bands were visualized with Pierce ECL Plus Western Blotting Substrate (Thermo Scientific, Rockford, IL) for α-tubulin, ECL Prime Western Blotting Detection System (GE Healthcare Life Sciences, Uppsala, Sweden) for myostatin. All blots were scanned, and the bands were analyzed with ImageJ software (http://rsbweb.nih.gov/ij/). The band densities were expressed relative to those obtained for the control. The number of mice for each group in this analysis was as follows: 5 for control, 6 for FL.

### 2.6. Statistical analysis

For CK and real-time PCR analyses, we used one-way ANOVA, followed by Tukey's post-hoc test. Data of western blotting were compared using unpaired Student's *t*-test. Data for and real-time PCR and western blotting were given as relative value to control with the data divided by the average value of control for normalization. The relative gene and protein levels of myostatin were calculated by means of comparison with the geometric mean of the translation of the internal control gene (GAPDH) and protein (α-tublin), respectively. For all statistical analyses, maximum and minimum values are excluded from each group. All data were presented as means ± SD. $P$ values of < 0.05 were considered statistically significant and the level of significance are expressed as follows in each figure: **, $P < 0.01$; ***, $P < 0.001$; NS, not significant.

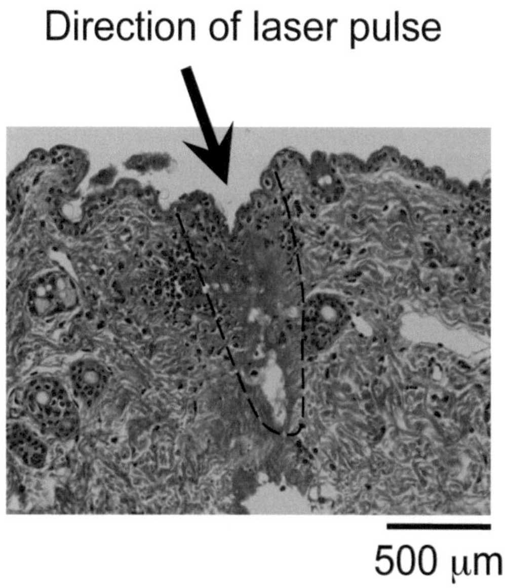


**Figure 2.** Histological microphotograph of the epidermis and dermis after single-shot irradiation with 300 uJ/pulse. The arrow indicates the direction of laser irradiation. The area within the dashed line was denatured by the laser irradiation. The skeletal muscle beneath the dermis was analyzed by real time-PCR and western blotting.

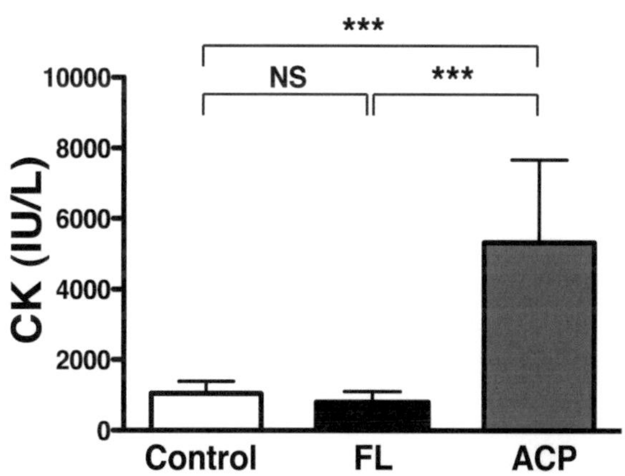


**Figure 3.** The serum creatine kinase after the femtosecond laser irradiation (FL) and common acupuncture stimuli (ACP).

## 3. Results and discussion

Figure 2b shows a representative histological microphotograph of epidermis and dermis with irradiation by a single-shot laser pulse with energy of 300 mJ/pulse. The microphotograph is a cross-section of a hind leg at a laser focal spot. The pulse energy was about 15 times larger than the ablation threshold (20 mJ/pulse). The diameter of the laser focal spot was about 30 μm, and we estimated the laser fluence and peak power density of the ablation threshold to be 0.7 $J/cm^2$ and $4.7x10^{12}$ $W/cm^2$, respectively. This is in rough agreement with the laser irradiation conditions reported as a threshold of the optical breakdown [8]. Under such conditions, the deposited laser energy is efficiently converted to shock and stress waves and propagates around the laser focal spot, as noted in the introduction. Along the axis of the laser irradiation and its surrounding area, the typical morphological pattern of the tissue was lost, indicating damage of the tissue. The diameter and depth of the damaged area were approximately 400 and 1100 μm, respectively (the area within the dashed line in (b)). Based on the depth, we estimated the absorption coefficient to be 10 $cm^{-1}$, which is reliable as an optical absorption property at 800 nm [9], though the absorption coefficient fluctuates greatly with the concentrations of melanin and hemoglobin. The diameter was larger than that of the laser focal spot size (about 30 μm), which means that the physical and/or physiological effects by the laser irradiation propagate from the area with the direct laser irradiation. Since a typical histological pattern due to heat denaturation was not observed in the damaged area, the damage was mainly induced by the photomechanical ablation. These results agree with those of previous studies [8,9]. Note that damage by the laser irradiation was not observed in the skeletal muscle (Figure 2a).

We evaluated the effects of laser on creatine kinase (CK) activity, because high level of CK means muscle damage [24]. Figure 3 indicates that the femtosecond laser irradiation (FL) dose not make injury in the muscle in contrast to ACP.

To reveal the muscle cell proliferation, the gene expression pattern of myostatin and GAPDH of the skeletal muscle after the laser irradiation was analyzed. The analysis was performed only for the skeletal muscle, from which epidermis and dermis were extracted. The expression of GAPDH, which is a kind of dehydrogenase, is not modulated by the environment surrounding changes in the tissue, the expression pattern was simultaneously monitored as an internal control of the gene expression of myostatin. Based on the ratio of the signal intensity of the pattern of myostatin to that of GAPDH, we can evaluate the gene expression of myostatin. Similarly, based on the ratio of the signal intensity of the pattern of myostatin to that of $\alpha$-tublin, we can evaluate the protein translation of myostatin because the translation of $\alpha$-tublin is stable in muscle.

Figure 4 shows the ratios after the femtosecond laser irradiation (FL) and common Acupuncture stimuli (ACP), which were normalized by the ratio of mouse hind leg muscle without laser irradiation (Control). An obvious suppression of myostatin gene expression was observed in case of laser irradiation and acupuncture. In addition, Figure 5 shows the myostatin translational ratios after the femtosecond laser irradiation (FL), which were normalized by the ratio of mouse hind leg muscle without laser irradiation (Control). An obvious suppression of myostatin protein translation was observed in case of laser irradiation, too.

In the ACP treatment, skeletal muscles of the hind leg were directly stimulated by punctured. On the other hand, although the stimulation by the femtosecond laser irradiation was limited to the epidermis and dermis, as shown in Figure 2, suppression of the myostatin gene and protein were observed for the bulk of the skeletal muscle (Figures 4 and 5). As mentioned in the introduction, the photon energy absorbed by the tissue is considered to be effectively converted to energy to generate shock and stress waves [8-10]. This fact suggests that the skeletal muscle is stimulated by the propagation of shock and stress waves though the laser irradiation to the epidermis and dermis. This mechanical stimulation of the muscle facilitates muscle cell proliferation. Such shock and stress waves are generated by picosecond or nanosecond laser irradiation. However, because a great deal of photon energy is required for the generation in these cases, not only the epidermis and dermis but also skeletal muscle would have critical damage.

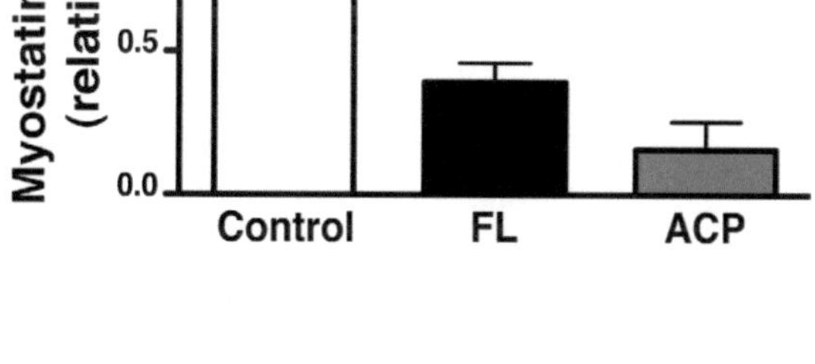


**Figure 4.** Real time-PCR analysis of myostatin gene expression after the femtosecond laser irradiation (FL) and common acupuncture stimuli (ACP). Relative transcript levels of myostatin were normalized with the signal intensity of the control. Glyceraldehyde-3-phosphate dehydrogenase (GAPDH) was used as an internal control.

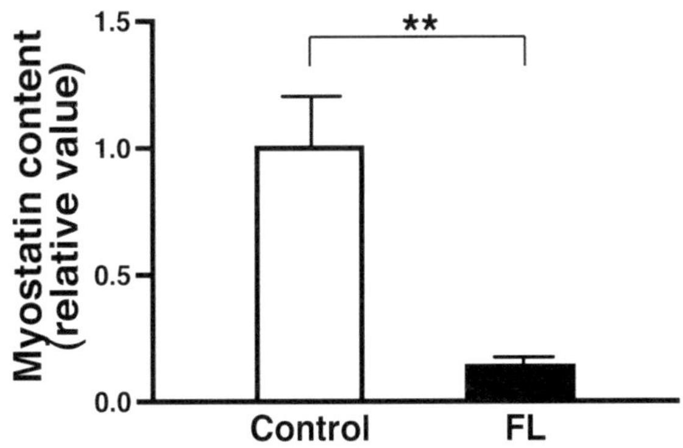


**Figure 5.** Western blotting analysis of myostatin translation under the femtosecond laser irradiation (FL) and common acupuncture (ACP). Relative protein levels of myostatin were normalized with the signal intensity of the control, and α-tublin was used as an internal control.

## 4. Conclusion

Photomechanical ablation due to femtosecond laser irradiation was induced on hind leg muscles of living mice. Although the epidermis and dermis were denatured by the laser irradiation, a direct influence due to the laser irradiation was not observed in the skeletal muscle beneath the dermis. The gene expression of myostatin of the skeletal muscle after the laser irradiation was evaluated by real time-PCR and western blotting, and obvious suppression of the myostatin were identified in the bulk of hind leg muscle. The suppression, meaning the facilitation of muscle cell proliferation, was comparable to or greater than that of the skeletal muscle after EA treatment, which is a conventional acupuncture technique. On the basis of these results, we recognize the potential of the femtosecond laser as a tool for noncontact acupuncture for the treatment of muscle disease. Since our FL technique does not require the use of needles, such infection can be avoided. Furthermore, because it is possible to scan the skin with the laser beam using an electric optical device such as a Galvano-mirror and acoustic-optical modulator, high-throughput, multipoint stimulation of muscle can be realized. We expect the present results will underscore the continuing potential of treatment by acupuncture.

## Acknowledgements

We thank Mr. Kenji Miura for his technical assistance. This work was partly supported by a Grant-in-Aid for Scientific Research (C) (grant number 22590653) and (grant number 24590884) from the Japan Society for the Promotion of Science to Y.T. and M.O.; Grant-in-Aid for Scientific Research (Innovative Areas) (grant number 22120010) from the Japan Min-

http://dx.doi.org/10.5772/54315

istry of Education, Culture, Sports, Science and Technology (MEXT) to Y.H.; a Grant-in-Aid for Challenging Exploratory Research (grant number 22657041) from MEXT to Y.H.

## Author details

Yutaka Takaoka[1,2*], Mika Ohta[1,2], Aki Sugano[1,2], Akihiko Ito[3] and Yoichiroh Hosokawa[4]

*Address all correspondence to: ytakaoka@med.kobe-u.ac.jp

1 Division of Medical Informatics and Bioinformatics, Kobe University Hospital, Chuo-ku, Kobe, Japan

2 Life Science Research Center, Kobe Tokiwa University, Nagata-ku, Kobe, Japan

3 Department of Pathology, Faculty of Medicine, Kinki University, Osaka-Sayama, Osaka, Japan

4 Graduate School of Materials Science, Nara Institute of Science and Technology (NAIST), Ikoma, Nara, Japan

## References

[1] Takaoka Y, Ohta M, Ito A, Takamatsu K, Sugano A, Funakoshi K, Takaoka N, Sato N, Yokozaki H, Arizono N, Goto S, Maeda E. Electroacupuncture suppresses myostatin gene expression: cell proliferative reaction in mouse skeletal muscle. Physiol Genomics 2007; 30: 102-110.

[2] Ohta M, Sugano A, Goto S, Yusoff S, Hirota Y, Funakoshi K, Miura K, Maeda E, Takaoka N, Sato N, Ishizuka H, Arizono N, Nishio H, Takaoka Y. Full-length sequence of mouse acupuncture-induced 1-L (aig1l) gene including its transcriptional start site. Evid Based Complement Alternat Med 2009; 2011: 249280.

[3] Ikemune S, Ohta M, Suzuki S, Machida M, Takemasa T, Takaoka Y, Miyamoto T. Electroacupuncture accelerates recovery of muscle atrophy induced by hindlimb suspension in mouse skeletal muscle (in Japanese). Journal of the Japan Society of Acupuncture and Moxibustion 2010; 60(4): 707-715.

[4] Ikemune S, Ohta M, Miyamoto T, Takaoka Y. Molecular Mechanisms of Inhibiting the Muscle Atrophy by Electroacupuncture (in Japanese). The Journal of the Japanese Society of Balneology, Climatology and Physical Medicine 2011; 74(2): 103-111.

[5] Zhang X. Acupuncture: Review and Analysis of Reports on Controlled Clinical Trials. http://apps.who.int/medicinedocs/en/d/Js4926e/ (accessed 12 August 2012)

[6] Culliton BJ. NIH says "yes" to acupuncture. Nat Med 1997; 3: 1307.

[7] Klein JL, Trachtenberg IA. Acupuncture. Current Bibliographies in Medicine 97-6 http://www.nlm.nih.gov/pubs/cbm/acupuncture.html (accessed 12 August 2012)

[8] Vogel A, Noack J, Hüttman G, Paltauf G. Mechanisms of femtosecond laser nanosurgery of cells and tissues. Applied physics B 2005; 81(8): 1015-1047.

[9] Vogel A, Venugopalan V. Mechanisms of pulsed laser ablation of biological tissues. Chem Rev 2003; 103(2): 577-644.

[10] Hosokawa Y, Yashiro M, Asahi T, Masuhara H. Photothermal conversion dynamics in femtosecond and picosecond discrete laser etching of Cu-phthalocyanine amorphous film analysed by ultrafast UV–VIS absorption spectroscopy. Journal of Photochemistry and Photobiology A: Chemistry 2001; 142: 197-207.

[11] Hosokawa Y, Takabayashi H, Miura S, Shukunami C, Hiraki Y, Masuhara H. Nondestructive isolation of single cultured animal cells by femtosecond laser-induced shockwave. Applied physics A 2004; 79(4-6): 795-798.

[12] Kaji T, Ito S, Miyasaka H, Hosokawa Y, Masuhara H, Shukunami C, Hiraki Y. Nondestructive micropatterning of living animal cells using focused femtosecond laser-induced impulsive force. Applied Physics Letters 2007; 91: 023904.

[13] Kuo Y, Wu C, Hosokawa Y, Maezawa Y, Okano K, Masuhara H, Kao F. Local stimulation of cultured myocyte cells by femtosecond laser-induced stress wave. Applied Physics A 2010; 101(4): 597-600.

[14] Hagiyama M, Furuno T, Hosokawa Y, Iino T, Ito T, Inoue T, Nakanishi M, Murakami Y, Ito A. Enhanced nerve-mast cell interaction by a neuronal short isoform of cell adhesion molecule-1. J Immunol 2011; 186(10): 5983-5992.

[15] Hosokawa Y, Hagiyama M, Iino T, Murakami Y, Ito A. Non-contact etimation of intercellular breaking force using a femtosecond laser impulse quantified by atomic force microscopy. Proceedings of the National Academy of Sciences 2011; 108: 1777-1782.

[16] Carlson CJ, Booth FW, Gordon SE. Skeletal muscle myostatin mRNA expression is fiber-type specific and increases during hindlimb unloading. Am J Physiol 1999; 277(2 Pt 2): R601-606.

[17] Trendelenburg AU, Meyer A, Rohner D, Boyle J, Hatakeyama S, Glass DJ. Myostatin reduces Akt/TORC1/p70S6K signaling, inhibiting myoblast differentiation and myotube size. Am J Physiol Cell Physiol 2009; 296(6): C1258-1270.

[18] Ministry of the Environment T, Japan. Standards Relating to the Care and Management, etc. of Experimental Animals. http://www.env.go.jp/nature/dobutsu/aigo/2_data/nt_h180428_88.html (accessed 12 August 2012)

[19] Takaoka Y, Ohta M, Miyakawa K, Nakamura O, Suzuki M, Takahashi K, Yamamura K, Sakaki Y. Cysteine 10 is a key residue in amyloidogenesis of human transthyretin Val30Met. Am J Pathol 2004; 164: 337-345.

[20] Morin LG. Creatine kinase: re-examination of optimum reaction conditions. Clin Chem 1977; 23(9): 1569-1575.

[21] Barber RD, Harmer DW, Coleman RA, Clark BJ. GAPDH as a housekeeping gene: analysis of GAPDH mRNA expression in a panel of 72 human tissues. Physiol Genomics 2005; 21: 389-395.

[22] Jemiolo B, Trappe S. Single muscle fiber gene expression in human skeletal muscle: validation of internal control with exercise. Biochem Biophys Res Commun 2004; 320: 1043-1050.

[23] Ochi E, Hirose T, Hiranuma K, Min SK, Ishii N, Nakazato K. Elevation of myostatin and FOXOs in prolonged muscular impairment induced by eccentric contractions in rat medial gastrocnemius muscle. J Appl Physiol 2010; 108(2): 306-313.

[24] Brancaccio P, Lippi G, Maffulli N. Biochemical markers of muscular damage. Clin Chem Lab Med 2010; 48(6): 757-767.

Section 3

# Acupuncture Therapy for Clinical Conditions

Chapter 11

# The Role of Acupuncture in Pain Management

Lucy Chen

Additional information is available at the end of the chapter

http://dx.doi.org/10.5772/

## 1. Introduction

Acupuncture is one of the most significant components of the healthcare system in China for more than 3,000 years. Over the last a few decades, acupuncture has garnered increasing popularity and scrutiny in Western nations. It was reported that office visits for alternative therapy were two times as many as the visits to primary care physicians in a nationwide survey in 1998. The total out-of-pocket expenditures relating to alternative therapies in 1997 were comparable to that for all US physician services, which was conservatively estimated at $27 billion [1]. This number has further increased to $33.9 billion in next 10 years [123]. Consistent with the ever-growing demand for acupuncture, an important component of complementary/ alternative medicine, FDA classified acupuncture needles as medical equipment, subject to the same strict standards for medical needles, syringes and surgical scalpels in 1996 [2]. The National Institutes of Health (NIH) organized a Consensus Development Conference on Acupuncture in 1997, which recognized that acupuncture has been extensively practiced by medical physicians, dentists, non-MD acupuncturists, and other practitioners. One of the reasons for patients seeking acupuncture treatment is the incidence of adverse effects is substantially lower than that of many drugs and commonly accepted medical procedures [3].

## 2. Traditional Chinese acupuncture theory

In the ancient theory of Chinese medicine, the human health is maintained through a delicate balance of two opposing but inseparable elements: *Yin* and *Yang*. Yin represents 'cold, slow, and passive elements', whereas Yang represents 'hot, exciting, and active elements'. Accordingly, the human internal "organs" are also divided into the Yin and Yang system. Health can be achieved by maintaining the human body in a 'balanced state of Yin and Yang'. Furthermore, this theory stipulates that *Qi* (pronounced as 'chee') is the life force or vital energy that influences health. *Qi* is thought to flow through specific pathways in a human body, so called meridians. Acupuncture involves the insertion of fine sterilized needles through the skin at specific points so-called Acupoints which mostly located in the meridians. Human body consists of 12 main meridians and 8 secondary meridians. There are also acupoints located beyond the meridians. Since the balance of the opposing forces of Yin and Yang is considered to be the basis for a healthy flow of *qi*, any imbalance would cause the disruption or blockage the flow of *qi* and lead to a state of disease or pain. Acupuncture treats a state of disease or pain through strengthening the weak *qi*; releasing the excessive *qi* or removing the blockage from the flow of qi in order to restore the normal balance of the Yin and Yang system.

## 3. Research in the mechanism of acupuncture

Although acupuncture has been used for thousands of years, its mechanism remains unclear. A large number of studies in humans and animals have demonstrated that acupuncture results in various biological effects on peripheral or central nerve system, neurohumoral factors neurotransmitters, and other chemical mediators.

*Peripheral nervous system* – Studies have showed that an intact peripheral nerve system appears to be necessary for the analgesic effects of acupuncture, because the analgesic effects can be abolished if the acupuncture site is affected by postherpetic neuralgia or intervened with local anesthetics [124,125].

*Central nervous system* -- Earlier studies showed that Electric Acupuncture (EA) at different frequencies could have different effects on the synthesis and release of neuropeptides, particularly synthesis of different opioid peptides in the central nervous system [11]. Moreover, an μ-opioid receptor antagonist or antiserum against endorphin blocked acupuncture analgesia induced by EA at 2 Hz but not at 100 Hz [12,13]. In addition, cholecystokinin-like immunoreactivity was increased within the medial thalamic area after EA [13], and EA enhanced or restored the activity of natural killer cells suppressed by the hypothalamic lesion [14].

The development in neuroimaging techniques such as functional magnetic resonance imaging (fMRI) and positron emission topographic (PET) scan has made it possible to further understand the acupuncture effects on human brain neuronal activity. Pain activates neuronal activity in periaqueductal gray (PAG), thalamus, hypothalamus, somatosensory cortex, and prefrontal cortex regions in the human brain [15], which appears to be attenuated by the sensation of 'de-qi' after acupuncture [16,17]. EA, particularly at a low frequency, produced more widespread fMRI signal changes in the anterior insula area (signal increases) as well as in the limbic and para-limbic structures (signal increases) than manual acupuncture. These findings are further supported by the data that different acupuncture points evoked a signal increase or decrease in specific areas within the central nerve system, suggesting that there might be a correlation between the effects of acupuncture and neuronal changes in the brain [18]. Other studies have also showed that neuronal responses to EA stimulation can be visualized in the rat primary somatosensory cortex using an optical imaging system [19]. This process may help understand the neural mechanisms of acupuncture treatment and Meridian phenomena [20]. Of interest to note is that using so-called 'Bi-digital O-ring Test Imaging Technique', researchers found that each meridian is connected to a representative area in the cerebral cortex, suggesting that the meridian system defined in the theories of Chinese medicine might overlap with distinct supraspinal regions [21].

*Humoral factors and Neurotransmitters* -- Scientists have found that acupuncture significantly increases the endogenous endorphin production and this effect can be blocked by the opioid receptor antagonist naloxone [4]. Humoral factors may mediate acupuncture analgesia by releasing substances into the cerebrospinal fluid after acupuncture. This notion was supported by a cross-perfusion experiment in which acupuncture-induced analgesic effects were replicated in the recipient rabbit which were not receiving acupuncture but received the cerebrospinal fluid from the donor rabbit with acupuncture treatment [5]. EA also has been shown to alter the condition of polycystic ovaries induced by steroids through the modulation of ovarian nerve growth factors [6].

In a study comparing with the sham group, EA increases the anandamide (an endogenous canabinoid) level in inflammatory skin tissues, and local pretreatment with a specific cannabinoid (CB2) receptor antagonist (AM630), significantly attenuated the antinociceptive effect of EA [7]. A presynaptic CB1 receptor likely contributes to the mechanism of the effects of EA modulating the sympathoexcitatory reflex responses in periaqueductal gray region of the brain by decreasing the release of gamma-aminobutyric acid (GABA, an inhibitory neurotransmitter), but not glutamate (an excitatory neurotransmitter) [8]. Animal study also showed that the N-Methyl-D-aspartic acid (NMDA) receptor subunit (NR2B or N-methyl D-aspartate receptor subtype 2B) was involved in the analgesic effects of EA in pain in the thyroid region by down regulating the NR2B phosphorylation level [9]. In a clinical randomized study, the local nitric oxide content in those subjects in acupuncture group was significantly higher than those in the non-acupuncture group, indicating that acupuncture stimulation can up-regulate nitric oxide content [10].

A large body of evidence indicates that acupuncture significantly affects the production and release of neurotransmitters including epinephrine, norepinephrine, dopamine, and 5-hydroxytryptamine [19]. Specifically, stress-induced increases in norepinephrine, dopamine, and corticosterone were inhibited after EA, a process that could be blocked by naloxone, suggesting that the EA effects on the release of neurotransmitters are likely to be mediated through endogenous opioids [22]. Similar results were observed in other animal studies of acupuncture analgesia [23-27]. The functional significance of acupuncture-induced changes in neurotransmitters was clearly indicated in a number of studies. For instance, EA at different frequencies (2, 10, or 100 Hz) elicited the analgesic effects and such effects could be at least partially blocked by a serotonin receptor antagonist [28]. Many brainstem regions could be selectively activated by EA at both 4 Hz and 100 Hz, whereas other regions could only be activated by EA at 4 Hz [29]. Importantly, the selective supraspinal activation by EA at difference frequencies may be related to the neurotransmitter release resulting from EA at a particular frequency. For instance, the analgesic effect from EA at 4 Hz was mediated through endogenous opioids [29], while the analgesic effect from EA at 2 Hz may involve substance P as its mediator [30].

Besides its effect on acupuncture analgesia, the EA-induced modulation of neurotransmitter release may also mediate other therapeutic effects of acupuncture. There is evidence that EA at 100Hz could protect axotomized dopaminergic neurons from degeneration by suppressing the axotomy-induced inflammatory response [31], raising the possibility that acupuncture may be used to treat certain neurological disorders such as Parkinson's disease [32]. Another example is that the excitatory effects on gastrointestinal mobility following EA or moxibustion in rats could be abolished by serotonin inhibitors [33], suggesting that serotonin may be a critical mediator of acupuncture regardless of its effects on gastric emptying or analgesia. Similarly, the reduced production of nitric oxide within the gracile nucleus after acupuncture has been considered to mediate the effect of acupuncture on reversing bradycardia [34].

## 4. Clinical research data on acupuncture

While acupuncture has become popular among patients and medical professionals, there is still debate regarding its application and overall efficacy. The challenges that we faced in clinical trials of the efficacy of acupuncture have their unique issues such as placebo controls, crossover design, and the individualization. It is encouraging to see that more controlled, randomize clinical studies of acupuncture have replaced the bulk of anecdotal case reports. The increasing numbers of clinical trials on acupuncture treatments have provided more information, particularly on the role of acupuncture in clinical pain management.

### 4.1. Low back pain

Chronic low back pain is a very common health problem associated with high medical expenses and disability. An estimated 70% of individuals in western countries have back pain sometime in their lifetime. Patients with back pain account for more than $90 billion in health care expenses every year [35]. Although there are many medical treatment options, long-term effects from these medical treatments remain limited. Recently, acupuncture has become one of the most frequently used alternative therapies in treating low back pain. In a randomized, placebo-controlled clinical trial with a 9 month follow up period, 131 patients with non-radiating low back pain for at least 6 months were divided into three groups for treatment of 12 weeks: control (only received physical therapy), acupuncture, or sham acupuncture (received 20 sessions of either acupuncture or sham acupuncture in addition to physical therapy. The results indicate that acupuncture was superior to physical therapy regarding pain intensity, pain-related disability, and psychological distress. When compared with sham acupuncture, acupuncture was also superior in the reduction of psychological stress [36].

In another study, the benefit from 8 weeks of acupuncture treatment on low back pain in 50 patients lasted up to 6 months in many aspects including returning to work, quality of sleep, and reduced use of analgesics [37]. The duration of acupuncture in a single session appeared to be an independent parameter to a treatment outcome. For example, a 30-min acupuncture session was more effective than a 15-min session, whereas a 45-min session did not further improve the outcome [38]. Similar finding was also been found in electrical acupuncture stimulation using percutaneously placed needles in 30-min and 45-min durations produced similar improvements in the visual analog pain scale, physical activity, quality of sleep scores, and a reduction in the oral analgesic requirements, which is better than 0 (no treatment) or 15-min duration [39]. Of interest to note is that both acupuncture and transcutaneous electrical stimulation (TENS) showed significant effects on pain reduction, although acupuncture appeared to be more effective than TENS in the improvement of lumbar spine range of motion [40].

In a recently conducted large study involved 1162 patients with chronic low back pain, acupuncture therapy improved low back pain for at least 6 months. The effectiveness of acupuncture, either verum (47.6%) or sham (44.2%), was almost twice that of conventional therapy (27.4%) [41]. In another large-scale clinical trial, 3,093 patients with chronic low back pain were recruited randomly into two groups: acupuncture and conventional medical care. Back function (Hannover Functional Ability Questionnaire), pain, and quality of life were assessed at the baseline and 3 and 6 months of duration. In addition, the cost-effectiveness was also analyzed. The results showed that acupuncture plus routine care was associated with a marked clinical improvement in these patients and was relatively cost-effective [42]. Overall, the clinical practice guideline from American College of Physicians and the American Pain Society for chronic low back pain patients recommend physicians to consider acupuncture as an addition of nonpharmacologic therapy with proven benefits for low back pain [43, 44].

### 4.2. Chronic neck and shoulder pain

There are promising results on the treatment of chronic neck and shoulder pain using acupuncture. In one study, the acupuncture treatment reduced chronic pain in neck and shoulders for at least three years with a concomitant improvement in depression, anxiety, sleep quality, pain-related activity impairment, and quality of life [39, 45, 46]. Several other clinical trials of acupuncture on chronic neck pain with sample sizes from 115 to 177 patients also have positive results. These studies demonstrated that acupuncture was superior to controls in reducing neck pain and improving the overall range of motion [47-51]. Moreover, in patients with balance disorders caused by cervical torsion after whiplash injuries, acupuncture has been shown to be effective in treating their symptoms [52].

Another study compared the treatment effect of acupuncture combining with physical therapy to that of acupuncture or physical therapy alone for patients with neck pain due to neck tension syndrome. All groups showed significant improvement after 10 weeks of treatment, but the group receiving a combination of acupuncture and physical therapy was superior in pain reduction and function disability improvement than other groups with acupuncture or physical therapy alone. The improvements of all groups were maintained ($p < 0.05$) at the 6 months of follow-up. The data suggest that acupuncture treatment may assist and/or enhance the physiotherapy effect on musculoskeletal rehabilitation for tension neck syndrome [53].

Chronic myofascial neck pain has been frequently treated with trigger point injection either with local anesthetics or using dry needling technique. One prospective, randomized, double-blind, sham-controlled crossover study compared acupuncture, sham acupuncture and dry needling of local myofascial trigger points in patients with chronic neck pain and limited cervical spine function. Acupuncture showed better results in reducing motion-related pain and improving range of motion [54]. For neck pain induced by cervical spondylosis, one study enrolled 106 subjects and randomly divided these subjects into real acupuncture group and control sham acupuncture group. The effective rate was 75.5% in the acupuncture group and 52.8% in the control group ($P<0.05$) [55]. To investigate the effectiveness of acupuncture in addition to routine care as compared to routine care alone in patients with chronic neck pain, a randomized controlled multi-center trial was conducted in Germany. A total of 14,161 patients with chronic neck pain (duration >6 months) were randomized to an acupuncture group (1,880 subjects; 15 acupuncture sessions over 3 months) or a control group receiving no acupuncture (1,886 subjects). In addition, 10,395 patients were included in a non-randomized acupuncture group. The results showed a significant improvement in neck pain and disability in the randomized acupuncture group ($P<0.001$). Of interest, patients in the non-randomized acupuncture group had more severe symptoms at baseline but showed more neck pain and disability improvement as compared to the randomized patients, suggesting a possible placebo effect. This large scale clinic trial demonstrates that integrating acupuncture with routine medical care in patients with chronic neck pain may result in both pain improvement and a reduction of disability [56].

In two meta-analysis studies with 10 to 14 clinical trials included, there was moderate evidence that acupuncture was more effective for pain relief than some types of sham controls or inactive, sham treatments, when measured immediately after the treatment and at short-term follow-up (pooled standardized mean differences, -0.37; 95% confidence interval, -0.61 to -0.12). There was limited evidence that acupuncture was more effective than massage at short-term follow-up. Overall, the short-term effectiveness and efficacy of acupuncture in the treatment of neck pain appear to be present [57, 58]. However, the cost-effectiveness of additional acupuncture treatment in patients with chronic neck pain as compared to patients receiving routine care alone remains to be determined. More interestingly, another study with a total of 3,451 patients (1,753 acupuncture-group, 1,698 control-group), acupuncture treatment was associated with higher costs over the first 3 months duration as compared to routine care. This cost increase was mainly due to the costs of acupuncture. Private medical expenses such as over the counter medication were not included. Beyond the 3 months study duration, acupuncture might be associated with further health economic effects. According to international cost-effectiveness threshold values, the conclusion of this study is that acupuncture is a cost-effective treatment strategy in patients with chronic neck Pain [59].

### 4.3. Headache

Even with the recent advancement in the diagnosis and treatment of different headache disorders, many patients with headaches are still suffering due to lack of effective treatment. Selective serotonin receptor agonists such as sumatriptan type medications have effectively treated millions migraine sufferers, there are still at least 30% of migraine patients who do not respond to such treatment. Alternatively, acupuncture has become a new modality of treatment for those patients suffering from tension headache, migraine, and other types of headaches [125]. In a multi-center study, 302 patients suffering from migraine headache were randomized into three groups (acupuncture, minimal acupuncture and waiting list). The trial found a significant effect of those treated with acupuncture and minimal acupuncture as compared to those on the waiting list for treatment [60]. Many other headache studies either with tension headache or migraine headache, with a sample size from 50 to 2,022 patients, also showed similar results [61-70]. According to international cost-effectiveness threshold values, acupuncture is a cost-effective treatment in patients with primary headache [71]. Moreover, the pediatric patient population also benefits from this alternative therapy for headache treatment [72]. For many patients, acupuncture not only has a similar, if not better, efficacy as compared with sumatriptan in preventing full migraine attack, acupuncture has unique benefits over sumatriptan-related medications because of its negligible side effects [67].

As a prophylactic measure of migraine without aura, acupuncture treatment for 2-4 months significantly reduced the number of migraine attacks comparing to oral therapy with flunarizine [73]. In a comprehensive review, 27 clinical trials were included to evaluate the efficacy of acupuncture in the treatment of primary headaches (migraine headache, tension headache, and mixed forms). The result revealed that the majority of trials (23 out of 27 trials) showed favorable outcomes in the treatment of headaches using acupuncture [74]. Another review included eleven trials with 2317 participants examined whether acupuncture is a) more effective than no prophylactic treatment/routine care only; b) more effective than 'sham' (placebo) acupuncture; and c) as effective as other interventions in reducing headache frequency in patients with episodic or chronic tension-type headache. The authors found that acupuncture treatment has statistically significant and clinically relevant short-term (up to 3 months) benefits over control in terms of the number of headache days and pain intensity. Small but statistically significant benefits of acupuncture over sham were also found. The authors conclude that acupuncture could be a valuable non-pharmacological tool in patients with frequent episodic or chronic tension-type headaches [75]. In another systemic review of 22 trials of 4,419 participants, there is consistent evidence that acupuncture provides additional benefit to treatment of acute migraine attacks as compared to routine care only [76]. However, more research is needed to investigate the treatment of specific tension-type headache subtypes [77].

## 5. Other pain conditions

Acupuncture has been used to treat many other pain conditions. Several studies have shown that patients who received acupuncture prior to operation had a lower pain level, reduced opioid requirement, a lower incidence of postoperative nausea and vomiting, and lower sympathoadrenal responses [78-81]. In another study of acupuncture treatment for labor pain, parturients who received acupuncture during labor significantly reduced the need of epidural analgesia with a better degree of relaxation but without a negative effect on delivery as compare with a control group [82-83]. Another active area of clinical acupuncture is the treatment of osteoarthritis of the knee. Acupuncture has been shown to provide some improvement in function and pain relief when compared with sham acupuncture or control groups using education [84]. In addition, the benefit of acupuncture treatment in fibromyalgia and rheumatoid arthritis is supported by several clinical trials, albeit in a small scale, suggesting that the large-scale clinical trials on these pain conditions may be warranted [85]. Similarly, chronic lateral epicondylitis (tennis elbow) may benefit from the acupuncture treatment in part due to the effect of acupuncture on the range of motion and reduction in pain on exertion [86]. In some cases, the effects of acupuncture on tennis elbow lasted up to one year after ten sessions of acupuncture [87].

## 6. Other uses of acupuncture

Besides its analgesic effects, acupuncture has been used for the treatment of many other conditions. For example, a number of clinical trials strongly support a therapeutic role of acupuncture (either needle acupuncture or applying acupressure to the relevant acupoints) in postoperative nausea and vomiting as compare with antiemetics such as droperidol and zolfran [88-94]. An increasing number of patients are turning to acupuncture either to supplement or replace their conventional treatments for many medical conditions including allergy, asthma, depression, anxiety, obesity, insomnia, cancer-related fatigue, premenstrual syndrome, menopause symptoms, assist conception and infertility, spinal cord injury, quitting smoking and detoxification from opioids or other drug addiction [95-117]. Table 1 lists a summary published in 2002 by the World Health Organization (WHO) for clinical pain conditions recommended for acupuncture [126].

## 7. Possible complications of acupuncture

Acupuncture has significantly lower complication rate comparing to many other medical treatment. The 1997 NIH consensus panel on acupuncture stated that the documented occurrence of adverse events in practice of acupuncture has been extremely low. The most commonly reported complication is bruising or bleeding at the needle insertion site, followed by the incidence of a transient vaso-vagal response. Other rare complications include infection, dermatitis and broken needle fragments. In one prospective large-scale survey with 34,407 acupuncture treatments in the UK, no serious adverse events were reported that required hospital admission, prolonging hospital stays, permanently disabling, or death. A total of 43 minor adverse events were reported (0.13%), including severe nausea and actual fainting, unexpected, severe and prolonged aggravation of symptoms, prolonged and unacceptable pain and bruising and psychological and emotional reactions [118]. Another survey conducted in the UK with a total of 31,822 acupuncture treatments also found only 43 minor adverse events, a rate of 14 per 10,000 treatments (0.14%). Other minor adverse events can be avoided such as patients being left unattended, needles being left in patients, cellulites and moxa burns [119]. When compared with medications routinely prescribed in the primary care setting, acupuncture is a relatively safe treatment modality. However, since acupuncture is an invasive medical intervention, serious complications such as pneumothorax, hemathorax, internal organ puncture, and pericardial effusion could happen if the treatment is not properly administered [120]. Some of these more serious complications generally occur in elderly and more fragile and debilitated patients with complex comorbidities or in the hands of less skilled practitioners. Thus, it is imperative that the acupuncture licensing and regulation mandate the use of standards of acupuncture training through adopting strict requirement for the knowledge of anatomy and sterile techniques.

## 8. Perspectives and future directions

Alone with the popularity of the acupuncture in recent years, an increasing number of physicians have integrated acupuncture into their practices. Many medical schools in the USA have already added topic courses of integrated medicine [121]. One recent survey of physicians regarding acupuncture use in their practice showed that an overwhelming majority of survey responders have a positive attitude and favorable experience with using acupuncture as an alternative modality for chronic pain management. However, the lack of insurance coverage and facility for acupuncture treatment are two primary barriers of acupuncture referrals. [122]. To face the ever-growing healthcare cost in the USA, more health insurance providers have begun to emphasize preventive and alternative measures. Third-party reimbursements for alternative therapies also have increased because of the demand from an increasing patient population. Accordingly, the National Center for Complementary and Alternative Medicine (NCCAM) has funded a good number of research projects related to acupuncture.

In the face of the positive development in the use of acupuncture as an alternative treatment modality, the current clinical research on acupuncture treatment is still challenged by a number of issues. First, although many studies on acupuncture treatment have been published, the scientific merits of these studies may be limited by the study design and non-standardized acupuncture practices. Second, it may be difficult to keep true blindness to patients in a clinical trial. Third, Non-specific needling (i.e. placing an acupuncture needle at an acupoint not intended for the treatment of the condition) or sham needling may elicit responses similar to responses to active acupuncture treatment, making it difficult to interpret the trial results. In this regard, it will be difficult to exclude a placebo effect in many clinical acupuncture trials. Fourth, in clinical setting, acupuncture treatment is often highly individualized for a given clinical condition, which varies from one practitioner to another. As such, it would be rather difficult to compare the treatment outcomes in different clinical trials if a given clinical condition were treated with various parameters including acupuncture points, needling techniques, electrical versus manual, duration of acupuncture in one session, and between-session intervals etc. Nonetheless, efforts should be made to standardize acupuncture clinical trials in order to improve the scientific merits of clinical trials. It can be anticipated that complementary medicine including acupuncture is likely to play a growing and positive role in pain management.

| Diseases, symptoms or conditions for which acupuncture has been shown to be effective | Diseases, symptoms or conditions for which the therapeutic effect of acupuncture remains to be determined |
|---|---|
| Headache | Abdominal pain (acute gastroenteritis or acute cute gastrointestinal spasm) |
| Knee pain | Cancer pain |
| Low back pain | Earache |
| Neck pain | Eye pain due to sub-conjunctival injection |
| Dental pain | Fibromyalgia and fasciitis |
| Facial pain and craniomandibular dysfunction | Labor pain |
| Postoperative pain | Pain due to endoscopic examination |
| Rheumatoid arthritis | Pain due to thrombtic angiitis obliteran |
| Periarthritis of shoulder | Chronic prostatitis |
| Renal colic | Pruritus |
| Tennis elbow | Radicular and pseudoradicular syndrome |
| Sciatica | Reflex sympathetic dystrophy |
| Sprain | Acute spine pain |
| | Stiff neck |
| | Temporomandibular dysfunction |

**Table 1.**

## Author details

Lucy Chen*

Address all correspondence to: llchen@partners.org

MGH Center for Translational Pain Research, MGH Center for Pain Medicine, Department of Anesthesia, Critical Care and Pain Medicine, Massachusetts General Hospital, Harvard Medical School, Boston, USA

## References

[1] Eisenberg DM, Davis RB, Ettner SL, et al. Trends in alternative medicine use in the united states, 1990-1997: Results of a follow-up national survey. JAMA. 1998;280(18): 1569-1575.

[2] Turner JS. The regulation of acupuncture needles by the united states food and drug administration. J Altern Complement Med. 1995;1(1):15-16.

[3] NIH consensus conference. acupuncture. JAMA. 1998;280(17):1518-1524.

[4] Mayer DJ, Price DD, Rafii A. Antagonism of acupuncture analgesia in man by the narcotic antagonist naloxone. Brain Res. 1977;121(2):368-372.

[5] Han JS, Terenius L. Neurochemical basis of acupuncture analgesia. Annu Rev Pharmacol Toxicol. 1982;22:193-220.

[6] Stener-Victorin E, Lundeberg T, Cajander S, et al. Steroid-induced polycystic ovaries in rats: Effect of electro-acupuncture on concentrations of endothelin-1 and nerve growth factor (NGF), and expression of NGF mRNA in the ovaries, the adrenal glands, and the central nervous system. Reprod Biol Endocrinol. 2003;1:33.

[7] Chen L, Zhang J, Li F, et al. Endogenous anandamide and cannabinoid receptor-2 contribute to electroacupuncture analgesia in rats. J Pain. 2009;10(7):732-739.

[8] Fu LW, Longhurst JC. Electroacupuncture modulates vlPAG release of GABA through presynaptic cannabinoid CB1 receptors. J Appl Physiol. 2009;106(6): 1800-1809.

[9] Gao YH, Chen SP, Wang JY, Qiao LN, Xu QL, Liu JL. Effects of electroacupuncture at different acupoints on the pain behavior and NMDA receptor 2 B subunit mRNA and protein expression and phosphorylation level in the cervical spinal cord in rats with thyroid regional pain. Zhen Ci Yan Jiu. 2009;34(6):376-382.

[10] Ben H, Li L, Gao XY, He W, Rong PJ. Comparison of NO contents and cutaneous electric conduction quantity at the acupoints and the non-acupoints. Zhen Ci Yan Jiu. 2009;34(6):383-6, 392.

[11] Guo HF, Wang XM, Tian JH, Huo YP, Han JS. 2 hz and 100 hz electroacupuncture accelerate the expression of genes encoding three opioid peptides in the rat brain. Sheng Li Xue Bao. 1997;49(2):121-127.

[12] Huang C, Wang Y, Chang JK, Han JS. Endomorphin and mu-opioid receptors in mouse brain mediate the analgesic effect induced by 2 hz but not 100 hz electroacupuncture stimulation. Neurosci Lett. 2000;294(3):159-162.

[13] Xu M, Aiuchi T, Nakaya K, et al. Effect of low-frequency electric stimulation on in vivo release of cholecystokinin-like immunoreactivity in medial thalamus of conscious rat. Neurosci Lett. 1990;118(2):205-207.

[14] Hahm ET, Lee JJ, Lee WK, Bae HS, Min BI, Cho YW. Electroacupuncture enhancement of natural killer cell activity suppressed by anterior hypothalamic lesions in rats. Neuroimmunomodulation. 2004;11(4):268-272.

[15] Hui KK, Liu J, Marina O, et al. The integrated response of the human cerebro-cerebellar and limbic systems to acupuncture stimulation at ST 36 as evidenced by fMRI. Neuroimage. 2005;27(3):479-496.

[16] Hsieh JC, Stahle-Backdahl M, Hagermark O, Stone-Elander S, Rosenquist G, Ingvar M. Traumatic nociceptive pain activates the hypothalamus and the periaqueductal gray: A positron emission tomography study. Pain. 1996;64(2):303-314.

[17] Napadow V, Makris N, Liu J, Kettner NW, Kwong KK, Hui KK. Effects of electroacupuncture versus manual acupuncture on the human brain as measured by fMRI. Hum Brain Mapp. 2005;24(3):193-205.

[18] Yan B, Li K, Xu J, et al. Acupoint-specific fMRI patterns in human brain. Neurosci Lett. 2005;383(3):236-240.

[19] Hou JG, Liu HL, He TX, et al. Study of the acupuncture effect on monoamine transmitters in rabbit plasma and brain tissue by high performance liquid chromatography with electrochemical detection. Se Pu. 2002;20(2):140-143.

[20] Chae Y, Park HJ, Hahm DH, Lee BH, Park HK, Lee H. Spatiotemporal patterns of neural activity in response to electroacupuncture stimulation in the rodent primary somatosensory cortex. Neurol Res. 2010;32 Suppl 1:64-68.

[21] Omura Y. Connections found between each meridian (heart, stomach, triple burner, etc.) & organ representation area of corresponding internal organs in each side of the cerebral cortex; release of common neurotransmitters and hormones unique to each meridian and corresponding acupuncture point & internal organ after acupuncture, electrical stimulation, mechanical stimulation (including shiatsu), soft laser stimulation or QI gong. Acupunct Electrother Res. 1989;14(2):155-186.

[22] Han SH, Yoon SH, Cho YW, Kim CJ, Min BI. Inhibitory effects of electroacupuncture on stress responses evoked by tooth-pulp stimulation in rats. Physiol Behav. 1999;66(2):217-222.

[23] Zhou Y, Wang Y, Fang Z, et al. Influence of acupuncture on blood pressure, contents of NE, DA and 5-HT of SHR and the interrelation between blood pressure and whole blood viscosity. Zhen Ci Yan Jiu. 1995;20(3):55-61.

[24] Wang H, Jiang J, Can X. Changes of norepinephrine release in rat's nucleus reticularis paragigantocellularis lateralis in acupuncture analgesia. Zhen Ci Yan Jiu. 1994;19(1):20-25.

[25] Wang Y, Wang S, Zhang W. Effects of naloxone on the changes of pain threshold and contents of monoamine neurotransmitters in rat brain induced by EA. J Tradit Chin Med. 1991;11(4):286-290.

[26] Zhu J, Xia Y, Cao X. Effects of noradrenaline and dopamine in preoptic area on acupuncture analgesia. Zhen Ci Yan Jiu. 1990;15(2):117-122.

[27] Zhu JM, He XP, Cao XD. Changes of releases of beta-endorphin-like immunoreactive substances and noradrenaline in rabbit's preoptic area during acupuncture analgesia. Sheng Li Xue Bao. 1990;42(2):188-193.

[28] Chang FC, Tsai HY, Yu MC, Yi PL, Lin JG. The central serotonergic system mediates the analgesic effect of electroacupuncture on ZUSANLI (ST36) acupoints. J Biomed Sci. 2004;11(2):179-185.

[29] Lee JH, Beitz AJ. The distribution of brain-stem and spinal cord nuclei associated with different frequencies of electroacupuncture analgesia. Pain. 1993;52(1):11-28.

[30] Shen S, Bian JT, Tian JB, Han JS. Frequency dependence of substance P release by electroacupuncture in rat spinal cord. Sheng Li Xue Bao. 1996;48(1):89-93.

[31] Liu XY, Zhou HF, Pan YL, et al. Electro-acupuncture stimulation protects dopaminergic neurons from inflammation-mediated damage in medial forebrain bundle-transected rats. Exp Neurol. 2004;189(1):189-196.

[32] Park HJ, Lim S, Joo WS, et al. Acupuncture prevents 6-hydroxydopamine-induced neuronal death in the nigrostriatal dopaminergic system in the rat parkinson's disease model. Exp Neurol. 2003;180(1):93-98.

[33] Sugai GC, Freire Ade O, Tabosa A, Yamamura Y, Tufik S, Mello LE. Serotonin involvement in the electroacupuncture- and moxibustion-induced gastric emptying in rats. Physiol Behav. 2004;82(5):855-861.

[34] Chen S, Ma SX. Nitric oxide in the gracile nucleus mediates depressor response to acupuncture (ST36). J Neurophysiol. 2003;90(2):780-785.

[35] Berman BM, Langevin HM, Witt CM, Dubner R. Acupuncture for chronic low back pain. N Engl J Med. 2010;363(5):454-461.

[36] Leibing E, Leonhardt U, Koster G, et al. Acupuncture treatment of chronic low-back pain -- a randomized, blinded, placebo-controlled trial with 9-month follow-up. Pain. 2002;96(1-2):189-196.

[37] Molsberger AF, Mau J, Pawelec DB, Winkler J. Does acupuncture improve the orthopedic management of chronic low back pain--a randomized, blinded, controlled trial with 3 months follow up. Pain. 2002;99(3):579-587.

[38] Grant DJ, Bishop-Miller J, Winchester DM, Anderson M, Faulkner S. A randomized comparative trial of acupuncture versus transcutaneous electrical nerve stimulation for chronic back pain in the elderly. Pain. 1999;82(1):9-13.

[39] Hamza MA, Ghoname EA, White PF, et al. Effect of the duration of electrical stimulation on the analgesic response in patients with low back pain. Anesthesiology. 1999;91(6):1622-1627.

[40] Carlsson CP, Sjolund BH. Acupuncture for chronic low back pain: A randomized placebo-controlled study with long-term follow-up. Clin J Pain. 2001;17(4):296-305.

[41] Haake M, Muller HH, Schade-Brittinger C, et al. German acupuncture trials (GERAC) for chronic low back pain: Randomized, multicenter, blinded, parallel-group trial with 3 groups. Arch Intern Med. 2007;167(17):1892-1898.

[42] Witt CM, Jena S, Selim D, et al. Pragmatic randomized trial evaluating the clinical and economic effectiveness of acupuncture for chronic low back pain. Am J Epidemiol. 2006;164(5):487-496.

[43] Chou R, Huffman LH, American Pain Society, American College of Physicians. Nonpharmacologic therapies for acute and chronic low back pain: A review of the evidence for an american pain Society/American college of physicians clinical practice guideline. Ann Intern Med. 2007;147(7):492-504.

[44] Chou R, Qaseem A, Snow V, et al. Diagnosis and treatment of low back pain: A joint clinical practice guideline from the american college of physicians and the american pain society. Ann Intern Med. 2007;147(7):478-491.

[45] He D, Veiersted KB, Hostmark AT, Medbo JI. Effect of acupuncture treatment on chronic neck and shoulder pain in sedentary female workers: A 6-month and 3-year follow-up study. Pain. 2004;109(3):299-307.

[46] He D, Hostmark AT, Veiersted KB, Medbo JI. Effect of intensive acupuncture on pain-related social and psychological variables for women with chronic neck and shoulder pain--an RCT with six month and three year follow up. Acupunct Med. 2005;23(2):52-61.

[47] White P, Lewith G, Prescott P, Conway J. Acupuncture versus placebo for the treatment of chronic mechanical neck pain: A randomized, controlled trial. Ann Intern Med. 2004;141(12):911-919.

[48] Blossfeldt P. Acupuncture for chronic neck pain--a cohort study in an NHS pain clinic. Acupunct Med. 2004;22(3):146-151.

[49] Konig A, Radke S, Molzen H, et al. Randomised trial of acupuncture compared with conventional massage and "sham" laser acupuncture for treatment of chronic neck pain - range of motion analysis. Z Orthop Ihre Grenzgeb. 2003;141(4):395-400.

[50] Giles LG, Muller R. Chronic spinal pain: A randomized clinical trial comparing medication, acupuncture, and spinal manipulation. Spine (Phila Pa 1976). 2003;28(14): 1490-502; discussion 1502-3.

[51] Irnich D, Behrens N, Molzen H, et al. Randomised trial of acupuncture compared with conventional massage and "sham" laser acupuncture for treatment of chronic neck pain. BMJ. 2001;322(7302):1574-1578.

[52] Fattori B, Ursino F, Cingolani C, Bruschini L, Dallan I, Nacci A. Acupuncture treatment of whiplash injury. Int Tinnitus J. 2004;10(2):156-160.

[53] Franca DL, Senna-Fernandes V, Cortez CM, Jackson MN, Bernardo-Filho M, Guimaraes MA. Tension neck syndrome treated by acupuncture combined with physiotherapy: A comparative clinical trial (pilot study). Complement Ther Med. 2008;16(5): 268-277.

[54] Irnich D, Behrens N, Gleditsch JM, et al. Immediate effects of dry needling and acupuncture at distant points in chronic neck pain: Results of a randomized, double-blind, sham-controlled crossover trial. Pain. 2002;99(1-2):83-89.

[55] Liang ZH, Yang YH, Yu P, et al. Logistic regression analysis on therapeutic effect of acupuncture on neck pain caused by cervical spondylosis and factors influencing therapeutic effect. Zhongguo Zhen Jiu. 2009;29(3):173-176.

[56] Witt CM, Jena S, Brinkhaus B, Liecker B, Wegscheider K, Willich SN. Acupuncture for patients with chronic neck pain. Pain. 2006;125(1-2):98-106.

[57] Fu LM, Li JT, Wu WS. Randomized controlled trials of acupuncture for neck pain: Systematic review and meta-analysis. J Altern Complement Med. 2009;15(2):133-145.

[58] Trinh K, Graham N, Gross A, et al. Acupuncture for neck disorders. Spine (Phila Pa 1976). 2007;32(2):236-243.

[59] Willich SN, Reinhold T, Selim D, Jena S, Brinkhaus B, Witt CM. Cost-effectiveness of acupuncture treatment in patients with chronic neck pain. Pain. 2006;125(1-2):107-113.

[60] Linde K, Streng A, Hoppe A, et al. Treatment in a randomized multicenter trial of acupuncture for migraine (ART migraine). Forsch Komplementmed. 2006;13(2): 101-108.

[61] Coeytaux RR, Kaufman JS, Kaptchuk TJ, et al. A randomized, controlled trial of acupuncture for chronic daily headache. Headache. 2005;45(9):1113-1123.

[62] Ebneshahidi NS, Heshmatipour M, Moghaddami A, Eghtesadi-Araghi P. The effects of laser acupuncture on chronic tension headache--a randomised controlled trial. Acupunct Med. 2005;23(1):13-18.

[63] Endres HG, Bowing G, Diener HC, et al. Acupuncture for tension-type headache: A multicentre, sham-controlled, patient-and observer-blinded, randomised trial. J Headache Pain. 2007;8(5):306-314.

[64] Endres HG, Diener HC, Molsberger A. Role of acupuncture in the treatment of migraine. Expert Rev Neurother. 2007;7(9):1121-1134.

[65] Facco E, Liguori A, Petti F, et al. Traditional acupuncture in migraine: A controlled, randomized study. Headache. 2008;48(3):398-407.

[66] Melchart D, Streng A, Hoppe A, et al. Acupuncture in patients with tension-type headache: Randomised controlled trial. BMJ. 2005;331(7513):376-382.

[67] Melchart D, Thormaehlen J, Hager S, Liao J, Linde K, Weidenhammer W. Acupuncture versus placebo versus sumatriptan for early treatment of migraine attacks: A randomized controlled trial. J Intern Med. 2003;253(2):181-188.

[68] Streng A, Linde K, Hoppe A, et al. Effectiveness and tolerability of acupuncture compared with metoprolol in migraine prophylaxis. Headache. 2006;46(10):1492-1502.

[69] Wang K, Svensson P, Arendt-Nielsen L. Effect of acupuncture-like electrical stimulation on chronic tension-type headache: A randomized, double-blinded, placebo-controlled trial. Clin J Pain. 2007;23(4):316-322.

[70] Melchart D, Weidenhammer W, Streng A, Hoppe A, Pfaffenrath V, Linde K. Acupuncture for chronic headaches--an epidemiological study. Headache. 2006;46(4): 632-641.

[71] Witt CM, Reinhold T, Jena S, Brinkhaus B, Willich SN. Cost-effectiveness of acupuncture treatment in patients with headache. Cephalalgia. 2008;28(4):334-345.

[72] Gottschling S, Meyer S, Gribova I, et al. Laser acupuncture in children with headache: A double-blind, randomized, bicenter, placebo-controlled trial. Pain. 2008;137(2):405-412.

[73] Allais G, De Lorenzo C, Quirico PE, et al. Acupuncture in the prophylactic treatment of migraine without aura: A comparison with flunarizine. Headache. 2002;42(9): 855-861.

[74] Manias P, Tagaris G, Karageorgiou K. Acupuncture in headache: A critical review. Clin J Pain. 2000;16(4):334-339.

[75] Linde K, Allais G, Brinkhaus B, Manheimer E, Vickers A, White AR. Acupuncture for tension-type headache. Cochrane Database Syst Rev. 2009;(1)(1):CD007587.

[76] Linde K, Allais G, Brinkhaus B, Manheimer E, Vickers A, White AR. Acupuncture for migraine prophylaxis. Cochrane Database Syst Rev. 2009;(1)(1):CD001218.

[77] Davis MA, Kononowech RW, Rolin SA, Spierings EL. Acupuncture for tension-type headache: A meta-analysis of randomized, controlled trials. J Pain. 2008;9(8):667-677.

[78] Kotani N, Hashimoto H, Sato Y, et al. Preoperative intradermal acupuncture reduces postoperative pain, nausea and vomiting, analgesic requirement, and sympathoadrenal responses. Anesthesiology. 2001;95(2):349-356.

[79] Lin JG, Lo MW, Wen YR, Hsieh CL, Tsai SK, Sun WZ. The effect of high and low frequency electroacupuncture in pain after lower abdominal surgery. Pain. 2002;99(3): 509-514.

[80] Sim CK, Xu PC, Pua HL, Zhang G, Lee TL. Effects of electroacupuncture on intraoperative and postoperative analgesic requirement. Acupunct Med. 2002;20(2-3):56-65.

[81] Wang SM, Kain ZN. P6 acupoint injections are as effective as droperidol in controlling early postoperative nausea and vomiting in children. Anesthesiology. 2002;97(2): 359-366.

[82] Ramnero A, Hanson U, Kihlgren M. Acupuncture treatment during labour--a randomised controlled trial. BJOG. 2002;109(6):637-644.

[83] Skilnand E, Fossen D, Heiberg E. Acupuncture in the management of pain in labor. Acta Obstet Gynecol Scand. 2002;81(10):943-948.

[84] Berman BM, Lao L, Langenberg P, Lee WL, Gilpin AM, Hochberg MC. Effectiveness of acupuncture as adjunctive therapy in osteoarthritis of the knee: A randomized, controlled trial. Ann Intern Med. 2004;141(12):901-910.

[85] Berman BM, Swyers JP, Ezzo J. The evidence for acupuncture as a treatment for rheumatologic conditions. Rheum Dis Clin North Am. 2000;26(1):103-15, ix-x.

[86] Tsui P, Leung MC. Comparison of the effectiveness between manual acupuncture and electro-acupuncture on patients with tennis elbow. Acupunct Electrother Res. 2002;27(2):107-117.

[87] Fink M, Wolkenstein E, Luennemann M, Gutenbrunner C, Gehrke A, Karst M. Chronic epicondylitis: Effects of real and sham acupuncture treatment: A randomised controlled patient- and examiner-blinded long-term trial. Forsch Komplementarmed Klass Naturheilkd. 2002;9(4):210-215.

[88] Alkaissi A, Evertsson K, Johnsson VA, Ofenbartl L, Kalman S. P6 acupressure may relieve nausea and vomiting after gynecological surgery: An effectiveness study in 410 women. Can J Anaesth. 2002;49(10):1034-1039.

[89] Allen DL, Kitching AJ, Nagle C. P6 acupressure and nausea and vomiting after gynaecological surgery. Anaesth Intensive Care. 1994;22(6):691-693.

[90] Belluomini J, Litt RC, Lee KA, Katz M. Acupressure for nausea and vomiting of pregnancy: A randomized, blinded study. Obstet Gynecol. 1994;84(2):245-248.

[91] Butkovic D, Toljan S, Matolic M, Kralik S, Radesic L. Comparison of laser acupuncture and metoclopramide in PONV prevention in children. Paediatr Anaesth. 2005;15(1):37-40.

[92] Ezzo J, Streitberger K, Schneider A. Cochrane systematic reviews examine P6 acupuncture-point stimulation for nausea and vomiting. J Altern Complement Med. 2006;12(5):489-495.

[93] Frey UH, Scharmann P, Lohlein C, Peters J. P6 acustimulation effectively decreases postoperative nausea and vomiting in high-risk patients. Br J Anaesth. 2009;102(5): 620-625.

[94] Gan TJ, Jiao KR, Zenn M, Georgiade G. A randomized controlled comparison of electro-acupoint stimulation or ondansetron versus placebo for the prevention of postoperative nausea and vomiting. Anesth Analg. 2004;99(4):1070-5, table of contents.

[95] Ashenden R, Silagy CA, Lodge M, Fowler G. A meta-analysis of the effectiveness of acupuncture in smoking cessation. Drug Alcohol Rev. 1997;16(1):33-40.

[96] Balk J, Day R, Rosenzweig M, Beriwal S. Pilot, randomized, modified, double-blind, placebo-controlled trial of acupuncture for cancer-related fatigue. J Soc Integr Oncol. 2009;7(1):4-11.

[97] Avis NE, Legault C, Coeytaux RR, et al. A randomized, controlled pilot study of acupuncture treatment for menopausal hot flashes. Menopause. 2008;15(6):1070-1078.

[98] Brinkhaus B, Witt CM, Ortiz M, et al. Acupuncture in seasonal allergic rhinitis (ACUSAR) - design and protocol of a randomised controlled multi-centre trial. Forsch Komplementmed. 2010;17(2):95-102.

[99] Biernacki W, Peake MD. Acupuncture in treatment of stable asthma. Respir Med. 1998;92(9):1143-1145.

[100] Bullock ML, Kiresuk TJ, Pheley AM, Culliton PD, Lenz SK. Auricular acupuncture in the treatment of cocaine abuse. A study of efficacy and dosing. J Subst Abuse Treat. 1999;16(1):31-38.

[101] Cao H, Pan X, Li H, Liu J. Acupuncture for treatment of insomnia: A systematic review of randomized controlled trials. J Altern Complement Med. 2009;15(11): 1171-1186.

[102] Chae Y, Kang OS, Lee HJ, et al. Effect of acupuncture on selective attention for smoking-related visual cues in smokers. Neurol Res. 2010;32 Suppl 1:27-30.

[103] Chen HY, Shi Y, Ng CS, Chan SM, Yung KK, Zhang QL. Auricular acupuncture treatment for insomnia: A systematic review. J Altern Complement Med. 2007;13(6): 669-676.

[104] Cheuk DK, Yeung WF, Chung KF, Wong V. Acupuncture for insomnia. Cochrane Database Syst Rev. 2007;(3)(3):CD005472.

[105] Cheong YC, Hung Yu Ng E, Ledger WL. Acupuncture and assisted conception. Cochrane Database Syst Rev. 2008;(4)(4):CD006920.

[106] El-Toukhy T, Sunkara SK, Khairy M, Dyer R, Khalaf Y, Coomarasamy A. A systematic review and meta-analysis of acupuncture in vitro fertilisation. BJOG. 2008;115(10): 1203-1213.

[107] Ernst E. Acupuncture for persistent allergic rhinitis: A randomised, sham-controlled trial. Med J Aust. 2008;188(1):64; author reply 64.

[108] Huang W, Kutner N, Bliwise DL. A systematic review of the effects of acupuncture in treating insomnia. Sleep Med Rev. 2009;13(1):73-104.

[109] Fung KP, Chow OK, So SY. Attenuation of exercise-induced asthma by acupuncture. Lancet. 1986;2(8521-22):1419-1422.

[110] Kokkotou E, Conboy LA, Ziogas DC, et al. Serum correlates of the placebo effect in irritable bowel syndrome. Neurogastroenterol Motil. 2010;22(3):285-e81.

[111] Lee MS, Shin BC, Ernst E. Acupuncture for treating menopausal hot flushes: A systematic review. Climacteric. 2009;12(1):16-25.

[112] Mora B, Iannuzzi M, Lang T, et al. Auricular acupressure as a treatment for anxiety before extracorporeal shock wave lithotripsy in the elderly. J Urol. 2007;178(1):160-4; discussion 164.

[113] Nir Y, Huang MI, Schnyer R, Chen B, Manber R. Acupuncture for postmenopausal hot flashes. Maturitas. 2007;56(4):383-395.

[114] Smith CA, Hay PP. Acupuncture for depression. Cochrane Database Syst Rev. 2005;(2)(2):CD004046.

[115] Smith CA, Hay PP, Macpherson H. Acupuncture for depression. Cochrane Database Syst Rev. 2010;(1)(1):CD004046.

[116] Wang SM, Kain ZN. Auricular acupuncture: A potential treatment for anxiety. Anesth Analg. 2001;92(2):548-553.

[117] Nayak S, Shiflett SC, Schoenberger NE, et al. Is acupuncture effective in treating chronic pain after spinal cord injury? Arch Phys Med Rehabil. 2001;82(11):1578-1586.

[118] MacPherson H, Thomas K, Walters S, Fitter M. A prospective survey of adverse events and treatment reactions following 34,000 consultations with professional acupuncturists. Acupunct Med. 2001;19(2):93-102.

[119] White A, Hayhoe S, Hart A, Ernst E, BMAS and AACP. British Medical Acupuncture Society and Acupuncture Association of Chartered Physiotherapists. Survey of adverse events following acupuncture (SAFA): A prospective study of 32,000 consultations. Acupunct Med. 2001;19(2):84-92.

[120] Melchart D, Weidenhammer W, Streng A, et al. Prospective investigation of adverse effects of acupuncture in 97 733 patients. Arch Intern Med. 2004;164(1):104-105.

[121] Brokaw JJ, Tunnicliff G, Raess BU, Saxon DW. The teaching of complementary and alternative medicine in U.S. medical schools: A survey of course directors. Acad Med. 2002;77(9):876-881.

[122] Chen L, Houghton M, Seefeld L, Malarick C, Mao J. A survey of selected physician views on acupuncture in pain management. Pain Med. 2010;11(4):530-534.

[123] National Health statistic report number 18, July 30 2009).

[124] Bowsher D. Mechanism of acupuncture. In: Filshie J, White A, eds. Medical acupuncture. Edinburgh, Scotland: Churchill Livingstone; 1998:69-80.

[125] Chiang CY, Chang CT. Peripheral afferent pathway for acupuncture analgesia. Sci Sin. 1973; 16:210-217.

[126] Alexander Mauskop. Alternative therapies in headache. Med Clinics of North America 2001 July; 85(4).

[127] WHO Acupuncture review and analysis of report on controlled clinical trials. 2002. www.who.int

Chapter 12

# Acupuncture in Cardiology

Tsung O. Cheng

Additional information is available at the end of the chapter

http://dx.doi.org/10.5772/55252

## 1. Introduction

Acupuncture combines the Latin *acus* (needle) and *punctum* (a prick) [1]. From the historical record of Huangdi Neijin (the Yellow Emperor's Classic), acupuncture has been used in China as a therapeutic tool for at least 2000 years [2]. In ancient China, soldiers noted, after being wounded by arrows, that their pain often eased for quite a while [3]. Therefore, a cause-and-effect relationship was assumed between the arrow wound and the unexpected diminution of pain. However, acupuncture has been little known in the Western world until 1970s after U.S. President Nixon's historic visit to China in 1972 [4]. Following the initial excitement engendered by the press reports [5], acupuncture becomes one of the most popular treatments in alternative medicine (Figure 1), and accounts for more than 10 million treatments given annually in the United States [6]. Much interest was further engendered by tales by subsequent visitors to China who witnessed surgical operations being successfully performed on conscious patients under acupunctural anesthesia [7-15]. Scientific studies using modern technology on acupuncture actually began in China in the late 1950s with further progress being made since the discovery of endogenous opioids in 1975 [2,16]. Much more advances have been made in more recent years in further understanding of the basic mechanisms underlying this millennium old medical treatment and its various clinical applications in the 21$^{st}$ century. This chapter reviews the current role of acupuncture in cardiology.

## 2. Hypercholesterolemia

Electro-acupuncture at "Fenglong" (ST 40) has some therapeutic effect on decreasing the content of total cholesterol and low-density-lipoprotein cholesterol in hyperlipidemic rats and improving the gene expression of ATP-binding cassette transporter A1, peroxisome proliferator-activated receptor alpha, liver X receptor alpha and retinoid X receptor-alpha mRNA, so

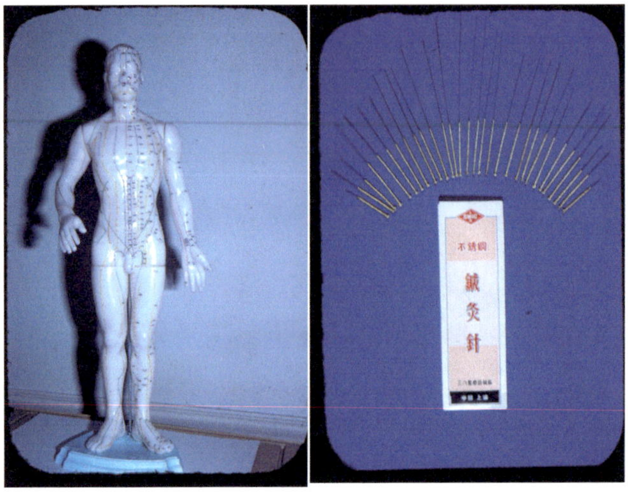


(A) (B)

**Figure 1.** A) An acupuncture manikin showing the location of the various acupoints along the meridians; (B) a complete set of acupuncture needles.

as to promote reverse cholesterol transport [17]. Furthermore, real-time PCR and western blot indicate that electroacupuncture at ST 40 induces the expression of nNOS and Mt1, two genes involved in NO signal transduction [18]. Acupuncture treatment for hypercholesterolemia thus involves the modulation of several biological pathways and provides a physiological link between NO signal transduction and the cholesterol-lowering effect of acupuncture [18].

## 3. Coronary artery disease

The effectiveness of acupuncture in treatment of angina has been well documented [19-21]. Its antianginal effect has been shown to be secondary to an antiischemic effect, which in turn is due to a decrease in heart rate and blood pressure and reduction in left ventricular afterload [22], a reduction in myocardial oxygen consumption, and a redistribution of coronary blood flow [23], myocardial release of β-endorphin [24], coronary vasodilatation [25], and increase in coronary collateral circulation [26]. Acupoint pressing has been shown to alleviate angina faster (2.45 +/- 1.67 min) than sublingual nitroglycerin (2.89 +/- 2.64 min) [27]. Transmyocardial acupuncture has also been used as a novel approach to myocardial revascularization [28,29], although its rationale has been questioned [30].

Acupuncture has been successfully used to improve microcirculation and left ventricular function in acute myocardial infarction [31-33]. Animal studies demonstrated that electroacupuncture could decrease the ST-segment elevation in ECG and reduce the infarct size following coronary ligation [34], although a recent study on rats failed to show a cardioprotective effect of electroacupuncture in terms of reduction of either infarct size or ventricular

http://dx.doi.org/10.5772/55252

arrhythmias [35]. Acupuncture has also been successfully employed to terminate nausea and vomiting [36] and intractable hiccup [37] complicating acute myocardial infarction.

## 4. Cardiac arrhythmias

Acupuncture has been employed to treat both experimental [38-40] and clinical arrhythmias. The latter included ventricular extrasystoles [41,42], sinus bradycardia [43], atrial fibrillation [44,45], decreased heart rate variability [46,47,48,49,50] and sudden death [51]. In the treatment of paroxysmal atrial fibrillation and atrial flutter, acupuncture at Neiguan, Shenmen, and Danzhong is more effective than intravenous amiodarone (conversion rate: 85% vs 67%, $p<0.01$; conversion time:39.6+/-13.7 min vs 50.1+/-14.8 min, $p<0.01$)[52]. Acupuncture at Neiguan, Shenmen and Xinshu also can prevent recurrences of atrial fibrillation after cardioversion in patients with persistent atrial fibrillation [53]. The advantage of acupuncture in treating atrial fibrillation is obvious, because it does not have any of the untoward effect of pharmacotherapy or ablation. Atrial fibrillation is the most common cardiac arrhythmia, and anxiety plays a significant role in either its initiation or its perpetuation [54]. Because acupuncture is very effective in treating anxiety, this therapeutic modality warrants further investigation as a promising therapeutic option.

A recently published systematic review of randomized controlled trials failed to provide conclusive evidence in support of acupuncture treatment for cardiac arrhythmias [55]. Furthermore, electro-acupuncture may interfere with demand pacemakers [56], although one recent case report from Greece indicated its safety [57]. Electo-acupuncture may also trigger inappropriate ICD discharges [58,59]. Therefore, extreme caution should be employed when electro-acupuncture is prescribed for patients with pacemakers and/or ICDs, and each patient should be considered individually with great care.

## 5. Congestive heart failure

In a Chinese echocardiographic study of patients with congestive heart failure due to dilated cardiomyopathy under maintenance doses of conventional drugs, including digitalis, diuretics and potassium supplements, acupuncture resulted in an increase in stroke volume [60]. Because patients with heart failure have increased sympathetic activity and acupuncture produces release of endogenous opioids in the central nervous system which would inhibit central sympathetic outflow, sympathetic activation during acute mental stress was markedly attenuated [61] or virtually eliminated [62] after acupuncture. This may explain why ear acupuncture has been used in treating chronic heart failure, because one of the acupuncture points stimulated by the needle in the ear corresponds to the closest position of the vagus nerve to the cutaneous surface (vide infra), and electrical vagus nerve stimulation has been advocated for patients with advanced heart failure [63].

Acupuncture may become an additional therapeutic strategy to improve the exercise tolerance of patients with chronic heart failure, potentially by improving skeletal muscle function [64].

The German researchers from the University Hospital of Heidelberg found a remarkable increase in 6-minute walk distance, improvement in ventilatory efficiency and post-exercise recovery, and increase in heart rate variability, despite a lack of improvement of the cardiac ejection fraction and peak oxygen uptake [64]. They recommended that further research be carried out to understand the beneficial mechanisms of acupuncture – in particular, its effects on neurohormonal balance and production of inflammatory cytokines [64].

In patients with chronic heart failure, acupuncture may reduce digitoxicity by regulating intracellular $Ca^{++}$, improving the function of $Ca^{++}$-ATPase in the sarcoplasmic reticulum, and increasing the calcium sensitivity of cardiac troponin [65]. These considerations may provide a novel clue for attenuating the toxicity of digitalis preparations given to patients with chronic heart failure.

## 6. Hypertension

Experimental studies have shown that acupuncture inhibits the reflex-induced hypertension by modulating the activity of cardiovascular parasympathetic neurons in the rostral ventrolateral medulla [66]. Activation of neurons in the arcuate nucleus of the hypothalamus, ventrolateral periaqueductal gray in the midbrain, and medullary nucleus raphé pallidus in the medulla by acupuncture can inhibit the activity of premotor sympathetic neurons in the rostral ventrolateral medulla. Glutamate, acetylcholine, opioids, gamma-aminobutyric acid, nociceptin, serotonin, nitric oxide and endocannabinoids in the brain all appear to participate in the antihypertensive response of acupuncture (Figure 2)[66]. Other possible mechanisms include decreases in plasma renin [67, 68], plasma neuropeptide Y [69], aldosterone [70] and angiotensin II activity [71,72]; increased excretion of sodium [73,74]; changes in plasma norepinephrine [75], serotonin [75] and endorphin levels [76,77]; and lowering of blood viscosity [75,78].

However, the Stop Hypertension with the Acupuncture Research Program (SHARP) pilot trial concluded that acupuncture provided no greater benefit than invasive sham acupuncture in controlling moderate hypertension [79]. Further research is obviously required to determine whether acupuncture can enhance clinical management of hypertension if used in combination with antihypertensive agents, over longer periods, or among specific subgroups of patients.

## 7. Stroke

Stroke should be considered as a coronary artery disease risk equivalent [80]. Acupuncture has useful applications in both the acute and chronic phases of a stroke. In ischemic stroke, acupuncture increases local cerebral blood flow as determined by single photon emission computed tomography [81] and near-infrared spectroscopy [82]. In rats with ischemic stroke, acupuncture has been shown to promote angiogenesis [83]. Acupuncture at Baihui and Fengchi is more effective than nimopidine in relieving cerebral vasospasm after embolization

http://dx.doi.org/10.5772/55252

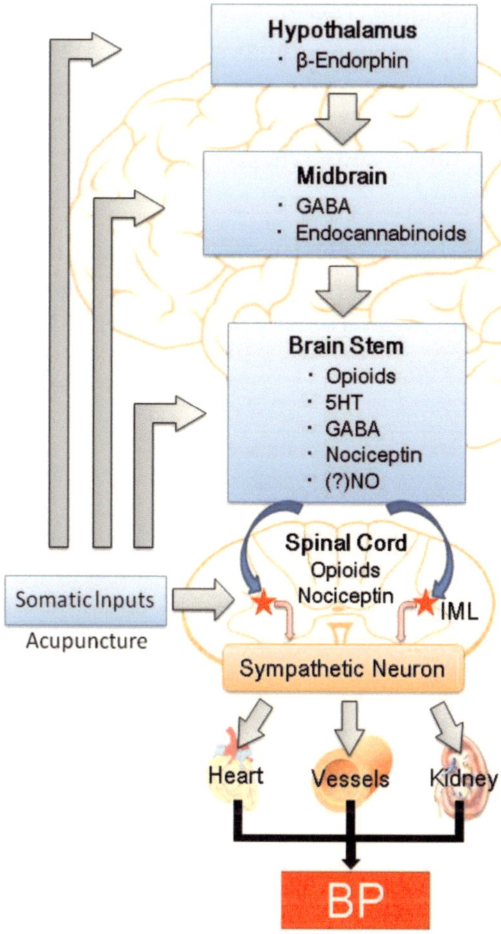


**Figure 2.** Neuroendocrine modulation of blood pressure by acupuncture. Abbreviations: GABA, γ-aminobutyric acid; 5HT, 5-hydroxytryptamine or serotonin; NO, nitric oxide; IML, intermediolateral column of the spinal cord. From Ref 66, courtesy W. Zhou.

of ruptured aneurysms in subarachnoid hemorrhage [84]. In a recent publication from Shanghai [85], the authors reviewed the progress of researches on the mechanism of acupuncture underlying improvement of acute cerebral hemorrhage from experimental studies and research methods. The effects of acupuncture mainly involve (1) lessening inflammatory reactions, (2) reducing impairment of free radicals and excitatory amino acids on cerebral neurons, (3) balancing release of vascular bioactive substances to increase regional cerebral blood flow, and (4) promoting repair and regeneration of the neural tissue. In regard to the research methods, many new biological techniques such as biological molecular approaches, neuro-cellular chemical methods, reverse transcription-polymerase chain reaction (RT-PCR) or quantitative real-time PCR, situ hybridization, western blotting, and electron microscopy have been extensively applied to researches on the underlying mechanisms of acupuncture therapy for cerebral infarction. In addition, the authors also pointed out that, in spite of achieving some greater progresses in experimental studies, most of the results basically reflect static, isolated and regional changes rather than dynamic and whole body changes. For these reasons, the authors recommended more in vivo research techniques and noninvasive research methods in the investigation of the underlying mechanisms of acupuncture therapy for acute cerebral ischemia [85].

Acupuncture has also been used successfully for post-stroke motor rehabilitation [86], behavioral recovery [87], aphasia [88], dysphasia [89], dysphagia [90], cognition disorders [91], depression [92], and urinary incontinence and urinary tract infection [93].

## 8. Smoking cessation

Cigarette smoking is prevalent in China; 67% of men [94] and 40% of male physicians [95] are smokers. It is a major cause of death in China and a principal cause of coronary heart disease in China [96]. In addition, secondhand smoke exposure (52% of nonsmokers in China are exposed to tobacco smoke for at least 15 minutes daily for >1 day per week [97]) was responsible for increased mortality due to coronary heart disease, ischemic stroke, lung cancer and chronic obstructive pulmonary disease in a recently published 17-year cohort study in China [98]. Another recently completed Chinese population study, the Kailuan community study, showed smoking cessation to be one of the seven key components of an essential population-wide strategy to reduce cardiovascular disease [99]. Although a 2012-15 blueprint on chronic disease prevention and control released by the Chinese Ministry of Health on May 21, 2012 set goals of reducing the adult smoking rate to below 25% among other goals [100], I have serious doubts as to how successful the Chinese Health Ministry's effort will be [101]. Nevertheless, any effective measure in curtailing cigarette smoking should be actively and urgently pursued.

Acupuncture has been found in a recently published review of smoking cessation intervention studies in China to yield a much higher abstinence rate than pharmacotherapy or counseling [102]. This observation was confirmed by two recently published meta-analyses of randomized controlled trials [103,104]. It has been postulated that, by increasing the levels of endorphin, enkephalin, epinephrine, norepinephrine, serotonin, and dopamine in the central nervous system and plasma, acupuncture provides the smoker with a deterioration in the taste of smoking, a decrease in the desire of smoking, and the obstruction of psychological symptoms resulting from smoking cessation [105]. The latest theory is that one of the acupuncture points stimulated by the acupuncture needle in the ear corresponds to the closest position of the vagus nerve to the cutaneous surface. Therefore, by stimulating this point, the acupuncturist blocks the outflow of withdrawal symptoms coming from the parasympathetic nervous system through the vagus nerve. However, more studies are needed to determine whether acupuncture is as efficacious as, or even more so than, pharmacotherapies.

## 9. Diabetes

Diabetes is associated with a marked increase in the risk of coronary artery disease, so much so that patients with diabetes shuld be treated as if they have existing coronary artery disease [106,107,108,109]. As a matter of fact, diabetes should be considered as a coronary artery disease equivalent [95,110]. The prevalence of diabetes is rising [108]. The main reasons for the rising prevalence of diabetes are smoking and obesity, which are certainly true for China [111,112]. A recent study from the University of North Carolina School of Global Public Health, using data from the China Health and Nutrition Survey, the longest ongoing study of its kind in China, reported that Chinese teenagers have a rate of diabetes nearly four to five times greater than their counterparts in the United States (1.9% vs 0.5% for boys and 0.4% for girls) [113]. Although acupuncture has been advocated for treatment of obesity (vide infra), a recent review of the literature questioned its validity owing to small sample size and low methodology quality of the studies [114].

On the other hand, acupuncture has been found to be effective in the management of patients with diabetes, by causing the release of endogenous opioid peptides such as β-endorphin from adrenal gland and thereby enhancing insulin secretion [115]. A recent literature review showed acupuncture to be effective in lowering blood glucose in both humans and rats [115]. Ear acupuncture in 45 diabetics in Peking University of Shenzhen Hospital, Shenzhen, Guangdong Province, China resulted in significant improvement in fasting plasma glucose, blood glucose load after 2-hour 75 gm oral glucose tolerance test and glycosylated hemoglobin [116]. Two recent studies from Beijing, China on patients with impaired glucose tolerance reported similar improvement in these parameters following electro-acupuncture, thus confirming its effectiveness in the prevention and treatment of diabetes at the early stage [117,118]. Another study from Nanjing, China reported acupuncture to be effective in lowering fasting blood leptin level, which may contribute to its clinical effect in improving diabetes [119]. Electro-acupuncture has also been used successfully for the treatment of diabetic peripheral neuropathy in rats [120] as well as in patients [121], although the quality of reports about randomized controlled trials is moderate to low [122]. Finally, acupuncture has been used in treating urinary tract infection in diabetic patients [123].

## 10. Obesity

Obesity is another risk factor for coronary artery disease, hypertension, chronic heart failure, stroke and diabetes [124]. It is increasing in prevalence worldwide, especially in developing countries like China [95,125,126]. Two recent systematic reviews, one published in 2009 [127] and the other in 2012 [114], both suggested that acupuncture is an effective treatment for obesity, with fewer adverse effects of the various dieting plans and Western anti-obesity drugs. A recent study in obese rats showed that electro-acupuncture led to a reduction of body weight, decrease in the plasma leptin levels, and an increase in leptin receptor expression in the hypothalamus, suggesting that regulating the expression of leptin and the leptin receptor might be one of the molecular mechanisms underlying the reduction of body weight in diet-induced obese rats by electro-acupuncture treatment [128]. Another human study reported in 2010 found that laser acupuncture exerted a therapeutic effect on simple obesity by reducing both body weight and body mass index [129]. However, the amount of evidence is not fully convincing, because of the small sample size and poor methodological quality of all the reported trials to date.

## 11. Acupunctural anesthesia for cardiac surgery

The most amazing application of acupuncture is acupunctural anesthesia. Skeptics who deny that acupunctural anesthesia can work have suggested that acupuncture is nothing more than an effective use of hypnosis or autosuggestion. I was also a skeptic until I witnessed with my own eyes several operative procedures performed on conscious patients under acupunctural anesthesia including those with acquired valvular and congenital heart diseases (Figures 3 and 4). Being a native-born Chinese, I was able to communicate directly with the patients, without going through any interpreters, who may either inadvertently or deliberately omit or distort any actual expressions from the patients, to find out what discomfort they might experience during the procedures. Of course, I was not the only physician who was impressed by cardiac surgery under acupunctural anesthesia. Other well-known surgeons around the world, such as DeBakey from the United States [130], Hollinger et al from Germany [131], and Caracausi from Italy [132] were too.

Acupuncture also has a cardioprotective effect as a pretreatment on patients undergoing heart valve replacement. Cardiac ischemia-reperfusion injury after cardiopulmonary bypass often contributes to postoperative morbidity and mortality in patients undergoing heart valve replacement. A randomized controlled trial, which was reported from Xi'an, China in 2010, showed that electro-acupuncture pretreatment significantly reduced overall serum troponin I release at 6 hours, 12 hours and 24 hours after aortic cross-clamping removal [133]. Meanwhile, electroacupuncture pretreatment also reduced the inotrope score at 12 hours, 24 hours, and 48 hours after the intensive care unit arrival and shortened intensive care unit stay time ($p<0.05$)[133]. The cardioprotective effect of transcutaneous electric acupoint stimulation was further confirmed recently in the pediatric cardiac patients with congenital heart disease [134].

After its initial enthusiasm in China in the 1970s, in the subequent years acupunctural anesthesia for open heart surgery gradually became less and less frequently used throughout China, because of its limitations and disadvantages [3,135]. Fortunately, with recent modification of the technique by combining acupuncture with conscious sedation, Zhou et al [135] were able to demonstrate its effectiveness again. This modification, which will be discussed bodes well for the future of acupunctural anesthesia for cardiac surgery, not only because of its sound physiological principles, simplicity in clinical application, significant benefit to the patient and favorable cost effectiveness, but also for its positive impact on healthcare cost.

http://dx.doi.org/10.5772/55252

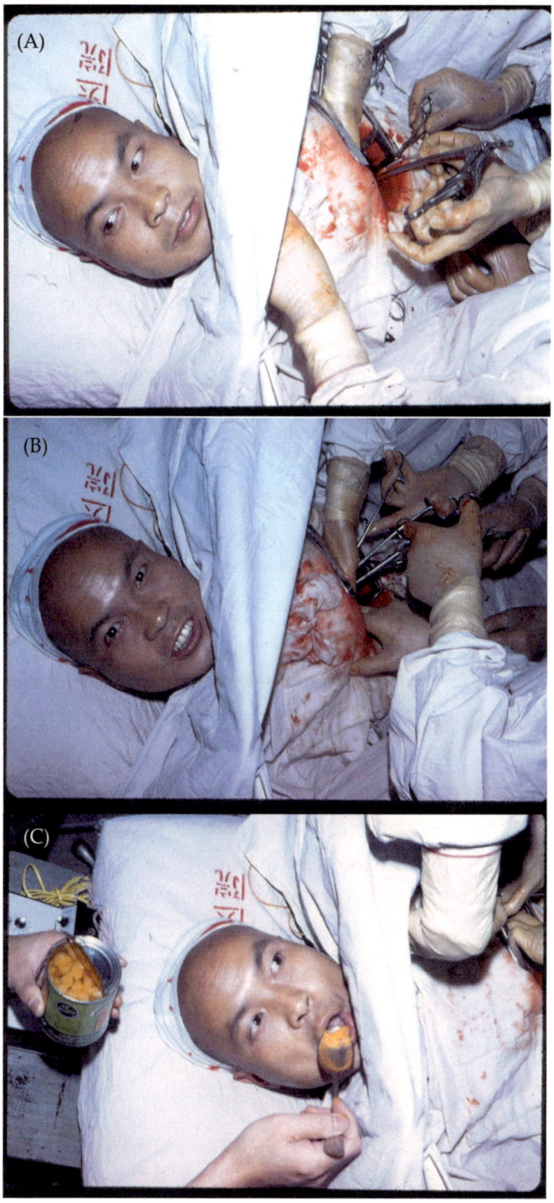

**Figure 3.** A man undergoing a closed transventricular mitral commissurotomy under acupunctural anesthesia in a hospital in Shanghai. (A) Patient fully awake and comfortable; (B) Patient smiling during the procedure; (C) Patient eating oranges during the operation. All photographs taken by the author during his 1972 visit to China.

## 12. Adverse effects and complications

Although acupuncture is extremely safe, adverse effects and sometimes serious complications have been reported. These include infective endocarditis [136,137,138], pericardial effusion

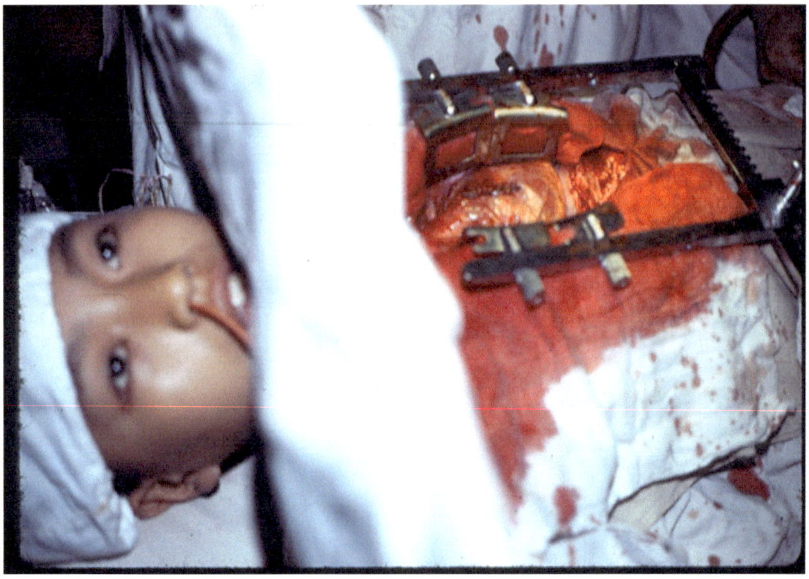

**Figure 4.** A child fully awake and comfortable while undergoing open heart surgical closure of a ventricular septal defect under acupunctural anesthesia. Photograph taken by the author during his 1972 visit to China.

[139], cardiac tamponade [138,140], pneumothorax [141] and AIDS [138,142]. However, infective endocarditis and AIDS are not due to acupuncture per se, but to the unsterile technique that was employed during acupuncture. Hundreds of thousands of acupuncturists worldwide perform millions of acupuncture procedures per year [143]. Considering the small number of reported complications in the literature, acupuncture is very safe indeed [143,144,145,146,147]. As a matter of fact, the recent report of the successful use of electro-acupuncture for treatment of arthritis in a patient with a total artificial heart is further testimonial to its safety [148].

## 13. Conclusion

Acupuncture has a definite place in cardiology. When performed by trained acupuncturists, it is safe, effective, cost-effective, and widely available. As more research evidence for acupuncture efficacy, including the application of functional magnetic resonance imaging technique in recent years [149], becomes available, it will be possible to increase physician knowledge and change attitudes towards acupuncture [150,151], as it was so predicted by the NIH Consensus Development Panel on Acupuncture convened a decade and a half ago [152]. When incorporated into conventional health care as an integrated approach, the future of this ancient Chinese therapeutic modality is bright. As a matter of fact, acupuncture should prove to be an attractive alternative to Western medicine in the current era of cost containment in healthcare [153]. Although Western medicine may be preferred in the management of some acute cardiac conditions, such as acute myocardial infarction or malignant arrhythmias, traditional Chinese medicine, of which acupuncture is an essential component, has a definite place in the management of various subacute and chronic cardiovascular disorders and risk factors. However, a recent systematic review showed that, in acute low back pain, acupuncture appears to be actually more effective than drugs for symptomatic improvement [154]. Therefore, more registered high-quality clinical trials need to be continued worldwide on this 2,000+-year-old ancient Chinese therapy [155].

## Author details

Tsung O. Cheng

Address all correspondence to: tcheng@mfa.gwu.edu

Department of Medicine, The George Washington University, Washington, D.C., USA

## References

[1] Haubrich WS: Medical Meanings. A Glossary of Word Origins. Philadelphia: American College of Physicians 1997:4.

[2] Han JS: Physiologic and neurochemical basis of acupuncture anesthesia. In: The International Textbook of Cardiology (Cheng TO, ed) New York/Oxford: Pergamon Press 1987:1124-1132.

[3] Cheng TO: Acupuncture anesthesia for open heart surgery: Past, present and future. Int J Cardiol 2011; 150:1-3.

[4] Cheng TO: Changes in China. N Engl J Med 1972; 287:259.

[5] Cheng TO: The evolution of cardiology in China. In: Cardiothoracic Surgery in China. Past, Present and Future (Wan S, Yim APC, eds). Hong Kong: The Chinese University Press, 2007: 204-305.

[6] Cheng TO: Acupuncture in cardiology. InCirculation.net February 7, 2007. http://www.incirculation.net/24174_84428.aspx Accessed February 7, 2007.

[7] Cheng TO: Acupuncture anesthesia. Science 1973; 179:521.

[8] Cheng TO: Medicine in China. J Am Geriatr Soc 1973; 21:289-313.

[9] Cheng TO: A view of modern Chinese medicine. Observations by a Shanghai-born physician during his recent visit after 22 years of absence. Ann Intern med 1973;78:285-290.

[10] Cheng TO: Future development of Chinese medical journals. Ann Intern Med 1973; 79:897-898.

[11] Cheng TO: China's "barefoot doctors". Prism (AMA) 1973; 1:16-18.

[12] Cheng TO: Cardiovascular diseases. In: China Medicine As We Saw It (Quinn JR, ed). Bethesda, Maryland: US Department of Health, Education, and Welfare, Public Health Service, National Institutes of Health, DHEW Publication No. (NIH) 75-684. 1974:261-288.

[13] Cheng TO: Cardiology in the People's Republic of China. In: New Horizons in Cardi ovascular Practice (Russek HI, ed). Baltimore: University Park Press, 1975:1-27.

[14] Cheng TO: Acupuncture anesthesia for open heart surgery. Am J Cardiol 1975; 36:411.

[15] Cheng TO: Stamps in cardiology. Acupuncture anaesthesia for open heart surgery. Heart 2000; 83:256.

[16] Han JS: Acupuncture and endorphins. Neurosci Letters 2004; 361:258-261.

[17] Zhang HX, Wang Q, Huang H, Yue W, Qin PF: Effect of electroacupuncture at "Fenglong" (ST 40) on rats with hyperlipidemia and its mechanism. Zhongguo Zhen Jiu 2012; 32:241-5.

[18] Li L, Tan GH, Zhang YZ: Modulated expression of genes associated with NO signal transduction contributes to the cholesterol-lowering effect of electro-acupuncture. Biotechnol Lett 2012 Mar 16 [Epub ahead of print]

[19] Cheng TO: Acupuncture treatment for angina. Cardiology 1998; 90:152.

[20] Cheng TO: Acupuncture for relief of angina. Circulation 1998; 98:2357-2358.

[21] Bueno EA, Mamtani R, Frishman WH: Alternative approaches to the medical management of angina pectoris: acupuncture, electric nerve stimulation, and spinal cord stimulation. Heart Disease 2001; 3:236-241.

[22] Diao LH, Yang ZB, Zhou GX, Chen Y, Fan LY, Zhang YY, Liu H, Liu ST: Observation on therapeutic effects of electroacupuncture at Neiguan (PC 6) on silent myocardial ischemia. Zhongguo Zhen Jiu 2011; 31:591-4.

[23] Mannheimer C, Eliasson T, Augustinsson L-E, Blomstrand C, Emanuelsson H, Larsson S, Norrsell H, Hjalmarsson A: Electrical stimulation versus coronary artery bypass surgery in severe angina pectoris. The ESBY study. Circulation 1998; 97:1157-1163.

[24] Eliasson T, Mannheimer C, Waagstein F, Andersson B, Bergh C-H, Augustinsson L-E, Hedner T, Larson G: Myocardial turnover of endogenous opioids and calcitonin-gene-related peptide in the human heart and the effects of spinal cord stimulation on pacing-induced angina pectoris. Cardiology 1998; 89:170-177.

[25] Kurono Y, Egawa M, Yano T, Shimoo K: The effect of acupuncture on the coronary arteries as evaluated by coronary angiography: a preliminary report. Am J Chin Med 2002; 30:387-396.

[26] Meng JB, Zhu GY, Fu WX, Song LM: Effect of acupuncture on the coronary collateral circulation of dogs suffering from experimental myocardial infarction. Zhen Ci Yan Jiu 1986; 11(3):196-197.

[27] Wang YM, Wang QY, Zhang J, Guo YL: Comparative study on acupoint pressing and medication for angina pectoris due to coronary heart disease. Zhongguo Zhen Jiu 2011; 31:595-8.

[28] Sen PK, Udwadia TE, Kinare SG, Parulkar GB: Transmyocardial acupuncture: a new approach to myocardial revascularization. J Thorac Cardiovasc Surg 1965; 50:181-189.

[29] Sen PK, Daulatram J, Kinare SG, Udwadia TE, Parulkar MS: Further studies in multiple transmyocardial acupuncture as a method of myocardial revascularization. Surgery 1968; 64:861-870.

[30] Pifarre R, Jasuja ML, Lynch RD, Neville WE: Myocardial revascularization by transmyocardial acupuncture. A physiologic impossibility. J Thorac Cardiovasc Surg 1969; 58:424-431.

[31] Zhu BJ, Bi L, Liang SY, Pang L, Wang SL, Liu JF, Jiang AP, Li CJ, Ye ZJ, Yang: Effect of acupuncture on left ventricular function, microcirculation, blood rheology and cyclic nucleotides in patients with acute myocardial infarction. J Tradit Chin Med 1989; 9:63-68.

[32] Zhu BJ, Liang SY: Effects of acupuncture on microcirculation of acute myocardial infarction patients. Zhen Ci Yan Jiu 1988;13:267-271.

[33] Li CJ, Bi LG, Zhu BJ, Qi MZ, Zhao CX, Xu YF, Yao ZL, Lu ZS, Sun SM, Dong H, et al: Effects of acupuncture on left ventricular function, microcirculation, cAMP and cGMP of acute myocardial infarction patients. J Tradit Chin Med 1986; 6:157-161.

[34] Meng J: The effects of acupuncture in treatment of coronary heart diseases. J Tradit Chin Med 2004;24:16-19.

[35] Dow J, Painovich J, Hale SL, Tien-A-Looi S, Longhurst JC, Kloner RA: Absence of actions of commonly used Chinese herbal medicines and electroacupuncture on myocardial infarct size. J Cardiovasc Pharmacol Ther 2012;17:403-411.

[36] Dent HE, Dewhurst NG, Mills SY, Willoughby M: Continuous PC6 wristband acupressure for relief of nausea and vomiting associated with acute myocardial infarction: a partially randomised, placebo-controlled trial. Complement Ther Med 2003; 11:72-77.

[37] Liu FC, Chen CA, Yang SS, Lin SH: Acupuncture therapy rapidly terminates intractable hiccups complicating acute myocardial infarction. South Med J 2005; 98:385-387.

[38] Xia Y, Guo XQ, Zhang AZ, Cao XD, Li P: Inhibitory effect of analogous electro-acupuncture on experimental arrhythmia. Acupunct Electrother Res 1985; 10:13-34.

[39] Fan W, Wu N, Fang C: Effect of acupuncture on ischemic ventricular tachyarrhythmia in experimental electrophysiology study. Zhonghua Xin Xue Guan Bing Za Zhi 1987; 15:285-288, 311.

[40] Zhang Y, Guo Y, Wang X, Shi L, Miao W, Xu T, Zhang C: Influence of changing $Ca^{++}$ concentration in neiguan (PC6) on the effect of acupuncture treating experimental arrhythmia of rabbits. Zhen Ci Yan Jiu 1995; 20:63-67.

[41] Liptak V, Habeler G, Egger J: Influence of acupuncture and electroacupuncture on heart rate and extrasystoles. Wien Med Wochenschr 1980; 130:668-670.

[42] Zhang J, Xu W: Frequent ventricular extrasystoles treated by needling neiguan (PC6) plus oral administration of mexiletine – a report of 30 cases. J Tradit Chin Med 2004; 24:40-41.

[43] Gao ZW, Yu XY, Shen AX, Bao LE, Lin XC, Qiu JH, Wang ZL, Hu ZG, Zhang SH: Acupuncture treatment of 54 cases of sinus bradycardia. J Tradit Chin Med 1987; 7:185-187.

[44] Berman RH: Acupuncture for cardioversion. Ann Intern Med 1973; 79:285.

[45] Lombardi F, Belletti S, Battezzati PM, Lomuscio A: Acupuncture for paroxysmal and persistent atrial fibrillation: An effective non-pharmacological tool? World J Cardiol 2012; 4(3):60-5.

[46] Shi X, Wang ZP, Liu KX: Effect of acupuncture on heart rate variability in coronary heart disease patients. Zhongguo Zhong Xi Yi Jie He Za Zhi 1995; 15:536-538.

[47] Litscher G, Cheng G, Cheng W, Wang L, Niu Q, Feng X, Gaischek I, Kuang H: Sino-European transcontinental basic and clinical high-tech acupuncture studies-part 2: acute stimulation effects on heart rate and its variability in patients with insomnia. Evid Based Complement Alternat Med 2012;2012:916085. Epub 2012 Mar 4.

[48] Litscher G, Cheng G, Wang L, Cheng W, Su H, Niu Q, Zou T, Wang Y, Feng X, Gaischek I, Sheng Z, Kuang H: Biomedical teleacupuncture between China and Austria using heart rate variability-Part 2: Patients with depression. Evid Based Complement Alternat Med 2012;2012:145904. Epub 2012 Apr 17.

[49] Anderson B, Nielsen A, McKee D, Jeffres A, Kligler B: Acupuncture and heart rate variability: a systems level approach to understanding mechanism. Explore (NY) 2012; 8(2):99-106.

[50] Gao XY, Liu K, Zhu B, Litscher G: Sino-European transcontinental basic and clinical high-tech acupuncture studies-part 1: auricular acupuncture increases heart rate var-

iability in anesthetized rats. Evid Based Complement Alternat Med 2012;2012:817378. Epub 2012 Feb 21.

[51] Tang ZL, Song XG, Zhou YP: A preliminary study on the prevention and cure of sudden death caused by coronary heart disease by acupuncture. Zhen Ci Yan Jiu 1985; 10:148-151,147.

[52] Xu HK, Zhang YF: Comparison between therapeutic effects of acupuncture and intravenous injection of amiodarone in the treatment of paroxysmal atrial fibrillation and atrial flutter. Zhongguo Zhen Jiu 2007; 27:96-8.

[53] Lomuscio A, Belletti S, Battezzati PM, Lombardi F: Efficacy of acupuncture in preventing atrial fibrillation recurrences after electrical cardioversion. J Cardiovasc Electrophysiol 2011; 22(3):241-7.

[54] Pozuelo L: Fine-tuning a heart-brain connection. Anxiety in atrial fibrillation. Circ Heart Fail 2012; 5:307-8.

[55] Kim TH, Choi TY, Lee MS, Ernst E: Acupuncture treatment for cardiac arrhythmias: A systematic review of randomized controlled trials. Int J Cardiol 2011; 149:263-5.

[56] Fujiwara H, Taniguchi K, Takeuchi J, Ikezono E: The influence of low frequency acupuncture on a demand pacemaker. Chest 1980; 78:96-97.

[57] Vasilakos DG, Fyntanidou BP: Electroacupuncture on a patient with pacemaker: a case report. Acupunct Med 2011; 29(2):152-3.

[58] Vlay SC: Electromagnetic interference and ICD discharge related to chiropractic treatment. Pacing Clin Electrophysiol 1998; 21:2009.

[59] Lau EW, Birnie DH, Lemery R, Tang AS, Green MS: Acupuncture triggering inappropriate ICD shocks. Europace 2005; 7:85-86.

[60] Huang DJ, Cheng DT, Das SK, Pitt, B: Effect of acupuncture on left ventricular size and function assessed by echocardiography in patients with stable dilated cardiomyopathy. J Tradit Chin Med 1985; 5:243-245.

[61] Middlekauff HR, Hui K, Yu JL, Hamilton MA, Fonarow GC, Moriguchi J, Maclellan WR, Hage A: Acupuncture inhibits sympathetic activation during mental stress in advanced heart failure patients. J Card Fail 2002; 8:399-406.

[62] Middlekauff HR: Acupuncture in the treatment of heart failure. Cardiol Rev 2004; 12(3):171-3.

[63] Sabbah HN: Electrical vagus nerve stimulation for the treatment of chronic heart failure. Cleveland Clin J Med 2011; 78 (Suppl 1):S24-S29.

[64] Kristen AV, Schuhmacher B, Strych K, Lossnitzer D, Friederich HC, Hilbel T, Haass M, Katus HA, Schneider A, Streitberger KM, Backs J: Acupuncture improves exercise

tolerance of patients with heart failure: a placebo-controlled pilot study. Heart 2010; 96:1396-400.

[65] Ma SH, Gao JH, Wang YM, Zhang M, Ma YY, Hu JJ, Fu WX, Cui HF, Yu XC: Considerations about study on mechanisms of acupuncture underlying efficacy-enhancement and toxicity-attenuation of digitalis drugs for heart failure. Zhen Ci Yan Jiu 2011; 36(3):225-9.

[66] Zhou W, Longhurst JC: Neuroendocrine mechanisms of acupuncture in the treatment of hypertension. Evid Based Complement Alternat Med 2012;878673. Epub 2011 Dec 18.

[67] Lee HS, Kim JY: Effects of acupuncture on blood pressure and plasma renin activity in two-kidney one clip Goldblatt hypertensive rats. Am J Chin Med 1994; 22:215-219.

[68] Chiu YJ, Chi A, Reid IA: Cardiovascular and endocrine effects of acupuncture in hypertensive patients. Clin Exp Hypertens 1997; 19:1047-1063.

[69] Zhang YL, Li CP, Peng M, Yang HS: Effect of acupuncture combined with medicine on neuropeptide Y in the patient of hypertension. Zhongguo Zhen Jiu 2005; 25:155-157.

[70] Anshelevich IuV, Merson MA, Afanas'eva GA: Serum aldosterone level in patients with hypertension during treatment by acupuncture. Ter Arkh 1985; 57(10):42-45

[71] Shen S, Li J, Wang XM, Han JS: Angiotensin II release and anti-electroacupuncture analgesia in spinal cord. Sheng Li Xue Bao 1996; 48:543-550.

[72] Huang H, Liang S: Acupuncture at otoacupoint heart for treatment of vascular hypertension. J Tradit Chin Med 1992; 12:133-136.

[73] Yao T: Acupuncture and somatic nerve stimulation: mechanism underlying effects on cardiovascular and renal activities. Scan J Rehabil Med Suppl 1993; 29:7-18.

[74] Lin MZ, Wei ZY: Effect of elctroacupuncture on the urine flow, sodium excretion and potassium excretion in the conscious dog. Zhen Ci Yan Jiu 1989; 143:365-369.

[75] Zhou Y, Wang Y, Fang Z, Xia C, Liu B, Chen Q, Zhang F: Influence of acupuncture on blood pressure, contents of NE, DA and 5-HT of SHR and the interrelation between blood pressure and whole blood viscosity. Zhen Ci Yan Jiu 1995; 20:55-61.

[76] Ulett GA, Han S, Han JS: Electroacupuncture: mechanisms and clinical application. Biol Psychiatry 1998; 44:129-138.

[77] Han JS: Acupuncture and endorphins. Neurosci Lett 2004; 361:258-261.

[78] Jin YX, Fu Q, Guo XQ: Effects of electroacupuncture of "zusanli" acupoint on high blood pressure and blood hyperviscosity in stress rats. J Tongji Med Univ 1992; 12:209-215.

[79] Macklin EA, Wayne PM, Kalish LA, Valaskatgis P, Thompson J, Pian-Smith MMC, Zhang Q, Stevens S, Goertz C, Prineas RJ, Buczynski B, Zusman RM: Stop Hyperten-

sion with the Acupuncture Research Program (SHARP): results of a randomized controlled clinical trial. Hypertension 2006; 48:838-845.

[80] Lackland DT, Elkind MSV, D'Agostino R Sr, Dhamoon MS, Goff DC Jr, Higashida RT, McClure LA, Nitchell PH, Sacco RL, Sila CA, Smith SC Jr, Tanne D, Tirschwell DL, Touzé E, Wechsler LR, on behalf of the American Heart Association Stroke Council, Council on Epidemiology and Prevention, Council on Cardiovascular Radiology and Intervention, Council on Cardiovascular Nursing, Council on Peripheral Vascular Disease, and Council on Quality of Care and Outcomes Research: Inclusion of stroke in cardiovascular risk prediction instruments: A statement for healthcare professionals From the American Heart Association/American Stroke Association. Stroke 2012; 43:1998-2027.

[81] Zhou HF, Wang J, Cao TJ, Ju QB, Huang CY, Feng Y, Li YM, Li XN, Qu F, Dou WB: Effects of eye acupuncture on SPECT-determined cerebral blood flow in patients with cerebral infarction. Zhongguo Zhen Jiu 2011; 31:391-4.

[82] Li H, Hou ZW, Bai YL, Gu SZ: Comparative study on curative effects of stroke treated with acupuncture by NIRS. Zhongguo Zhen Jiu 2011; 31:998-1002.

[83] Du Y, Shi L, Li J, Xiong J, Li B, Fan X: Angiogenesis and improved cerebral blood flow in the ischemic boundary area were detected after electroacupuncture treatment to rats with ischemic stroke. Neurol Res 2011; 33;101-7.

[84] Jiang YZ, Li C, Xu JY, Lu YZ, Xu R, Han B, Lu WH: Observation of clinical efficacy of acupuncture for cerebral vasospasm after embolization of ruptured aneurysms. Zhongguo Zhen Jiu 2012; 32:193-7.

[85] Wang F, Wang HQ, Dong GR: Progress of researches on mechanism of acupuncture therapy underlying improvement of acute cerebral hemorrhage. Zhen Ci Yan Jiu 2011; 36(2):145-9.

[86] Fu QH, Pei J, Jia Q, Song Y, Gu YH, You XX: Acupuncture treatment programs for post-stroke motor rehabilitation in community hospitals: study protocol of a multicenter, randomized, controlled trial. Zhong Xi Yi Jie He Xue Bao 2012; 10(5):516-24.

[87] Lu T, Luo Y, Sun H, Qin W, Li Y: Electroacupuncture improves behavioral recovery and increases SCF/c-kit expression in a rat model of focal cerebral ischemia/reperfusion. Neurol Sci 2012 Apr 13 [Epub ahead of print].

[88] Li G, Yang ES: An fMRI study of acupuncture-induced brain activation of aphasia stroke patients. Complement Ther Med 2011; 19 Suppl 1:S49-59.

[89] Zheng H, Zhu SW, Yang F, Huang XM, Wang Z, Cui FF, Zhang DB: Efficacy observation of Thoroughfare Vessel theory in acupuncture for post-stroke dysphasia. Zhongguo Zhen Jiu 2011; 31:1067-70.

[90] Sun XR, Fan GQ, Dai XZ: Primary optimization of acupuncture program for dysphagia after cerebral infarction. Zhongguo Zhen Jiu 2011; 31:879-82.

[91] Li W, Cheng YH, Yu XG: Observation on therapeutic effect of acupuncture combined with medicine on mild cognition disorders in patients with post-stroke. Zhongguo Zhen Jiu 2012; 32:3-7.

[92] Zhang GC, Fu WB, Xu NG, Liu JH, Zhu XP, Liang ZH, Huang YF, Chen YF: Meta analysis of the curative effect of acupuncture on post-stroke depression. J Tradit Chin Med 2012; 32:6-11.

[93] Chu JM, Bao YH, Zou C, Zhao HL, Gong Y, Wang CM: Randomized controlled clinical trials for electroacupuncture treatment of urinary incontinence in stroke patients. Zhen Ci Yan Jiu 2011; 36(6):428-32.

[94] Cheng TO: The current state of cardiology in China. Int J Cardiol 2004; 96:425-439.

[95] Cheng TO: Cardiovascular health, risks and diseases in contemporary China. Int J Cardiol 2012; 154:233-242.

[96] Cheng TO: Prevention of cardiovascular disease in modern China: Utile or futile? CVD Prevention and Control 2009; 4:1-7.

[97] Jiang Y, Elton-Marshall T, Fong GT, Li Q: Quitting smoking in China: findings from the ITC China survey. Tobacco Control 2010; 19(Suppl 2):i12-i17.

[98] He Y, Jiang B, Li LS, Li LS, Ko L, Wu L. Sun DL, He SF, Liang BQ, Hu FB, Lam TH: Secondhand smoke exposure predicted chronic obstructive pulmonary disease and other tobacco related mortality in a 17-year cohort study in China. Chest 2012 May 24. [Epub ahead of print]

[99] Wu S, Huang Z, Yang X, Zhou Y, Wang A, Chen L, Zhao H, Ruan C, Wu Y, Xin A, Li K, Jin C, Cai J: Prevalence of ideal cardiovascular health and its relationship with the 4-year cardiovascular events in a northern Chinese industrial city. Circ Cardiovasc Qual Outcomes 2012; 5:487-493.

[100] Anonymous: Chronic disease challenge. Beijing Review May 31, 2012; 55(22):5.

[101] Cheng TO: Is China finally going to ban cigarette smoking? Int J Cardiol 2010; 145:1-2.

[102] Kim SS, Chen W, Kolodziej M, Wang X, Wang VJ, Ziedonis D: A systematic review of smoking cessation intervention studies in China. Nicotine Tob Res 2012;14:891-

[103] Tahiri M, Mottillo S, Joseph L, Pilotee L, Eisenberg MJ: Alternative smoking cessation aids: a meta-analysis of randomized controlled trials. Am J Med 2012;125:576-584

[104] Cheng HM, Chung YC, Chen HH, Chang YH, Yeh ML: Systematic review and meta-analysis of the effects of acupoint stimulation on smoking cessation. Am J Chin Med 2012; 40(3):429-442.

[105] Cabioglu MT, Ergene N, Tan U: Smoking cessation after acupuncture treatment. Int J Neurosci 2007; 117(5):571-8.

http://dx.doi.org/10.5772/55252

[106] Kannel WB, McGee DL: Diabetes and cardiovascular disease. The Framingham study. JAMA 1979; 241:2035-2038.

[107] Haffner SM, Lehto S, Ronnemaa T, Pyörälä K, Laakso M: Mortality from coronary heart disease in subjects with type 2 diabetes and in nondiabetic subjects with and without prior myocardial infarction. N Engl J Med 1998; 339:229-34.

[108] Gregg EW, Cheng YJ, Saydah S, Cowie C, Garfield S, Geiss L, Barker L: Trends in death rates among U.S. adults with and without diabetes between 1997 and 2006: findings from the national health interview survey. Diabetes Care 2012; 35:1252-7.

[109] Benn M, Tybjærg-Hansen A, McCarthy MI, Jensen GB, Grande P, Nordestgaard BG: Nonfasting glucose, ischemic heart disease, and myocardial infarction. A Mendelian randomization study. J Am Coll Cardiol 2012; 59:2356-65.

[110] Hu DY, Pan CY, Yu JM, for the China Heart Survey Group: The relationship between coronary artery disease and abnormal glucose regulation in China: the China Heart Survey. Eur Heart J 2006; 27: 2573-79.

[111] Cheng TO: Smoking and diabetes in Chinese men. Postgrad Med J 2001; 77:551.

[112] Cheng TO: Diabetes epidemic in China and its economic impact. Int J Cardiol 2011; 149:1-3.

[113] Yan S, Li J, Li S, Zhang B, Du S, Gordon-Larsen P, Adair L, Popkin B: The expanding burden of cardiometabolic risk in China: the China Health and Nutrition Survey. Obes Rev 2012;13:810-821

[114] Sui Y, Zhao HL, Wong VCW, Brown N, Li XL, Kwan AKL, Hui HLW, Ziea ETC, Chan JCN: A systematic review on use of Chinese medicine and acupuncture for treatment of obesity. Obes Rev 2012; 13(5):409-30.

[115] Peplow PV, Baxter GD: Electroacupuncture for control of blood glucose in diabetes: literature review. J Acupunct Meridian Stud 2012; 5:1-10.

[116] Ju YL, Chen ML, Wang L, Lan W, Chi X, Liu JX, Zhang HL: Effects of stimulating in the cavum concha on glucometabolism in patients with diabetes. Zhongguo Zhen Jiu 2012; 32:198-200.

[117] Meng H, Zhai X, Hao JD, Wang HC: Intervention of electroacupuncture for patients with impaired glucose tolerance. Zhongguo Zhen Jiu 2011; 31:971-3.

[118] Meng H, Hao JD, Wang HC, Zhao JY, Zhao CL, Zhai X: Effects of different frequencies of electroacupuncture on blood glucose level in impaired glucose tolerance patients. Zhen Ci Yan Jiu 2011; 36(3):220-3.

[119] Cai H, Zhao LJ, Zhao ZM, Guo JH, Yuan AH: Effect of acupuncture on serum leptin level in patients with type II diabetes mellitus. Zhen Ci Yan Jiu 2011; 36(4):288-91.

[120] Hwang HS, Yang EJ, Lee SM, Lee SC, Choi SM: Antiallodynic effects of electroacupuncture combined with MK-801 treatment through the regulation of p35/p25 in experimental diabetic neuropathy. Exp Neurobiol 2011; 20(3):144-52.

[121] Jin Z, Zhang BF, Shang LX, Wang LN, Wang YL, Chen J, Jiang SS: Clinical observation on diabetic peripheral neuropathy treated with electroacupuncture and acupoint injection. Zhongguo Zhen Jiu 2011; 31:613-6.

[122] Bo C, Xue Z, Yi G, Zelin C, Yang B, Zixu W, Yajun W: Assessing the quality of reports about randomized controlled trials of acupuncture treatment on diabetic peripheral neuropathy. PLoS One 2012; 7(7):e38461.

[123] Luo YX: Acupuncture for 62 cases of urinary infection of diabetes. Zhongguo Zhen Jiu 2011; 31:702.

[124] Roger VL, Go AS, Lloyd-Jones DM, Benjamin EJ, Berry JD, Borden WB, Bravata DM, Dai S, Ford ES, Fox CS, Fullerton HJ, Gillespie C, Hailpern SM, Heit JA, Howard VJ, Kissela BM, Kittner SJ, Lackland DT, Lichtman JH, Lisabeth LD, Makuc DM, Marcus GM, Marelli A, Matchar DB, Moy CS, Mozaffarian D, Mussolino ME, Nichol G, Paynter NP, Soliman EZ, Sorlie PD, Sotoodehnia N, Turan TN, Virani SS, Wong ND, Woo D, Turner MB; American Heart Association Statistics Committee and Stroke Statistics Subcommittee: Heart disease and stroke statistics—2012 update: a report from the American Heart Association. Circulation 2012; 125:e2-e220.

[125] Xu H, Li Y, Liu A, Zhang Q, Hu X, Fang H, Li T, Guo H, Li Y, Xu G, Ma J, Du L, Ma G: Prevalence of the metabolic syndrome among children from six cities of China. BMC Public Health 2012; 12:13. http://www.biomedcentral.com/1471-2458/12/13

[126] Cheng TO: Childhood obesity in modern China. Int J Cardiol 2012; 157:315-7.

[127] Cho S-H, Lee J-S, Thabane L, Lee J: Acupuncture for obesity: a systematic review and meta-analysis. Int J Obesity 2009; 33:183-196.

[128] Gong M, Wang X, Mao Z, Shao Q, Xiang X, Xu B: Effect of electroacupuncture on leptin resistance in rats with diet-induced obesity. Am J Chin Med 2012; 40:511-20.

[129] Hu WL, Chang CH, Hung YC: Clinical observations on laser acupuncture in simple obesity therapy. Am J Chin Med 2010; 38(5):861-7.

[130] DeBakey ME: A Surgeon's Diary of a Visit to China. Phoenix, Arizona: Phoenix Newspapers, Inc. 1974:31-33.

[131] Hollinger I, Richter JA, Pongratz W, Baum M: Acupuncture anesthesia for open heart surgery: a report of 800 cases. Am J Chin Med 1979; 7:77-90.

[132] Caracausi SR: Electro-acupuncture in thoracic and cardiovascular surgery. Minerva Med 1979; 70:3857-3860.

[133] Yang L, Yang J, Wang Q, Chen M, Lu Z, Chen S, Xiong L: Cardioprotective effects of electroacupuncture pretreatment on patients undergoing heart valve replacement surgery: a randomized controlled trial. Ann Thorac Surg 2010; 89:781-6.

[134] Ni X, Xie Y, Wang Q, Zhong H, Chen M, Wang F, Xiong L: Cardioprotective effect of transcutaneous electric acupoint stimulation in the pediatric cardiac patients: a randomized controlled clinical trial. Paediatr Anaesth 2012;22:805-811.

[135] Zhou J, Chi H, Cheng TO, Chen TY, Wu YY, Zhou WX, Shen WD, Yuan L: Acupuncture anesthesia for open heart surgery in contemporary China. Int J Cardiol 2011; 150:12-16.

[136] Cheng TO: Acupuncture needles as a cause of bacterial endocarditis. Br Med J 1983; 287:689.

[137] Cheng TO: Subacute bacterial endocarditis following ear acupuncture. Int J Cardiol 1985; 8:97.

[138] Cheng TO: Infective endocarditis, cardiac tamponade, and AIDS as serious complications of acupuncture. Arch Intern Med 2004; 164:1464.

[139] Cheng TO: Pericardial effusion from self-inserted needle in the heart. Eur Heart J 1991; 12:958.

[140] Cheng TO: Cardiac tamponade following acupuncture. Chest 2000; 118:1836-1837.

[141] Andersen SA: Bilateral pneumothorax associated to acupuncture. Uqeskr Laeger 2011; 173:2724-5.

[142] Cheng TO: acupuncture and acquired immunodeficiency syndrome. Am J Med 1989; 87:489.

[143] Ernst E, White A: Life-threatening adverse reactions after acupuncture? A systematic review. Pain 1997; 71:123-126.

[144] Ernst E, White AR: Prospective studies of the safety of acupuncture: a systematic review. Am J Med 2001; 110:481-5.

[145] Melchart D, Weidenhammer W, Streng A, Reitmayr S, Hoppe A, Ernst E, Linde K: Prospective investigation of adverse effects of acupuncture in 97733 patients. Arch Intern Med 2004; 164:104-105.

[146] Endres HG, Molsberger A, Trampisch HJ: Adverse events in acupuncture: a prospective survey of adverse events after acupuncture treatment of 190,000 chronic pain patients. J Alternative Complementary Med 2004; 10:212.

[147] MacPherson H, Scullion T, Thomas K, Walters S: Patient reports of adverse events associated with acupuncture: a large scale prospective survey. J Alternative Complementary Med 2004; 10:215.

[148] Gopalan R, Scott R, Arabia F, Chandrasekaran K: Electro-acupuncture therapy in a patient with a total artificial heart. Acupunct Med 2011; 29:302-3.

[149] Zhong HZ, Chang JL, Zhu D, Gao Y: An overview of researches on underlying mechanisms of acupuncture therapy by functional magnetic resonance imaging in recent 5 years. Zhen Ci Yan Jiu 2012; 37(2):161-7.

[150] Hewson MG, Copeland HL, Mascha E, Arrigain S, Topol E, Fox JE: Integrative medicine: implementation and evaluation of a professional development program using experiential learning and conceptual change teaching approaches. Patient Educ Couns 2006; 62:5-12.

[151] Park JJ, Beckman-Harned S, Cho G, Kim D, Kim H: The current acceptance, accessibility and recognition of Chinese and Ayurvedic medicine in the United States in the public, governmental, and industrial sectors. Chin J Integr Med 2012; 18:405-8.

[152] NIH Consensus Development Panel on Acupuncture. NIH Consensus Conference. Acupuncture. JAMA 1998; 280:1518-1524.

[153] 2007 national health interview survey. http://nccam.nih.gov/about/plans/2011/introduction.htm.

[154] Lee JH. Choi TY, Lee MS, Lee H, Shin BC, Lee H: Acupuncture for acute low back pain: a systematic review. Clin J Pain 2013;29:172-185.

[155] Li ZJ, Liu ML, Wang JN, Liang FR: Method and current situations on acupuncture clinical trial registration in the world. Zhen Ci Yan Jiu 2012; 37:86, inside back cover.

Chapter 13

# Acupuncture for Cancer Patients: Practice and Research

Lizhen Wang and Ting Bao

Additional information is available at the end of the chapter

http://dx.doi.org/10.5772/54005

## 1. Introduction

Acupuncture is a traditional Chinese medicine technique that involves inserting and manipulating filiform needles in predefined points on the skin (i.e., *acupuncture points*) to achieve therapeutic effect. Although studies have not been able to fully explain the mechanism of acupuncture, it has been proposed that acupuncture worked through its effect on neurotransmitters and neurohormones. [1, 2]

Acupuncture points can be stimulated in various ways. With manual acupuncture, the filiform acupuncture needle is inserted in an acupuncture point and manually rotated to stimulate the point. With electroacupuncture, acupuncture points are stimulated by passing electrical current through inserted needles. Electrical current may also be passed through an electrode on the skin without inserting acupuncture needles, a technique called *noninvasive electrostimulation*. Acupressure is a form of modified acupuncture that replaces needles with physical pressure generated with either a finger or device such as an embedded stud in an elastic wrist band.

Acupuncture and acupuncture point stimulation have been widely used as a complementary therapy to treat wide range of illnesses by many patients, especially cancer patients. Growing evidence suggests that acupuncture is beneficial for cancer pain, chemotherapy-induced nausea, vomiting, and may be beneficial for symptoms such as radiation therapy-induced xerostomia, fatigue, hot flashes, depression, anxiety, and insomnia. This chapter provides an overview of the role of acupuncture in alleviating cancer patients' symptoms, with focus on the scientific evidence behind the practice.

## 2. Acupuncture to treat cancer pain

Cancer pain is the most common and one of the most distressing and feared symptoms among cancer patients. It is estimated that up to two thirds of patients with metastatic cancer suffered from cancer related pain.[3] More than 75% of hospitalized oncology patients experienced cancer related pain.[4-6] Due to its importance, pain is often referred to as the fifth vital sign of oncology patients. Cancer pain varies both by types of malignancy, and sites of cancer involvement.[7] The majority of cancer pain is caused by direct effect of cancer as a result of visceral involvement, bony metastasis, soft tissue invasion, or infiltration to the nerve or nerve plexus.[8] Cancer treatments such as chemotherapy, radiation and surgery may also cause treatment-induced cancer pain.

Cancer pain has traditionally been treated with opioids and interventional anesthetic or neurosurgical procedures. Despite maximal use of pain medications and application of interventional procedures, a significant portion of cancer patients still suffer from pain. In addition, the undesired side effects of long term usage of opioid pain medication, particularly change of mental status, constipation, nausea, fear of dependence, could be an issue. As a result, cancer patients often seek help in complementary alternative medicine, including acupuncture in an attempt to control their pain.

Even though acupuncture has been widely used among oncology patients to control cancer pain, the role of acupuncture in controlling cancer pain has not been clearly established through well-designed clinical trials. Many clinical trials suffered from methodological flaws such as poor study design, small sample size and lack of statistical analysis.[11] As a result, two recent Cochrane systematic reviews of randomized controlled clinical trials on the role of acupuncture to treat cancer pain showed no strong evidence for the effectiveness of acupuncture in reducing cancer pain. Another Cochrane systematic review assessed the value of Transcutaneous Electrical Nerve Stimulation (TENS) in the management of cancer-related pain in adults and remained inconclusive due to lack of suitable RCTs.[14]

On the other hand, a number of recent well-designed Randomized Controlled Trials (RCTs) have been conducted to study the role of acupuncture in treating cancer pain and are summarized in table 1.[15-23] Among them, four RCTs studied the efficacy of different types of acupuncture in controlling postoperative pain and presented mixed results. Deng et al's RCT on 106 cancer patients experiencing post-thoracotomy pain showed no statistical difference between the real versus sham acupuncture groups in patient's pain scores measured by Brief Pain Inventory at the 30-, 60-, and 90 days follow-ups.[15] The efficacy of the unique intradermal needles used in this study was questionable. Wong et al's smaller RCT (N=27) showed a trend of lower Visual Analog Scale (VAS) pain scores in patients receiving electro-acupuncture when compared to patients receiving sham acupuncture on post-operative days 2 and 6; and a statistically significant lower cumulative dose of Patient Controlled Analgesia (PCA) on postop day 2 ($p < 0.05$).[16] This study was, however, limited by its small sample size. Mehling et al's RCT (N=93) compared acupuncture plus massage therapy with usual care in controlling postoperative pain, nausea, vomiting and depressive moods.[17] It showed that postop acupuncture and massage in addition to usual care significantly improved pain control when compared to usual care alone. Lastly, Pfister et al's study showed that four weekly acupuncture treatments significantly reduced pain and improved function in cancer patients with chronic pain or dysfunction due to neck dissection than standard care alone.[24] However, with no sham therapy group in the last two studies, it is difficult to tease out the placebo effect, and leave the question that if the professionally trained acupuncturists and massage therapists and real acupuncture needles are required in the intervention remained unanswered.

| Reference/ Sample size | Type of Pain | Treatment Groups | Treatment Duration | Evaluation Method | Results |
|---|---|---|---|---|---|
| Deng et al 2008[15] N=106 | Post-thoracotomy pain | Group 1: intradermal acupuncture; 2: sham acupuncture | 1 month | Brief pain inventory | No difference between the two groups |
| Wong et al 2006[16] N=27 | Post-thoracotomy pain | Group1:electroacupuncture, 2: sham acupuncture | 7 days | VAS and medication quantification | Lower cumulative dose of patient controlled analgesic morphine used on postop day 2 in EA group (P < 0.05) |
| Mehling et al 2007[17] N=45 | Post-op pain | Group 1: acupuncture and massage; 2: usual care | 2 days | Pain numeric rating scale | The treatment group has less pain P = 0.038 |
| Pfister et al 2010[24] N=58 | pain and dysfunction in patients with cancer with a history of neck dissection | 1.acupuncture (N=28) 2. usual care (N=30) | Weekly for 4 weeks | Constant-Murley score, a composite measure of pain, function, and activities of daily living | Constant-Murley scores improved more in the acupuncture group (adjusted difference between groups = 11.2; 95% CI, 3.0 to 19.3; P = .008). |
| Alimi et al 2003[19] N=90 | Peripheral or central neuropathic pain arising after cancer treatment | Group 1: auricular acupuncture; 2: sham control; 3: control | 2 month | VAS | The acupuncture group had a significant decrease (P < 0.01) in pain intensity after 2 months (35% decrease) compared with the control groups |
| Dang et al 1998[22] N=48 | Stomach Cancer Pain | Group 1: acupuncture; 2:acupuncture point injection; 3: western analgesics | 2 months | WHO pain scale | No difference among the three groups in long-term effective rate of analgesia, 81% in all groups. |

| Reference/ Sample size | Type of Pain | Treatment Groups | Treatment Duration | Evaluation Method | Results |
|---|---|---|---|---|---|
| He et al 1999[21] N=80 | Post-operative pain in breast cancer patients | Group 1: acupuncture; 2: usual care | Post-op days 3, 5, 7 and day of discharge | VAS and range of movement | The acupuncture group had an improved post-op pain (p≤0.01) and range of movement (p<0.001) |
| Crew et al 2010[27] N=38 | Aromatase inhibitor-induced joint muscle pain | Group 1: acupuncture 2: sham acupuncture | Twice per week for 6 weeks | Brief Pain Inventory–Short Form (BPI-SF) | Significantly less pain (p=0.003) and pain-related interference (p=0.002) at week 6 in acupuncture arm than sham acupuncture arm |

**Table 1.** Summary of Randomized Control Trials on Acupuncture for Cancer Pain Relief

There have been a number of clinical trials showing the effect of acupuncture in reducing neuropathic pain in cancer patients. Among them, one clinical trial showed the effectiveness of auricular acupuncture in treating cancer treatment induced neuropathy.[19] This was a randomized, blinded, controlled trial conducted on 90 cancer patients with peripheral or central neuropathic pain arising after cancer treatment. The patients were randomized into one of three arms. One arm received real auricular acupuncture at real ear acupuncture points, which is defined as points where the electrodermal signal is being detected. The other two arms were placebo arms. The second arm received real auricular acupuncture at the placebo points. The third arm received sham acupuncture through auricular seeds at the placebo points.[19] All patients received two courses of real or placebo auricular acupuncture in two months, one month apart. The needles were left in place until they fell out or were removed at a follow up appointment. Their pain intensity measured by VAS at the end of the second month was used to measure the treatment efficacy. This study showed that in the group that received real acupuncture, pain intensity decreased by 36% at the end of 2 months when compared with baseline, whereas it only decreased by 2% in the placebo groups ($P < 0.0001$).[19 A recent acupuncture versus best medical care to treat peripheral neuropathy study showed that 76% patients in the acupuncture group had improvement in symptoms and nerve conduction studies whereas only 15% in the best medical care group did.[26] In addition, this study showed full correlation between the improvement in symptoms and nerve conduction studies.[26] Lastly, a recent randomized controlled clinical trial demonstrated that acupuncture significantly reduced aromatase inhibitor-associated joint pain and stiffness than sham acupuncture.[27]

These studies suggest that acupuncture may be a valuable alternative modality within a comprehensive program of cancer pain management. With minimal side effects reported, acupuncture remains a viable option for patients suffering from cancer pain. Further research should focus on using rigorous scientific methodology and an effective protocol based on a sound, evidence-based rationale.

## 2. Acupuncture to treat cancer therapy induced nausea and vomiting

Chemotherapy-Induced Nausea and Vomiting (CINV) is one of the most common and feared treatment-related side effects among patients with cancer. As a result, nutritional status, quality of life, and treatment adherence may be severely compromised in patients.[28] Over the past 20 years, better understanding of the physiology of CINV and the subsequent development of modern pharmacologic antiemetic agents have substantially improved the control of CINV. However, study suggests that CINV remains a significant problem among these patients.[29]

CINV can either be acute, delayed, or anticipatory. Acute CINV occurs within 24 hours of chemotherapy, usually beginning within 2 to 4 hours and peaking in the first 4 to 6 hours.[30] Delayed CINV occurs from day 2 to 6 of chemotherapy.[30] Anticipatory CINV occurs before chemotherapy treatments in patients who have previously experienced significant CINV.[30] Most antiemetic research focuses on reducing acute and delayed CINV, with the understanding that this would result in better control of anticipatory CINV. Despite recent advances in pharmacologic antiemetic therapy, additional treatment for breakthrough CINV is needed. Several randomized controlled clinical trials suggested the efficacy of acupuncture in controlling this side effect.

A meta-analysis of 11 RCTs on 1247 cancer patients with CINV showed that the proportion of acute vomiting episodes was significantly lower in the acupuncture point stimulation group than the control group (22% vs. 31%, p=0.04). Those trials, however, did not show that acupuncture significantly alleviate acute chemotherapy-induced nausea or delayed CINV.[35,36] The clinical relevance of these results were limited by the fact that those clinical trials predated the use of aprepitant and that only 1 or 2 acupuncture points were stimulated during acupuncture treatment. More clinical trials to study the effect of acupuncture with additional antiemetic acupuncture points in adjunct to modern pharmacologic antiemetic therapy are needed.

In addition to acupuncture, acupressure has been demonstrated to effectively reduce CINV. In a single-arm prospective study on 100 metastatic solid tumor patients experiencing persistent CINV despite standard antiemetic agents, 68% of patients' emetic symptoms improved after being treated with acupressure at PC6 point.[33] A RCT on 160 breast cancer patients who experienced moderate nausea during previous chemotherapy cycles and were getting ready to begin their 2$^{nd}$ or 3$^{rd}$ cycle of chemotherapy showed that acupressure at PC6 through a wrist device significantly decreased the amount of delayed vomiting and the intensity of nausea over time when compared with placebo acupressure and usual care groups.[34] The authors concluded that acupressure was safe and effective for cancer patients to manage delayed CINV and should be offered to breast cancer patients during chemotherapy. [34]

There has been a number of RCTs studying the effect of acupuncture in reducing Radiation-Induced Nausea and Vomiting (RINV), and showed that even though there is no statistically significant difference between real and sham acupuncture, both treatments were significantly more effective than standard care alone in reducing the frequency and severity of RINV (table 2). Over 90% patients in both treatment groups believed that acupuncture has been effective against radiation-induced nausea.[35]

| Reference/ Sample size | Treatment Groups | Treatment Duration | Primary end point | Results |
|---|---|---|---|---|
| Enblom et al 2012[35] N=215 | 1. verum acupuncture (penetrating and causing 'deqi' sensation) (n = 109) 2. sham acupuncture (use non-penetrating sham needles) (n = 106) | two to three times per week during radiation | % of patients with at least 1 emesis episode during radiation | 70% patients in the verum acupuncture group and 62% in the sham acupuncture group experienced nausea at least 1 emesis during radiation. No significant difference between two groups. |
| Enblom et al 2011[36] N=262 | 1.verum acupuncture (n=109; 99 provided data) 2. sham acupuncture (n=106; 101 provided data) 3. standard care alone (n=62; 62 provided data) | 2-3 times per week during radiation | Occurrence of nausea and emesis in each group was after a mean dose of 27 Gray. | Verum group: 37% experienced nausea, 8% vomiting; Sham group: 37% experienced nausea, 7% vomiting; Standard care group: 65% experienced nausea, 15% vomiting. |

**Table 2.** Summary of Randomized Control Trials on Acupuncture for the Relief of radiation induced nausea and vomiting

These studies suggest that acupuncture and acupressure are effective in reducing cancer treatment-induced nausea and vomiting in cancer patients. Most studies were conducted on break through CINV after the patients failed conventional anti-emetic medication. Further research needs to be conducted to determine if the combination of antiemetics and P6 acupoint stimulation works better than each component alone. Indeed, an animal study showed that combination therapy of electroacupuncture (EA) at P6 acupoint with ondansetron, droperidol or metoclopramide prevented emesis more significantly than EA or any of the medications alone.[37] These data suggested that EA and anti-emetic medication work synergistically.

## 3. Acupuncture to treat cancer fatigue

Fatigue is a common symptom in patients with cancer and a frequent side effect of chemo and radiation therapy, with no effective treatment exists. Several prospective pilot studies have suggested that acupuncture may benefit patients suffering from cancer fatigue (table 3). These studies were limited by their small sample size, but have provided encouraging information for further lare sample sized RCTs.

| Reference/ Sample size | Treatment Groups | Treatment | Evaluation Method | Results |
|---|---|---|---|---|
| Molassiotis et al 200738 (N=47) | 1.acupuncture: six 20-min sessions over 2 week 2.acupressure: massage acupoints daily 3.sham acupressure: massage none acupoints daily | Two weeks | Multidimensional Fatigue Inventory | Both acupuncture and acupressure significantly reduced cancer fatigue. Acupuncture was a more effective method than acupressure or sham acupressure. |
| Johnston et al. 2011[68] (N=50) | 1. education integrated with acupuncture 2. usual care | improve self-care + weekly 50-minute acupuncture sessions | Brief Fatigue Inventory (BFI) | A 2.38-point decline in fatigue as measured by the BFI when compared to usual care control (90% Confidence Interval from 0.586 to 5.014; p <0.10). |
| Balk et al. 2009[69] (N=23) | 1.real acupuncture 2.sham acupuncture | once to twice per week during the 6-week course of radiation therapy | Functional Assessment of Chronic Illness Therapy-Fatigue Subscale | Both groups had improvement in fatigue, fatigue distress, quality of life and depression from baseline to week 10, but no statistically significant intergroup difference. |
| Mao et al. 2009[39] (N=16) | 1. acupuncture: 12 treatments | 12 treatments during the course of radiation therapy | The Lee Fatigue Scale (LFS), the Patient Global Impression of Change (PGIC). | Average fatigue and energy domains of the LFS remained stable during and after RT, without any expected statistical decline owing to RT. |

**Table 3.** Summary of Pilot Studies on Acupuncture for Cancer Fatigue

Among these pilot studies, Molassiotis et al's pilot three-arm RCT was the most telling. In this trial, 47 cancer patients experiencing moderate to severe cancer fatigue were randomized into three groups: acupuncture (n = 15), acupressure (n = 16), and sham acupressure (n = 16). Patients in the acupuncture group received six 20-minute acupuncture sessions over two weeks, whereas patients in the two acupressure groups were taught to massage real versus sham acupuncture points daily for two weeks. [38] The Multidimensional Fatigue Inventory was used to assess their responses at baseline, week 2 and week 4 follow up. At the end of week two, general fatigue, physical fatigue, activity, and motivation significantly improved in the acupuncture and acupressure groups when compared to baseline.[38] At the end of week 2, fatigue level improved by 36% in the acupuncture group, 19% in the acupressure group and 0.6% in the control group. Moreover, the improvement maintained at the week 4 follow-up.[38] Acupuncture was found to be a more effective method than acupressure or sham acupressure. The authors concluded that acupuncture showed great potential to manage cancer-related fatigue and should be tested further with larger sample size and multi-center RCT. [38]

In addition to treating cancer fatigue, pilot study has also suggested the effect of acupuncture in preventing radiation-induced fatigue. A single-arm acupuncture trial conducted on 16 cancer patients undergoing radiation showed that 12 acupuncture treatment during radiation resulted in a stable average fatigue score during radiation therapy and 87% patients reported either stable or improved fatigue during radiation. [39] These findings invite further research to study the role of acupuncture in preventing the development of cancer fatigue.

These pilot clinical trials encourages further large sample sized randomized controlled trials to evaluate the effect of acupuncture on treating and preventing fatigue in cancer patients.

## 4. Acupuncture to treat hot flashes in cancer patients

Vasomotor symptoms (hot flashes, night sweats) are common complaints among breast cancer survivors. These symptoms are usually the result of breast cancer related treatment such as chemotherapy-induced menopause or estrogen deprivation therapy. Management of hot flashes among breast cancer survivors is challenging as the most effective treatment, hormone replacement therapy, is associated with increased risk of breast cancer recurrence and development of new breast cancer. Acupuncture shows promise as a therapeutic approach for hot flashed with minimal side effects. The role of acupuncture in reducing hot flashes in women with breast cancer has been studied in a number of well-designed RCTs (table 4).

In 2007, Deng et al reported results from a randomized, sham-controlled trial on the effect of acupuncture in treating breast cancer patients who experienced three or more hot flashes per day.[40] Seventy-two women were randomized to 8 sessions (4 weeks biweekly) real versus sham acupuncture. The primary end point was hot flash frequency at week 6. Patients randomized to the sham acupuncture arm were crossed over to receive real acupuncture at week 7 and were evaluated 6 weeks later. All patients were also evaluated at 6 months. The investigators reported that the mean number of hot flashes per day at week 6 changed from 8.7 to 6.2 in the real acupuncture arm, and from 10.0 to 7.6 in the sham acupuncture arm. The difference between real and sham acupuncture arm was not statistically significant ($p = 0.3$). When patients in the sham acupuncture arm were crossed over to receive real acupuncture, their hot flash frequency further reduced from 7.6 to 5.8. The reduction in hot flashes in all patients persisted during the 6 months follow up (real acupuncture arm down to 6.1 per day and sham acupuncture arm to 6.8 per day). The authors concluded that acupuncture reduced hot flash frequency as it was reduced significantly in both treatment arms, even though there was no statistically significant difference between real versus sham acupuncture.[40] Importantly, only fourteen minor adverse events, such as mild bleeding and bruising that did not require medical intervention were reported from the 560 acupuncture sessions.[40] Similar results were demonstrated in other RCT studying the effect of acupuncture to treat hot flashes in perimenopausal women.[41]

| Reference/ Sample size | Treatment Groups | Treatment Duration | Evaluation Method | Results |
|---|---|---|---|---|
| Deng et al. 2007[40] (N=72) | 1. real acupuncture 2. sham acupuncture | 4 weeks | Hot flash frequency | True acupuncture was associated with 0.8 fewer hot flashes per day than sham at 6 weeks, but the difference did not reach statistical significance |
| Hervik et al. 2009[42] (N=59) | 1. real acupuncture 2. sham acupuncture (SA) | 10 weeks | Mean number of hot flashes at day and night, and Kupperman index. | During the treatment period mean number of hot flashes at day and night was significantly reduced by almost 60%, respectively from baseline in the acupuncture group, and was further reduced by 30% both at day and night during the next 12 weeks. Kupperman index was reduced by 44% from baseline to the end of the treatment period in the acupuncture group, and largely maintained 12 weeks after treatment ended. |
| Frisk et al. 2008[43] (N=45) | 1. electro-acupuncture (EA) 2.hormone therapy (HT) | 24 months | Number of hot flashes per day | In the EA group, the median number of hot flushes/24 h decreased from 9.6 at baseline to 4.3 at 12 weeks of treatment ($p < 0.001$). In the HT group, the median number of hot flushes/24 h decreased from 6.6 at baseline to 0. |
| Walker et al. 2010[44] (N=50) | 1. acupuncture 2. venlafaxine | 12 weeks | Hot flashes frequency and severity | acupuncture was as effective as venlafaxine |

**Table 4.** Summary of Randomized Control Trials on Acupuncture for hot flashes in breast cancer patients

In 2008, Hervik et al reported another randomized, sham acupuncture-controlled trial on the effect of acupuncture in treating breast cancer patients suffering from hot flashes following at least 3 months tamoxifen.[42] Fifty-nine women were randomized to 15 sessions (5 weeks biweekly followed by 5 weeks weekly) real versus sham acupuncture. The authors measured mean number of hot flashes at baseline, at the end of the treatment period, and 12 weeks after treatment to assess the treatment effect. They reported that at the end of the treatment period, mean number of daytime hot flashes reduced significantly from 9.5 to 4.7 ($p=0.001$) in the real acupuncture arm, and from 12.3 to 11.7 ($p=0.382$) in the sham acupuncture arm. At 12 weeks follow up, further reduction was observed in real acupuncture arm (from 4.7 to 3.2) but not in sham acupuncture arm (from 11.7 to 12.1). A similar pattern was observed in night-time hot flashes as the number of hot flashes reduced from 6 to 2.6 in the real acupuncture arm and from 7.2 to 5.4 in the sham acupuncture arm at the end of the treatment period, with further reduction in the real acupuncture arm (from 2.6 to 1.7) but not sham acupuncture arm (from 5.4 to 6.1) at the 12 weeks follow up. The difference between the real and sham acupuncture arms was statistically significant ($p < 0.001$). The authors concluded that acupuncture provided effective relief from hot flashes in breast cancer patients suffering from hot flashes while taking tamoxifen.[42] The evidence generated from these two trials suggests that acupuncture effectively decreases hot flashes frequency, although it is not clear whether it is superior to sham acupuncture.

In addition, another clinical trial compared the effects of electro-acupuncture (EA) with hormonal therapy in breast cancer survivors with vasomotor symptoms and showed that in the 19 out of 27 women who completed 12 weeks of EA treatment, the number of hot flashes significantly reduced from 9.6 per day to 4.3 per day. The improvement persisted at month 12 follow up.[43] In the hormonal treatment group, the median hot flashes number dropped from 6.6 at baseline to 0 at week 12. Although flushes decreased less in the EA group than in the HT group, HRQoL improved at least to the same extent. It suggests that EA should be further evaluated as treatment for women with breast cancer and climacteric complaints, since HT is no longer recommended for breast cancer survivors. [43]

Lastly, in 2010, Walker et al reported another RCT comparing the effect of acupuncture with venlafaxine in treating vasomotor symptoms in breast cancer patients suffering from greater than 13 hot flashes per week.[44] Changes in hot flash frequency from baseline to 3, 6, 9 and 12 month follow up were used as the primary outcome. Fifty patients were randomized to 12 weeks (biweekly for 4 weeks, followed by weekly for 8 weeks) of acupuncture versus daily venlafaxine (37.5mg for one week, then 75 mg for 11 weeks). The investigators observed a significant reduction in hot flashes frequency and severity in both groups. In addition, two weeks after treatments were stopped, those randomized to venlafaxine reported increased in hot flash frequency, whereas the acupuncture group remained at low level of hot flashes. There was no significant difference between acupuncture arm and venlafaxine arm. There were 18 reported adverse events (i.e. nausea, dizziness, headache) in the venlafaxine arm and none in the acupuncture arm. The authors concluded that acupuncture appears as effective as venlafaxine and is a safe and durable treatment option for breast cancer patients experiencing vasomotor symptoms.[44]

A systematic review of six RCTs showed further research is needed to determine whether acupuncture produces specific effects that alleviate hot flashes in patients with breast cancer.[45] Lastly, hot flashes are also common side effects of hormonal therapy for prostate cancer patients. A pilot study showed that when 25 prostate cancer patients receiving androgen deprivation therapy (ADT) were treated with electroacupuncture biweekly for 4 weeks, then weekly for 6 weeks 9 out of 22 evaluable patients (41% ) had >50% reduction in the hot flash score at week 4, and 12 patients(55%) had clinically significant reduction in hot flashes during the treatment course, and none had a significant increase in hot flashes during therapy.[46] This pilot study provided promising preliminary data to further study the role of acupuncture in treating hot flashes in prostate cancer patients.

http://dx.doi.org/10.5772/54005

## 5. Acupuncture to treat and prevent xerostomia

Xerostomia, or dry mouth, is caused by the dysfunction of parotid glands damaged by radiation therapy and is considered a significant factor underlying dysphasia. Patients with xerostomia lose their taste and have difficulty speaking and swallowing. Several pilot clinical studies suggest that acupuncture may improve xerostomia symptoms caused by radiation therapy in patients who have head and neck cancers.[47-50] In addition, one clinical case series, seven xerostomia patients treated with acupuncture reported increase in salivary flow and ability to eat and speak.[51] Another study showed that after 12 session of acupuncture during 6 weeks, 12 patients with severe xerostomia had statistically significant improvement in salivary flow rates on both subjective and objective evaluations.[52]

Since then, a number of RCTs have been conducted to study the effect of acupuncture in treating and preventing radiation-induced xerostomia and are summarized in table 5. One study showed that even though both real and sham acupuncture increased the whole salivary flow rate with no significant difference between the two groups, it was only the real acupuncture that markedly increased the unstimulated salivary flow rates.[54] Moreover, real acupuncture significantly improved the dry mouth score when compared to sham acupuncture control.[54]

There has been a number of RCTs studying the effect of acupuncture in preventing xerostomia in head/neck patients undergoing radiotherapy. One study randomized 23 patients with nasopharygeal carcinoma to real acupuncture (N=11) and sham acupuncture (N=12) with three times/week treatment during radiation therapy. [55] Starting from week 3, xerostomia symptoms were significantly better in the real acupuncture group than sham acupuncture group, however, there was no significant difference in salivary flow rate. [55] The same group of investigators concurrently conducted another RCT that used standard care alone as control and showed that xerostomia symptoms was significantly better in the acupuncture group than standard care group starting in week 3 during radiation therapy through 6 months follow up. Interestingly, there was statistically significant greater saliva flow in the acupuncture group at week 7, 11 and 6 month follow up than in the standard care group. [56] Similar findings of acupuncture increased salivary flow when compared to standard care were reported in a smaller sample sized RCT.[57]

As exciting as these results were a recent systematic review on the preventive and therapeutic effect of acupuncture for radiation-Induced xerostomia in patients with head and neck cancer reported that because of the significant variation among the existing RCTs, meta-analysis was not possible. In the RCTs used placebo (sham acupuncture) control, no significant differences were noted between the two treatments with regard to increasing salivary flow. It was important to note that no significant side effects were reported due to acupuncture. The authors concluded that there was insufficient evidence available to judge if acupuncture is more effective than sham acupuncture in treating xerostomia and further research is needed.[58]

| Reference/ Sample size | Treatment Groups | Treatment | Evaluation Method | Results |
|---|---|---|---|---|
| | | *Treatment Trials* | | |
| Blom et al 1996[53] N=38 | 1.acupuncture (N=20) 2.superficial acupuncture (N=18) | Twice per week | salivary flow rates | In both groups the patients showed significantly increased salivary flow rates after the acupuncture treatment. |
| Cho et al. 2008[54] (N=12) | 1.real acupuncture (N=6) 2.sham acupuncture (N=6) | twice weekly for 6 weeks | whole salivary flow rates (stimulated and unstimulated) and questionnaire-based assessment of subjective symptoms | Both groups showed a slight increase in whole salivary flow rates, with no significant difference between them. However, real acupuncture markedly increased unstimulated salivary flow rates, and improved the score for dry mouth according to the xerostomia questionnaire, by 2.33 points versus 0.33 in the controls. |
| Pfister et al 2010[24] N=58 | 1.acupuncture (N=28) 2. usual care (N=30) | Once per week | Xerostomia Inventory (although Xerostomia was secondary end point) | Acupuncture produced greater improvement in reported xerostomia compared to usual care(adjusted difference in Xerostomia Inventory = -5.8; 95% CI, -0.9 to -10.7; P = .02). |
| | | *Prevention Trials* | | |
| Meng et al. 2012[55] (N=23) | 1.real acupuncture (N=11) 2.sham acupuncture (N=12) | 3/week during radiation therapy | Xerostomia Questionnaire (XQ), MD Anderson Symptom Inventory for Head and Neck Cancer (MDASI-HN). Unstimulated whole salivary flow rates (UWSFR) and stimulated salivary flow rates (SSFR). | XQ, MDASI-HN scores for acupuncture were significantly lower than sham controls starting in week 3 and lasted through the 1-month follow-up. No group differences for UWSFR and SSFR. |
| Meng et al. 2012[56] (N=86) | 1.acupuncture (N=40) 2.standard care (N=46) | 3/week during radiotherapy | | XQ, MDASI-HN scores for acupuncture were significantly lower than standard care control starting in week 3 and lasted through the 6-month follow-up. Greater saliva flow in the acupuncture group at week 7, 11, 6-month follow-up than standard care control. |
| Braga et al. 2011[57] (N=24) | 1. acupuncture (N=12) 2. standard care (N=12) | treated with acupuncture before and during RT | Syalometry, measuring the resting (RSFR) and stimulated (SSFR) salivary flow rates, and visual analogue scale (VAS) regarding dry mouth-related symptoms | Patients in the acupuncture group showed improved salivary flow rates (RSFR, SSFR; $p < 0.001$) and decreased xerostomia-related symptoms (VAS, $p < 0.05$) compared with patients in the control group. |

**Table 5.** Summary of Randomized Control Trials on Acupuncture for Xerostomia

http://dx.doi.org/10.5772/54005

## 6. Acupuncture to treat other cancer or cancer treatment-related symptoms

### 6.1. Depression and insomnia

Acupuncture has been reported to reduce depression and improve sleep quality. There has not been extensive research conducted in this area. One recent RCT on 80 cancer patients suffering from cancer related depression and sleep disorder showed that acupuncture was more effective than fluoxetine in reducing depression and improving sleep quality.[59] Further study is warranted.

### 6.2. Dysphagia

Dysphagia is a common side effect from chemoradiation therapy (CRT) in patients with head and neck cancer (HNC). In a retrospective case series, 10 patients with HNC were treated with weekly acupuncture for radiation-induced dysphagia and xerostomia. Ninety percent patients reported subjective improvement and 86% Percutaneous Endoscopic Gastrostomy (PEG)-tube dependent patients had their PEG-tube removed after acupuncture treatments.[60] The same group of researchers are conducting a randomized, sham acupuncture controlled clinical trial on 42 squamous cell carcinoma HNC patients to study the effect of acupuncture in treating dysphagia in HNC patients after chemoradiation.[61]

### 6.3. Dyspnea

Dyspnea is one of the most distressing symptoms experienced by end stage cancer patients. Pharmacologic management has proven yet limited benefit. Additional treatments are needed. Anecdotally, acupuncture has helped patients to breathe better. A pilot RCT on 47 lung and breast cancer patients, however, failed to show that.[62] Further study is needed.

### 6.4. Lymphedema

Lymphedema is a distressing symptom among cancer patients, especially breast cancer patients, with no effective treatment. There have been a number of observational studies showing the feasibility, safety and efficacy of acupuncture in reducing lymphedema in cancer patients.[63-66] Among them, one pilot study on 9 breast cancer patients with chronic lymphedema showed that 4 women had greater or equal to 30% reduction in the extent of lymphedema after 4 weeks biweekly acupuncture treatments. Importantly, no serious side effect from acupuncture was reported.[65]

## 7. Discussion

This chapter summarized the current practice and clinical research on acupuncture for cancer patients. It is important to note that with the use of acupuncture being more and more accepted by cancer patients and oncologists, there have been an increasing number of well-designed clinical trials to support the practice. These trials have shown that there have been minimal side effects associated with acupuncture. When compared to standard care alone, acupuncture is superior in reducing both subjective and objective symptoms. However, when compared to placebo control (usually sham acupuncture), the benefit of acupuncture became less obvious. This may be due to the fact that sham acupuncture also has physiological effects. Indeed, one study already showed that both real and sham acupuncture significantly reduced patients' serum cortisol concentration.[67] Despite that the majority of RCTs showed no significant difference between real and sham acupuncture, acupuncture has been used more often by cancer patients in the clinical setting. This is mainly because of its minimal side effect and potential significant benefit. Further research needs to be conducted to study the mechanism of acupuncture and identify the population that may benefit most from acupuncture, and the conditions that acupuncture may be most helpful.

## Author details

Lizhen Wang[1,2] and Ting Bao[2,3]

1 Shanghai University of Traditional Chinese Medicine, College of Acupuncture-Moxibustion and Tuina, Shanghai, P.R. China

2 Center for Integrative Medicine, University of Maryland School of Medicine, Baltimore, Maryland, U.S.A.

3 The University of Maryland Marlene and Stewart Greenebaum Cancer Center, University of Maryland School of Medicine, Baltimore, Maryland, U.S.A.

## References

[1] C T. Mechanism of acupuncture analgesia based on animal experiments. In: Pomerantz B SG, eds., ed. Scientific Bases of Acupuncture. Berlin, Germany: Springer-Verlag; 1989.

[2] Lee BY LP, Newberg AB. Acupuncture in theory and practice. Hospital Physician 2004;40:11-8.

[3] Cleeland CS, Gonin R, Hatfield AK, et al. Pain and its treatment in outpatients with metastatic cancer. N Engl J Med 1994;330:592-6.

[4] Brescia FJ, Portenoy RK, Ryan M, Krasnoff L, Gray G. Pain, opioid use, and survival in hospitalized patients with advanced cancer. J Clin Oncol 1992;10:149-55.

[5] Wells N. Pain intensity and pain interference in hospitalized patients with cancer. Oncol Nurs Forum 2000;27:985-91.

[6] McMillan SC, Tittle M, Hagan S, Laughlin J. Management of pain and pain-related symptoms in hospitalized veterans with cancer. Cancer Nurs 2000;23:327-36.

[7] Foley K. Pain syndromes in patients with cancer. in Advances in Pain Research and Therapy. New York: Raven Press; 1979.

[8] Banning A, Sjogren P, Henriksen H. Pain causes in 200 patients referred to a multidisciplinary cancer pain clinic. Pain 1991;45:45-8.

[9] Coyle N, Adelhardt J, Foley KM, Portenoy RK. Character of terminal illness in the advanced cancer patient: pain and other symptoms during the last four weeks of life. J Pain Symptom Manage 1990;5:83-93.

[10] Zech DF, Grond S, Lynch J, Hertel D, Lehmann KA. Validation of World Health Organization Guidelines for cancer pain relief: a 10-year prospective study. Pain 1995;63:65-76.

[11] Lee H, Schmidt K, Ernst E. Acupuncture for the relief of cancer-related pain--a systematic review. Eur J Pain 2005;9:437-44.

[12] Choi TY, Lee MS, Kim TH, Zaslawski C, Ernst E. Acupuncture for the treatment of cancer pain: a systematic review of randomised clinical trials. Support Care Cancer 2012;20:1147-58.

[13] Paley CA, Johnson MI, Tashani OA, Bagnall AM. Acupuncture for cancer pain in adults. Cochrane Database Syst Rev 2011:CD007753.

[14] Hurlow A, Bennett MI, Robb KA, Johnson MI, Simpson KH, Oxberry SG. Transcutaneous electric nerve stimulation (TENS) for cancer pain in adults. Cochrane Database Syst Rev 2012;3:CD006276.

[15] Deng G, Rusch V, Vickers A, et al. Randomized controlled trial of a special acupuncture technique for pain after thoracotomy. J Thorac Cardiovasc Surg 2008;136:1464-9.

[16] Wong RH, Lee TW, Sihoe AD, et al. Analgesic effect of electroacupuncture in post-thoracotomy pain: a prospective randomized trial. Ann Thorac Surg 2006;81:2031-6.

[17] Mehling WE, Jacobs B, Acree M, et al. Symptom management with massage and acupuncture in postoperative cancer patients: a randomized controlled trial. J Pain Symptom Manage 2007;33:258-66.

[18] Crew KD, Capodice JL, Greenlee H, et al. Pilot study of acupuncture for the treatment of joint symptoms related to adjuvant aromatase inhibitor therapy in postmenopausal breast cancer patients. J Cancer Surviv 2007;1:283-91.

[19] Alimi D, Rubino C, Pichard-Leandri E, Fermand-Brule S, Dubreuil-Lemaire ML, Hill C. Analgesic effect of auricular acupuncture for cancer pain: a randomized, blinded, controlled trial. J Clin Oncol 2003;21:4120-6.

[20] Alimi D, Rubino C, Leandri EP, Brule SF. Analgesic effects of auricular acupuncture for cancer pain. J Pain Symptom Manage 2000;19:81-2.

[21] He JP, Friedrich M, Ertan AK, Muller K, Schmidt W. Pain-relief and movement improvement by acupuncture after ablation and axillary lymphadenectomy in patients with mammary cancer. Clin Exp Obstet Gynecol 1999;26:81-4.

[22] Dang W, Yang J. Clinical study on acupuncture treatment of stomach carcinoma pain. J Tradit Chin Med 1998;18:31-8.

[23] Li QS, Cao SH, Xie GM, et al. Combined traditional Chinese medicine and Western medicine. Relieving effects of Chinese herbs, ear-acupuncture and epidural morphine on postoperative pain in liver cancer. Chin Med J (Engl) 1994;107:289-94.

[24] Pfister DG, Cassileth BR, Deng GE, et al. Acupuncture for pain and dysfunction after neck dissection: results of a randomized controlled trial. J Clin Oncol 2010;28:2565-70.

[25] Minton O, Higginson IJ. Electroacupuncture as an adjunctive treatment to control neuropathic pain in patients with cancer. J Pain Symptom Manage 2007;33:115-7.

[26] Schroder S, Liepert J, Remppis A, Greten JH. Acupuncture treatment improves nerve conduction in peripheral neuropathy. Eur J Neurol 2007;14:276-81.

[27] Crew KD, Capodice JL, Greenlee H, et al. Randomized, blinded, sham-controlled trial of acupuncture for the management of aromatase inhibitor-associated joint symptoms in women with early-stage breast cancer. Journal of clinical oncology : official journal of the American Society of Clinical Oncology 2010;28:1154-60.

[28] Naeim A, Dy SM, Lorenz KA, Sanati H, Walling A, Asch SM. Evidence-based recommendations for cancer nausea and vomiting. J Clin Oncol 2008;26:3903-10.

[29] Hickok JT, Roscoe JA, Morrow GR, King DK, Atkins JN, Fitch TR. Nausea and emesis remain significant problems of chemotherapy despite prophylaxis with 5-hydroxytryptamine-3 antiemetics: a University of Rochester James P. Wilmot Cancer Center Community Clinical Oncology Program Study of 360 cancer patients treated in the community. Cancer 2003;97:2880-6.

[30] Hesketh PJ. Chemotherapy-induced nausea and vomiting. N Engl J Med 2008;358:2482-94.

[31] Ezzo J, Streitberger K, Schneider A. Cochrane systematic reviews examine P6 acupuncture-point stimulation for nausea and vomiting. J Altern Complement Med 2006;12:489-95.

[32] Ezzo JM, Richardson MA, Vickers A, et al. Acupuncture-point stimulation for chemotherapy-induced nausea or vomiting. Cochrane Database Syst Rev 2006:CD002285.

[33] Gardani G, Cerrone R, Biella C, et al. A progress study of 100 cancer patients treated by acupressure for chemotherapy-induced vomiting after failure with the pharmacological approach. Minerva Med 2007;98:665-8.

[34] Dibble SL, Luce J, Cooper BA, et al. Acupressure for chemotherapy-induced nausea and vomiting: a randomized clinical trial. Oncol Nurs Forum 2007;34:813-20.

[35] Enblom A, Johnsson A, Hammar M, Onelov E, Steineck G, Borjeson S. Acupuncture compared with placebo acupuncture in radiotherapy-induced nausea--a randomized controlled study. Ann Oncol 2012;23:1353-61.

[36] Enblom A, Lekander M, Hammar M, et al. Getting the grip on nonspecific treatment effects: emesis in patients randomized to acupuncture or sham compared to patients receiving standard care. PLoS One 2011;6:e14766.

[37] Lao L, Zhang G, Wong RH, Carter AK, Wynn RL, Berman BM. The effect of electroacupuncture as an adjunct on cyclophosphamide-induced emesis in ferrets. Pharmacol Biochem Behav 2003;74:691-9.

[38] Molassiotis A, Sylt P, Diggins H. The management of cancer-related fatigue after chemotherapy with acupuncture and acupressure: a randomised controlled trial. Complement Ther Med 2007;15:228-37.

[39] Mao JJ, Styles T, Cheville A, Wolf J, Fernandes S, Farrar JT. Acupuncture for nonpalliative radiation therapy-related fatigue: feasibility study. J Soc Integr Oncol 2009;7:52-8.

[40] Deng G, Vickers A, Yeung S, et al. Randomized, controlled trial of acupuncture for the treatment of hot flashes in breast cancer patients. Journal of clinical oncology : official journal of the American Society of Clinical Oncology 2007;25:5584-90.

[41] Vincent A, Barton DL, Mandrekar JN, et al. Acupuncture for hot flashes: a randomized, sham-controlled clinical study. Menopause 2007;14:45-52.

[42] Hervik J, Mjaland O. Acupuncture for the treatment of hot flashes in breast cancer patients, a randomized, controlled trial. Breast Cancer Res Treat 2009;116:311-6.

[43] Frisk J, Carlhall S, Kallstrom AC, Lindh-Astrand L, Malmstrom A, Hammar M. Long-term follow-up of acupuncture and hormone therapy on hot flushes in women with breast cancer: a prospective, randomized, controlled multicenter trial. Climacteric 2008;11:166-74.

[44] Walker EM, Rodriguez AI, Kohn B, et al. Acupuncture versus venlafaxine for the management of vasomotor symptoms in patients with hormone receptor-positive breast cancer: a randomized controlled trial. Journal of clinical oncology : official journal of the American Society of Clinical Oncology 2010;28:634-40.

[45] Lee MS, Kim KH, Choi SM, Ernst E. Acupuncture for treating hot flashes in breast cancer patients: a systematic review. Breast Cancer Res Treat 2009;115:497-503.

[46] Beer TM, Benavides M, Emmons SL, et al. Acupuncture for hot flashes in patients with prostate cancer. Urology 2010;76:1182-8.

[47] Johnstone PA, Peng YP, May BC, Inouye WS, Niemtzow RC. Acupuncture for pilocarpine-resistant xerostomia following radiotherapy for head and neck malignancies. Int J Radiat Oncol Biol Phys 2001;50:353-7.

[48] Johnstone PA, Niemtzow RC, Riffenburgh RH. Acupuncture for xerostomia: clinical update. Cancer 2002;94:1151-6.

[49] Simcock R, Fallowfield L, Jenkins V. Group acupuncture to relieve radiation induced xerostomia: a feasibility study. Acupunct Med 2009;27:109-13.

[50] Garcia MK, Chiang JS, Cohen L, et al. Acupuncture for radiation-induced xerostomia in patients with cancer: a pilot study. Head Neck 2009;31:1360-8.

[51] Morganstein WM. Acupuncture in the treatment of xerostomia: clinical report. Gen Dent 2005;53:223-6; quiz 7.

[52] Braga FP, Sugaya NN, Hirota SK, Weinfeld I, Magalhaes MH, Migliari DA. The effect of acupuncture on salivary flow rates in patients with radiation-induced xerostomia. Minerva Stomatol 2008;57:343-8.

[53] Blom M, Dawidson I, Fernberg JO, Johnson G, Angmar-Mansson B. Acupuncture treatment of patients with radiation-induced xerostomia. Eur J Cancer B Oral Oncol 1996;32B:182-90.

[54] Cho JH, Chung WK, Kang W, Choi SM, Cho CK, Son CG. Manual acupuncture improved quality of life in cancer patients with radiation-induced xerostomia. J Altern Complement Med 2008;14:523-6.

[55] Meng Z, Kay Garcia M, Hu C, et al. Sham-controlled, randomised, feasibility trial of acupuncture for prevention of radiation-induced xerostomia among patients with nasopharyngeal carcinoma. Eur J Cancer 2012;48:1692-9.

[56] Meng Z, Garcia MK, Hu C, et al. Randomized controlled trial of acupuncture for prevention of radiation-induced xerostomia among patients with nasopharyngeal carcinoma. Cancer 2012;118:3337-44.

[57] Braga FP, Lemos Junior CA, Alves FA, Migliari DA. Acupuncture for the prevention of radiation-induced xerostomia in patients with head and neck cancer. Braz Oral Res 2011;25:180-5.

[58] Zhuang L, Yang Z, Zeng X, et al. The Preventive and Therapeutic Effect of Acupuncture for Radiation-Induced Xerostomia in Patients With Head and Neck Cancer: A Systematic Review. Integr Cancer Ther 2012.

[59] Feng Y, Wang XY, Li SD, et al. Clinical research of acupuncture on malignant tumor patients for improving depression and sleep quality. J Tradit Chin Med 2011;31:199-202.

[60] Lu W, Posner MR, Wayne P, Rosenthal DS, Haddad RI. Acupuncture for dysphagia after chemoradiation therapy in head and neck cancer: a case series report. Integr Cancer Ther 2010;9:284-90.

[61] Lu W, Wayne PM, Davis RB, et al. Acupuncture for dysphagia after chemoradiation in head and neck cancer: rationale and design of a randomized, sham-controlled trial. Contemp Clin Trials 2012;33:700-11.

[62] Vickers AJ, Feinstein MB, Deng GE, Cassileth BR. Acupuncture for dyspnea in advanced cancer: a randomized, placebo-controlled pilot trial [ISRCTN89462491]. BMC Palliat Care 2005;4:5.

[63] Kanakura Y, Niwa K, Kometani K, et al. Effectiveness of acupuncture and moxibustion treatment for lymphedema following intrapelvic lymph node dissection: a preliminary report. Am J Chin Med 2002;30:37-43.

[64] Yang XH, Liu H, Chai JH, Zhao XC. [Observation on 27 elderly women in britain with lymphedema syndrome treated by acupuncture combined with medicine]. Zhongguo Zhen Jiu 2009;29:998-1000.

[65] Cassileth BR, Van Zee KJ, Chan Y, et al. A safety and efficacy pilot study of acupuncture for the treatment of chronic lymphoedema. Acupunct Med 2011;29:170-2.

[66] de Valois BA, Young TE, Melsome E. Assessing the feasibility of using acupuncture and moxibustion to improve quality of life for cancer survivors with upper body lymphoedema. Eur J Oncol Nurs 2012;16:301-9.

[67] So EW, Ng EH, Wong YY, Yeung WS, Ho PC. Acupuncture for frozen-thawed embryo transfer cycles: a double-blind randomized controlled trial. Reprod Biomed Online 2010;20:814-21.

[68] Johnston MF, Hays RD, Subramanian SK, et al. Patient education integrated with acupuncture for relief of cancer-related fatigue randomized controlled feasibility study. BMC Complement Altern Med 2011;11:49.

[69] Balk J, Day R, Rosenzweig M, Beriwal S. Pilot, randomized, modified, double-blind, placebo-controlled trial of acupuncture for cancer-related fatigue. J Soc Integr Oncol 2009;7:4-11.

Chapter 14

# Acupuncture for Addictions

P.C. Leung, L. Zhang, L.Y. Eliza Wong and
S.Y. Ellie Pang

Additional information is available at the end of the chapter

http://dx.doi.org/10.5772/54788

## 1. Introduction

### 1.1. Heroin addiction

For centuries opiate addiction has been a difficult health and social problem. The morbidity and mortality related to such addiction affect not only the individual but also bring disastrous effects to the affected families and their communities [1, 2]. Based on Quoting epidemiological data in social surveys done in the last decade, over 13 million opium addicts are living in different countries, while Asia has the largest number. Heroin addiction gives the most severe affections and the number might be exceeding 9 millions [3, 4]. In the city of Hong Kong alone, about 16,000 heroin addicts have registered with the Central Registry of Drug Abuse [5].

Before we consider various means that can be used to counteract opium addiction, we need to know how the addiction affects the individuals.

### 1.2. Health hazards related to opiate addiction

Opiate and its derivatives depress the central nervous system activities which can last up to six hours after opiates have been consumed. Moreover, there is a subjective effect, which persists for another 5-6 hours. Once the opiate tolerance developed, the opiate consumer tends to require higher and higher doses to avoid the withdrawal symptoms. Apart from the central nervous system, there are severe gastro-intestinal upsetsand disturbances to other physiological systems [6].

Opiate or heroin is commonly taken together with alcohol, barbiturates and/or other abusive drugs, resulting in life-threatening morbidities such as respiratory distress, serious infections etc. The application of injections introduces viral infections like hepatitis and AIDS [7].

The intolerability and the degree of withdrawal symptoms are so severe that addicts tend to experience a change of personality and their daily activities are focused on the acquisition of the drug. The direct outcome is the rapid development of anti-social behaviour. The abrupt or gradually loss of harmony in the families of the addicts merge into difficult anti-social problems, often involving crimes. The general health deteriorations and anti-social tendencies make this group of people particularly prone to addiction related infections like HIV. Statistics have already indicated that about 80% HIV infections are related to heroin injections [7].

### 1.3. Treatment available for withdrawal symptoms

Opiate physical dependence can berapidly developed after only 2 to 10 days of continuous consumption of opiates, particularly with heroin. When the drug is stopped, a complex system of symptoms consisting of diffuse pain autonomic disturbances i.e. diarrhea, rhinorrhea, nausea and vomiting, and central nervous system irritations may be presented in these addicts with rapidly increased intensities.

The treatment for Heroin Addiction include detoxification, substitutional therapy and symptom control. Detoxification includes weaning off the opiate with the use of adrenergic antagonistic drugs (like clonidine), pain-killers, and sedatives to minimize the withdraw symptoms, improve sleep and anxiety. Detoxification medication may help during the urgent need for relief of the withdrawal syndrome, but the overall effectiveness has not been satisfactory [8].

The disappointment with detoxification therapy has led to the introduction and later adoption of substitutional therapy. SinceHeroin is producing such severe withdrawal syndrome which are difficult to control, one way to manage the heroin addiction is to replace with a less addicting, more tolerable opiate, as a step towards the ultimate removal. Methadone has been accepted world-wide as a suitable opiate that satisfies the need of substitution because it has an oral preparation with stable effects and long half-life of 18 to 24 hours. Withdrawal symptoms arising from Methadone are not as severe as compared to heroin and other opiates. Methadone has therefore been popularly used as a substitute, when problems in personality, family and/or community are hindering the proper arrangements for a total withdrawal. In the latter situation, a special term "Methadone Maintenance Treatment" (MMT) has been created. In some cases a single dose of around 80 mgm MMT,would be sufficient for a day [9].

One disadventage of Methadone and MMT is that adverse effects are still prominent which include nausea, vomiting, dizziness, gastro-intestinal symptoms, respiratory symptoms and even haematological disturbances. Long term methadone users have tendency to develop depression [10].

Opiate addiction is such a long medical and social problem. Although therapeutic means are available, none of them is considered satisfactory. Further exploration on other alternative ways is needed for therapeutic control. The heavy influence of personality and socio-psychological interactions contributing towards the occurrence of addiction naturally call for special psychological therapy, which has been adopted as standard therapeutic measures for addicts in well-established centers. Other alternative treatment includes the application of traditional Chinese medicine [11].

http://dx.doi.org/10.5772/54788

### 1.4. Acupuncture as treatment for withdrawal symptoms

Acupuncture is well-known for the control of pain and some autonomic symptoms like nausea, vomiting and dizziness. In China, the application of acupuncture for opiate withdrawal is therefore a logical historical attempt. Now acupuncture as a treatment option for difficult pain related conditions, is increasing its popularity over the world. In 1998, the National Institutes of Health of the US, held a Consensus Conference which endorsed Acupuncture as the therapeutic measure to be recommended for pain, as well as nausea and vomiting control [12].

Looking through the available literature from 1976 to 2006, more than 70 clinical trials on the use of acupuncture for heroin addiction have been published in the Chinese and English language journals, involving more than 5,000 cases [13]. Summarizing the reports about the results of treatment, the suggestions include the following:

- **i.** Acupuncture gives rapid and efficient effects against the withdrawal symptoms when used as detoxification agent [14].
- **ii.** Acupuncture works well together with Methadone in the MMT scheme [15].
- **iii.** The newer form of auricular acupuncture shows good responses [16].
- **iv.** Herbal medicine can be used together with acupuncture for additional effects and acupuncture has better individual effect when compared with the use of herbal medicine alone [17].
- **v.** A special meridian and acupuncture points have been identified as particularly effective for withdrawal therapy [18].
- **vi.** Electrical stimulation in Acupuncture might have better results [19].
- **vii.** Acupuncture is found to be useful not only as a detoxification agent, but might help preventing relapses [20].

Given all the positive indications revealed in the literature search, it might be interesting to compare the observations made in properly organized reviews with reference to the conventional therapeutic measures of opioid detoxification. A Cochrane review done in 2006 [8] on the effectiveness of adrenergic antagonists showed the following:

- **i.** The effects of clonidine were obvious although side effects of hypotension and dizziness were frequent.
- **ii.** No other adrenergic antagonist seemed to work better than clonidine.
- **iii.** Addicts on the MMT regime experienced better effects with adrenergic-antagonists.

On the other hand, looking through some of the details of the acupuncture records, the following facts could further support its applications [14-20]:

- **a.** Most of the acupuncture treatments were given in hospital or retention home settings.
- **b.** The form of acupuncture included simple needling, electrical stimulation or together with moxibustion.

c. The duration of acupuncture treatment lasted 1-3 weeks.

d. The assessments included the Standard Withdrawal Symptom Score (WSS) the Patients' Detoxificated Number (PDN); adverse effects incidence; relapse rate; anxiety and long term effects. These data tended to be complicated and only simple observations could be made on the preferential choices of different forms of treatment. However, it is obvious that safety is not an issue at all.

e. Only a few trials attempted to go long term. One trial indicated a 28% relapse rate for the combined treatment of Methadone with acupuncture, compared with a 57% relapse in Methadone alone.

An analysis of the acupuncture meridian and acupoints used is useful. The following should be noted:

a. Most acupoints used fell within the Du Mai channel (24%), Urinary bladder channel (15%) and Ren Mai channel (9%).

b. Commonly used body acupoints included:

c. Neignan (PC 6), Zusanli (ST 36), Hegu (LI 4), Sanyinjiao (SP 6), Laogong (PC 8), Shemen (HT 7) Waignan (SJ 5), Shenshu (BL 23), Baihui (DU 20), Dazhui (DU I4).

d. Commonly used auricular acupoints included:

e. Liver, Kidney, Endocrine, Lung, Heart, Brainstem, usually together with body points. Auricular points were either punctured with short needles which could be retained. Alternatively, small hard beads could be taped onto the ear-lobe for self-pressure manipulations [16].

f. Duration of puncture varied from 15 to 60 minutes.

### 1.5. Mechanism of action of acupuncture as means of detoxification

Heroin addicts have acquired high concentrations of exogenous opiates which in turn inhibit the bioactivities of endogenous opioid peptides in the central nervous system. Once the exogenous opiate level declines, the endogenous system fails to adapt to the normal needs for homeostasis. The resulting dysfunction initiates the withdrawal symptoms and yearning desire for exogenous 'refill' of opiates [21].

1. Acupuncture helps to regulate the normal bodily function through the following mechanisms:Endorphin release: Acupuncture increases the release of endogenous opiate like substances, including endorphin, enkephalin, dynorphin in the cerebral tissues and nerve cells.

2. 5 hydroxy tryptamine release: With acupuncture stimulation, the 5 hydroxy tryptamine pathway in the hypothalamus is stimulated to release dopamine which is related to the feeling of euphoria with which the withdrawal syndrome is counteracts [22].

While the modern neuro-physiology and related humoral theories could throw some light into the scientific mechanism of acupuncture and withdrawal symptoms, they are yet insufficient

http://dx.doi.org/10.5772/54788

to offer the comprehensive explanations. The traditional theories of acupuncture, however, could supplement some basic understandings.

The Du Mai and Ren Mai, are Extraordinary Channels, governing, connecting and regulating the Twelve Ordinary meridians, running through the human body, harmonizing physiological functions to maintain homeostasis. The Urinary Bladder Channel on the other hand, connects the kidney with the Urinary Bladder and it is the most important system coupling the interior to the exterior according to the classical theory in Chinese Medicine. In particular, the Du Mai has the principal role for the treatment of mental diseases, febrile illnesses, and musculo-skeletal problems. Clinical observations showed that the acupoint-stimulation on the Du Mai effectively alleviates the withdrawal symptoms, such as muscularskeletal pain, perspiration and anxiety. Acupuncture using points located on Du Mai tonifies the Qi which maintains normal functional activities of the body [23, 24].

The Ren Mai is described as a sea of Yin which regulates metabolisms and blood function in the human body. It maintains the connection among the other organ's function including Lung, Heart, Liver, Spleen and Kidneys [25]. The selected acupoints for detoxification purposes within these three popular meridians are mainly those related to pain control, the nervous system, cardiovascular system and digestive system.

### 1.6. Discussion

Detoxification is a treatment offered to opiate addicts in support of their attempts to withdraw from addicted drug. There is obviously a need in medical and health services in response to the rising challenges of drug abuses in modern sociaty. However, using traditional medicine or acupuncture in Detoxification, has not been a serious consideration.. Traditional Chinese Medicine practitioners might have used herbs or acupuncture for the relief of symptoms of pain, nausea and vomiting when the need arises among the few opiate abusers. The first properly recorded application of acupuncture used systematically for withdrawal symptoms might have been originated in Hong Kong in the 1970's when a neurosurgeon used auricular acupuncture for this purpose [26, 27]. Subsequently using acupuncture to treat symptoms addicts invited more and more medical and community interests, so that more and more trials were initiated.

Up to today, there is yet no treatment program that guarantees the success of detoxification and subsequent total withdrawal from opiate/heroin addiction with no relapses. Methadone substitution is accepted as a standard offer while the limitations remain. Alternative treatment like acupuncture, could be considered a valid option of detoxification using with methadone or alone. Evidence of using acupuncture for pain, nausea and vomiting, and some other withdrawal symptoms has been accumulating and the treatment is easy, cheap and safe. We are not yet clear, whether the long term results, including relapses, are favourable. Given the complexity of drug abuse includepersonality, psychosocial influences, and health related etiologies, it is hard to establish simple solution to this problem. Acupunctures, with the adventage of least investment and highest safety, could be accepted as a favourable option and research could concentrate on the modalities of combined treatment which might give better chances of cure.

## 2. Cigarette addiction

Smoking has developed gradually from a fashionable social activity to a hateful anti social behaviour in recent years. Those who are addicted to Cigarette smoking might be facing bitter pressure to seriously engage in quitting attempts. The most determined individuals might find little difficulties in the quitting endeavours. There are however, personal and social reasons barring the success of such quitting determinations [28].

This section describes the use of self-administered acupressure as a means to help quitting smoking, through the experience of a pilot study on the same subject completed in Hong Kong.

### 2.1. Introduction

According to the information gathered by the Hong Kong Census and Statistics Department in a thematic household survey during December 2007 to March 2008 [29], there were 679,500 daily smokers, accounting for 11.8% of all persons aged 15 years and older in Hong Kong. Among them, 99.6% were cigarette smokers, consuming an average of 14 cigarettes per day. A third of daily smokers had tried but failed to quit smoking. The 3 most commonly cited reasons for failure were "not determined enough", "cigarette smoking had formed a favorite habit", and "friends/colleagues were also smokers".

The new amendment of the Smoking (Public Health) Ordinance [30] became effective January 1, 2007; no-smoking areas have been extended by law to cover the indoor areas of all restaurant premises, indoor workplaces, public indoor places, and also some public outdoor places. On July 1, 2009, the no-smoking area was further extended to recreational venues to provide protection against "secondhand smoking" in indoor workplace and public places. Through public education, health campaigns, and government legislation, smoking has become less socially acceptable as people become more health conscious. The service to aid smoking cessation thus becomes highly significant and demanding.

There are a number of ways to help smokers stop this habit such as anti-smoking advice given by physicians, self-help materials, behavioral therapy, nicotine substitutes (nicotine replacement therapy), and other adjuvant therapy including hypnosis, smoking deterrents, nicotine gum, etc [31]. However, the efficacy of such therapies in terms of cost, adherence, side effects, and personal preference varies. Acupuncture has been used to treat drug and alcohol dependence since the 1970s. Acupuncture has also been used to help cigarette consumers quit smoking; the specific aim is to reduce withdrawal symptoms [32-34]. While acupuncture is gaining worldwide popularity, health clinics and natural healing clinics in various countries have started to provide acupuncture as a treatment for smoking cessation.

In this pilot study, a prospective method using auricular acupressure was established to investigate the outcome on smoking cessation among community smokers in Hong Kong. Acupressure, an alternative maneuver to acupuncture, is a simple and easy technique. Instead of using needles to deeply stimulate selected acupoints on the external ear, small hard beads were attached with adhesive tapes and placed against the points so that patients could apply

http://dx.doi.org/10.5772/54788

pressure on the beads at regular intervals. Acupressure has the additional advantage of avoiding bleeding and infection of the punctured sites.

## 2.2. Methods

### *2.2.1. Design*

The smoking cessation study was approved by the Clinical Research Ethics Committee of the Chinese University of Hong Kong. All participants were required to give written informed consent before the trial started. The blocked randomization scheme was used to allocate participants in equal proportions to the active treatment or sham groups. Participants were recruited from outpatient clinics and the community through poster advertisements. Eligible individuals had to be aged 18 years or older, have a daily cigarette smoking habit, and be motivated to quit smoking. They could not use other smoking cessation therapy simultaneously.

### *2.2.2. Intervention*

Auricular acupressure was introduced via hard beads fixed with adhesive against the selected acupoints to provide continuous stimulation. Four acupoints on the external ear—Shenmen, Lung, Mouth, and Brain—were used [35]. In addition, 2 more acupoints on the hand—Hegu and Neiguan—were similarly taped with hard beads. For the sham group, non-specific non-meridian points were chosen away from those selected for the treatment group. Figure 1 shows the positions of the acupoints.

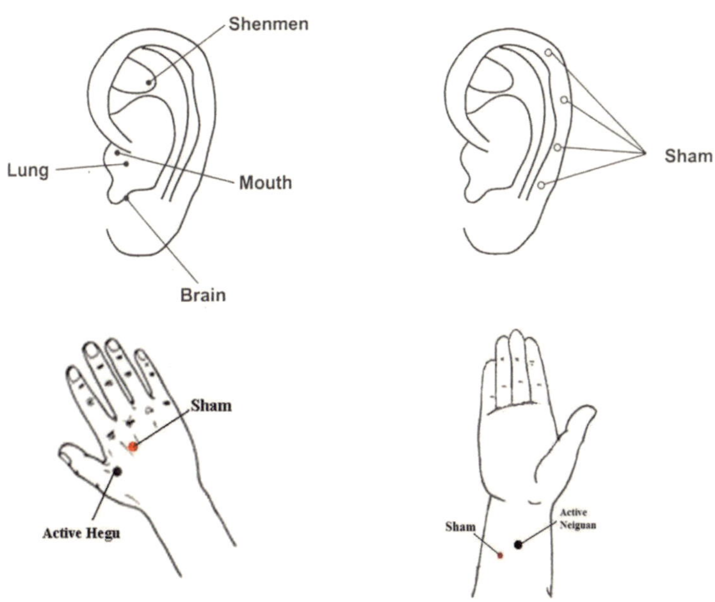


**Figure 1.** Active auricular points and sham points.

Participants were instructed to press on the beads repeatedly at least 3 times a day or whenever they desired to smoke during the 3 weeks of treatment. They were then followed up weekly during the treatment period, 7 days after treatment was completed, and 3 months after treatment via phone interview.

#### 2.2.3. *Assessments*

Baseline characteristics and participants' smoking history were collected. A Chinese version of the Fagerstrom Test was administered to measure the magnitude and profile of nicotine dependence [36]. Participants' attitude toward smoking cessation was assessed by a validated questionnaire (Contemplation Ladder) [37].

Individual cigarette withdrawal symptoms were assessed by Mood and Physical Symptoms Scale (MPSS) [38 - 40], which was developed in the early 1980s and variants of it have been used for 20 years. It is composed of 2 parts: the first part rates the severity of depressed mood, irritability, restlessness, hunger, difficult concentrating, and constipation (5 points); the second part rates smoking urges by "time spent in urge to smoke" and "strength of urge to smoke" (6 points). Other physical illnesses were also recorded weekly. The participants' cigarette consumption was obtained by daily selfreports and also objectively verified through breath carbon monoxide monitor (Bedfont Micro Smokerlyzer, United Kingdom) [41]. The measurement of exhaled carbon monoxide levels in parts per million (ppm) was based on the conversion of carbon monoxide to carbon dioxide over a catalytically active electrode. Data of ≥10 ppm of carbon monoxide indicated smokers; 6–10 ppm indicated sporadic smokers, and <6 ppm indicated non-smokers [42, 43]. Participants could not smoke at least an hour before taking the breath test.

### 2.3. Statistical analysis

The data analysis was based on intention-to-treat. Comparisons were performed using the t-test and paired t-test for continuous variables; Pearson's test and Fisher's exact test were used to compare categorical variables. A 2-tailed P value <.05 was considered significant. All statistical analyses were performed using SPSS version 16.0 (SPSS Inc., Chicago, IL).

### 2.4. Results

From November 2007 to March 2009, 70 eligible participants were enrolled in the pilot trial. The participants were predominantly men (70%). The mean age was 46.5 years with a mean smoking period of 27.8 years (range, 5-50 years). The mean (SD) cigarette consumption was 16 (7.19) per day. The mean (SD) breath carbon monoxide level was 15.06 (7.56) ppm at the start of the study. Past quitting attempt was 0.94 times.

According to the Fagerstrom nicotine dependence test, 33% of participants were severe, 36% were moderate, and 31% mild. For the degree of motivation to quit smoking, 32.9% of participants were either prepared or determined to take action. There were no major differences between the active and sham groups at baseline level (Table 1).

http://dx.doi.org/10.5772/54788

Participant adherence to the intervention was as follows: 87% (61) attended the first visit, 80% (56) the second visit, 76% (53) the third visit, and 73% (51) kept all 4 appointments. Participants manipulated the acupressure points on average 4.22 times a day in the active group and 5.12 times a day in the sham group.

| | | Active | Sham | Total | P |
|---|---|---|---|---|---|
| | | N = 38 | N= 32 | N= 70 | value |
| Sex | Male(%) | 26 (68.4) | 23 (71.9) | 49 (70) | 0.753 |
| | Female(%) | 12 (31.6) | 9 (28.1) | 21 (30) | |
| Age | Mean (SD) | 46.5 (12.36) | 16.4 (11.36) | 46.5 (11.82) | 0.958 |
| | 30 or Less(%) | 5 (13.2) | 4 (12.5) | 9 (12.9) | 0.707 |
| | 31-60(%) | 27 (71.1) | 25 (78.1) | 52 (74.3) | |
| | 61 or Above(%) | 6(15.8) | 3(9.4) | 9 (12.9) | |
| Smoking History | Mean Smoke Yr (SD) | 27.11 (11.39) | 28.53 (11.50) | 27.76 (11.38) | 0.605 |
| | Range | 6 - 46 | 5 - 50 | 5 - 50 | |
| Cigarettes per day | Mean Stick(s)/day(SD) | 14.50 (6.33) | 17.94 (7.77) | 16.07 (7.19) | 0.045 |
| | Range | 5 - 33 | 5 - 50 | 5 - 50 | |
| Contemplation Ladder | Less Determination(%) | 28 (73.7) | 19 (59.4) | 47 (67.1) | 0.204 |
| | More Determination(%) | 10 (26.3) | 13 (40.6) | 23 (32.9) | |
| Fagerstrom Score | Low (0-3)(%) | 15 (39.5) | 7 (21.9) | 22 (31.4) | 0.244 |
| | Moderate (4-5)(%) | 11 (28.9) | 14 (43.8) | 25 (35.7) | |
| | Severe (6-10)(%) | 12 (31.6) | 11 (34.4) | 23 (32.9) | |
| | Mean Score(SD) | 4.0 (2.48) | 4.75(2.50) | 4.34(2.50) | 0.214 |
| CO level | Mean CO ppm (SD) | 13.68 (7.13) | 16.69 (7.84) | 15.06 (7.56) | 0.098 |
| | Range | 1, 31 | 2,36 | 1, 36 | |

SD, standard deviation; ppm, parts per million.

**Table 1.** Participant Characteristics

Three individuals dropped out because of skin irritations under the adhesive tapes. Other reasons for discontinuation included external appearance of the tapes, busy working schedules, and other personal matters.

The effectiveness of acupressure was free of smoking by end of treatment and point prevalence of smoking cessation at 7 days following treatment completion. Success in quitting was defined as discontinuation of the smoking habit and the breathing test for carbon monoxide level showing less than 6 ppm. Failure was defined as a continuation of the smoking habit or absence from follow-up [43].

The successful rate of discontinuation at the end of treatment was 2.6% (1) and 9.4% (3) (P =. 33); 7 days post treatment it was 5.3% (2) and 6.2% (2) (P =.86), and 3 months post treatment it was 7.9% (3) and 3.1% (1) (P =.62) for the active and sham group, respectively. For the breathing test, only 65 individuals whose carbon monoxide level at pretreatment was higher than 6 ppm were analyzed. At the end of treatment, 18.2% (6) of the active group and 16.7% (5) of the sham group showed carbon monoxide levels of less than 6 ppm (P =.87); at 7 days post treatment, the active group was 25.8% (8) and sham group was 16.1% (5) (P =.35). There was no statistically significant difference between the groups.

Although some participants could not quit smoking completely, 30.9% (21) of them (35.1% (13) of the active group and 25.8% (8) of the sham group) succeeded in reducing 50% of their daily cigarette consumption at 7 days following treatment. The mean number of cigarettes smoked daily and the carbon monoxide expiration level decreased significantly from pre-treatment values in both groups (Figure 2 and 3). The mean cigarette reduction was 45.9% for the active group and the 43.7% for sham group. There was no statistically significant difference between the groups.

At 3 months post treatment, 25 of 51 participants were reached via phone interview. Twenty of them smoked less than at baseline; those belonging to the active group were smoking less (–9.17±7.5) than the sham group (–3.5±7.4; P =.07; Figure 4).

Cigarette withdrawal symptoms were measured, including depressed mood, irritability, restlessness, hunger, difficulty concentrating, and constipation along with the urge and the strength of urge to smoke. During the 3-week treatment period, more than 60% of individuals experienced more than 1 withdrawal symptom and most of them had the problem of hunger. The overall mean score was around 8 to 10 (score range, 6–30), meaning that the participants were tolerating the withdrawal symptoms reasonably well. The mean of the total urges was around 5; (Figure 5) demonstrates the pattern of the scoring. There were no statistical differences between the 2 groups in the withdrawal symptoms and urges (Table 2).

Subgroup analyses (Table 3) were performed with respect to the amount of cigarette consumption, attitude toward quitting (Contemplation Ladder), and dependence of nicotine (Fagerstrom score). None of the outcomes including successful rate of discontinuation of smoking, cigarette reduction, and withdrawal symptoms reached statistical significance between the active and sham group at 7 days post treatment. However, the participants with more determination to stop smoking achieved the greatest magnitude in success rate and percentage of cigarette reduction. At 3 months post treatment, the active group showed a more significant reduction of cigarette consumption than baseline in heavy cigarette consumption subgroup (–13±7.5 vs -3±8.1, *P*<.05), and in high Fagerstrom score subgroup (–10.3±7.6 vs -2.26±6.0, *P*<.05).

Apart from 3 participants who experienced skin allergy at the site of the adhesive tapes, there was no adverse event reported.

http://dx.doi.org/10.5772/54788

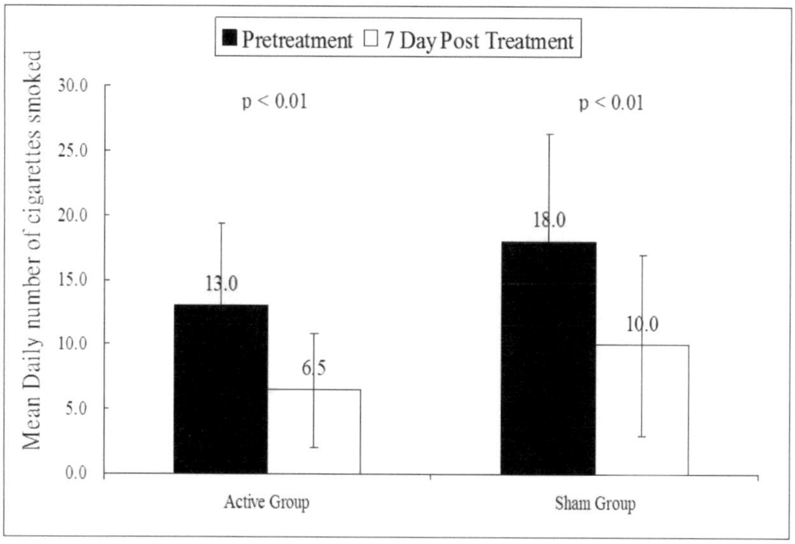


**Figure 2.** Cigarette consumption at 7 days post treatment.

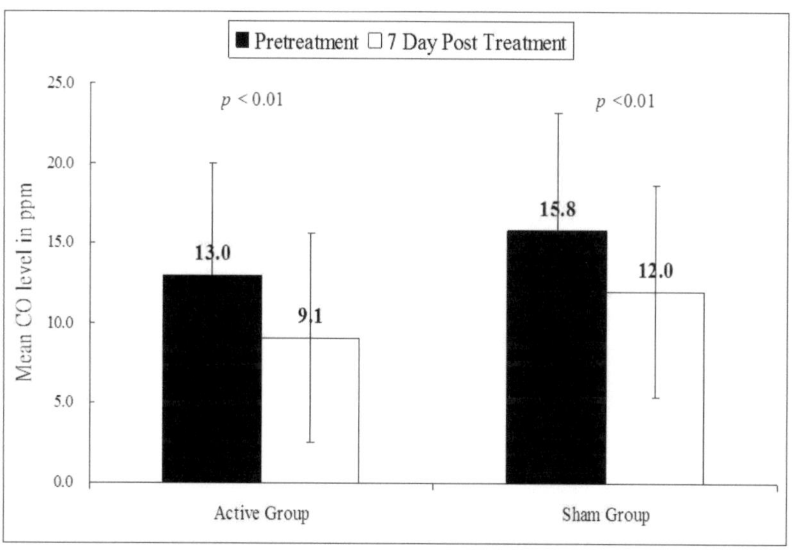


**Figure 3.** Carbon monoxide expiration at 7 days post treatment.

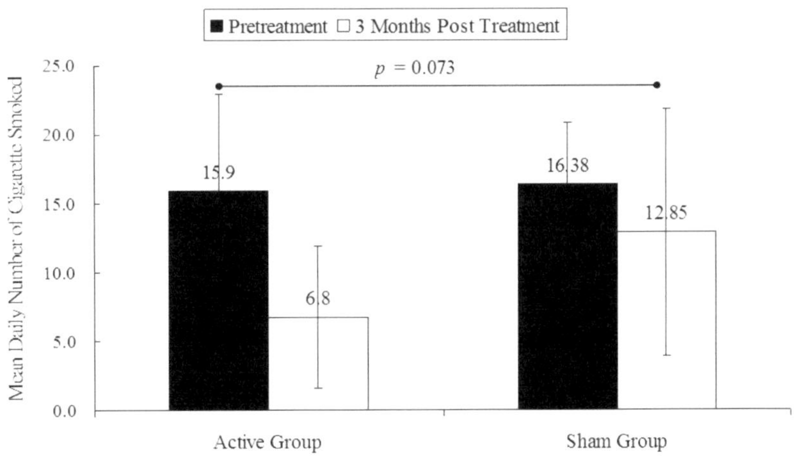


**Figure 4.** Cigarette consumption at 3 months post treatment.

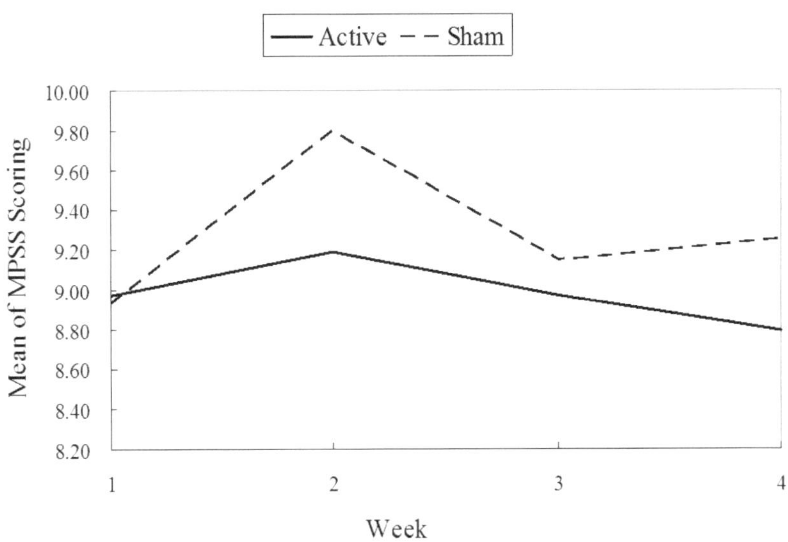


**Figure 5.** Withdrawal symptoms scoring pattern.

http://dx.doi.org/10.5772/54788

| | Week after first treatment | | Second Week | | Third Week | | 7 days post treatment | |
|---|---|---|---|---|---|---|---|---|
| | Active | Sham | Active | Sham | Active | Sham | Active | Sham |
| Overall Score Mean (SD) † | 8.97 (3.06) | 8.93 (3.65) | 9.19 (3.35) | 9.80 (4.39) | 8.97 (3.64) | 9.15 (3.77) | 8.79 (2.91) | 9.25 (4.05) |
| Total Urge Score Mean(SD)‡ | 4.26 (1.64) | 3.89 (1.74) | 4.03 (1.51) | 4.24 (1.56) | 3.95 (1.51) | 3.92 (1.84) | 3.79 (1.60) | 3.92 (1.84) |
| Any Withdrawal Symptom | 27 (79.4%) | 17 (63.0%) | 22 (68.8%) | 19 (73.1%) | 19 (61.3%) | 21 (80.8%) | 22 (79.6%) | 20 (83.3%) |
| Depressed | 1 (2.9%) | 4 (14.8%) | 4 (12.5%) | 6 (24.0%) | 4 (12.9%) | 5 (19.2%) | 3 (10.7%) | 5 (20.8%) |
| Irritability | 5 (14.7%) | 3 (11.1%) | 3 (9.4%) | 3 (12.0%) | 5 (16.1%) | 4 (15.4%) | 4 (14.3%) | 4 (16.7%) |
| Restlessness | 4 (11.8%) | 5 (18.5%) | 6 (18.8%) | 6 (24.0%) | 3 (9.7%) | 4 (15.4%) | 3 (10.7%) | 3 (12.5%) |
| Hungry | 11 (32.4%) | 6 (22.2%) | 11 (34.4%) | 7 (28.0%) | 9 (29.0%) | 5 (19.2%) | 6 (21.4%) | 5 (20.8%) |
| Difficult in Concentration | 3 (8.8%) | 5 (18.5%) | 4 (12.5%) | 6 (24.0%) | 5 (16.1%) | 6 (23.1%) | 2 (7.1%) | 5 (20.8%) |
| Constipation | 3 (8.8%) | 1 (3.7%) | 4 (12.5%) | 2 (8.0%) | 3 (9.7%) | 0 (0%) | 1 (3.6%) | 3 (12.5%) |

†Overall Score Range 6 to 30 ; ‡Total Urge Score Range 0 to 10.

**Table 2.** Mood and Physical Symptoms Scale overall scoring and proportion with severity rated moderate to severe.

| | **Cigarette Consumption** | | **Readiness to Quit** | | **Fagerstrom Score** | |
|---|---|---|---|---|---|---|
| | **Less than 15 sticks** | **Above 15 sticks** | **Less Determination** | **More Determination** | **Low** | **Moderate to Severe** |
| | A vs S | A vs S | A vs S | A vs S | A vs S | A vs S |
| At 7 days Post Treatment | n = 25 | n = 45 | n = 47 | n = 23 | n = 22 | n = 48 |
| Successful Rate | 5.0% vs 0% | 5.6% vs 7.4% | 3.6% vs 5.3% | 10.0% vs 7.7% | 6.7% vs 14.3% | 4.3% vs 4.0% |
| Cigarette Reduction | 38% vs 32.9% | 60.2% vs 45.9% | 38.8% vs 39.4% | 61% vs 49.1% | 49.4% vs 54.6% | 43.3% vs 41.3% |
| Overall Withdrawal Symptom Score Mean ± SD | 8.89±3.03 vs 9.5±2.38 | 8.6±2.84 vs 9.2±4.35 | 8.37±2.50 vs 9.31±3.92 | 9.67±3.64 vs 9.18±4.38 | 8.33±2.64 vs 7.60±1.14 | 9.13±3.14 vs 9.68±4.43 |
| Total Urge Score Mean ± SD | 3.67±1.78 vs 3.75±2.06 | 4.0±1.25 vs 3.95±1.85 | 3.79±1.40 vs 4.15±1.57 | 3.78±2.05 vs 3.64±2.16 | 3.08±1.68 vs 2.80±1.30 | 4.31±1.35 vs 4.21±1.87 |
| At 3 Months Post Treatment N=25 | n=8 | n=17 | n=14 | n=11 | n=4 | n=21 |
| Cigarette Reduction Compared with Pre-treatment Mean ± SD | -5.33±5.79 vs -4.5±2.12 | -13±7.46 vs -3±8.10† | -8.14±8.15 vs -4.29±1.38 | -10.6±7.16 vs -2.67±11.34 | 3.5±4.94 vs 10±14.14 | 10.3±7.6 vs 2.36±6.04† |

A, Active group; S, Sham Group; † $P < 0.05$.

**Table 3.** Subgroup Analyses on Cigarette Consumption, Readiness to Quit and Fagerstrom Score

### 2.5. Discussion

This pilot study sought to determine whether auricular acupressure could be an effective anti-smoking intervention and if it could help with the relief of withdrawal symptoms. Although there was a lack of statistical evidence to support the efficacy of the active treatment, both active and sham groups revealed a large reduction in the number of cigarettes consumed, confirmed by a substantial reduction of the carbon monoxide level in the breathing tests. As revealed from the Contemplation Ladder estimation at pretreatment, 67% of participants were still in the precontemplation and contemplation stage (i.e., they were not yet totally committed to quit smoking). For such participants, counseling programs could help achieve better results. The low absolute cessation rate in our study may be related to the relative lack of determination among our patients.

Although withdrawal symptoms were commonly experienced by chronic smokers who wanted to quit, our participants' withdrawal symptoms were not severe and did not increase as time elapsed.

A report given by the Smoking Cessation Health Centre in Hong Kong 2001 [44] revealed that by providing individual counseling and nicotine replacement therapy (nicotine gum, patch, or inhaler) to participants, after 1 month, 26% of participants successfully quit smoking, 48% reduced their average consumption of cigarettes, and 18% did not change their smoking habits at all. Compared with our completed study at 7 days post treatment, 30.9% of participants halved their daily cigarette consumption, but only 5.7% successfully discontinued smoking. In another survey done in 2001 [45] with regard to the determination to quit smoking, the proportion of pre-contemplation and contemplation decreased from 71% at baseline to 42% at 3-month follow-up. This observation perhaps demonstrated the effects of individualized behavioral counselling. Four weeks of nicotine replacement therapy provided in one other study resulted in only 16% adherence [28]. In our auricular acupressure study, patients' adherence was encouraging and reached 73%. The positive attitude of the participants on acupressure supports further exploration of its use as an option for smoking control.

The sham points chosen for the control group were meant to be really inert to stimulation. However, this sham group also showed a prominent reduction in cigarette consumption as did the active treatment group using known acupoints with targets. It is uncertain, whether the sham points also elicite stimulation on applying pressure. One has to realize that the sham points are in fact very near the target points. The Cochrane review on acupuncture and related intervention for smoking cessation done in 2005 revealed that there was no consistent evidence that acupuncture was superior to no treatment, and there was no evidence that the effects of acupuncture were different from that of other anti-smoking interventions, or that any particular related technique was superior to other techniques [34]. Our study did not show significant results between the acupressure and sham group.

As in other reported studies, we had difficulty getting the absolute results of the smoking cessation attempts [46]. To evaluate the effectiveness of smoking cessation, interventions neither participants self-report on cigarette consumption nor carbon monoxide breath test is absolutely reliable. The result may be biased due to faulty memory or intentional biases. Moreover, the carbon monoxide breath test only indicates recent exposures of smoking (it has only, 6–9 hours short half-life, and faces rapid disposition). Each individual breath test taken during follow-up visits varied from participant to participant, i.e. the test could be taken in the morning or after a meal, which give lower readings. Other more reliable approaches such as plasma and urine nicotine concentrations, which are more reliable indications of longer exposures of smoking (5–7 days with longer half-life) are available [47]. However, the high costs did not allow their inclusion in our study.

Given that perfect choices are not available, the majority of smoking cessation studies used breath tests instead of a plasma cotinine concentration test, which was also invasive and more expensive. Participants' self-reports on cigarette consumption verified by their carbon monoxide breath tests could therefore be practical means for the evaluation of the effectiveness of acupuncture in smoking cessation.

In conclusion, acupressure on the external auricle is a simple maneuver and taking acupoints and sham points together, the positive results reached promising levels. Acupressure is a safe technique for all smokers who want to quit smoking, including pregnant and breastfeeding women, while nicotine replacement therapy might not be as safe and acceptable. Acupressure as a means to help stop smoking may therefore be recommended as a valid option.

## Acknowledgements

Authors are grateful to Dr. Xu Min who is mainly responsible for a meta analysis on the use of acupuncture for Heroin withdrawal syndrome, quoted in Section I of this manuscript. The review project was supported by the "Beat-drug Fund" of the Hong Kong Government. The review was started when Dr. Xu Min worked under the Institute of Chinese Medicine at The Chinese University of Hong Kong.

## Author details

P.C. Leung[1*], L. Zhang[1], L.Y. Eliza Wong[2] and S.Y. Ellie Pang[1]

*Address all correspondence to: pingcleung@cuhk.edu.hk

1 Institute of Chinese Medicine, The Chinese University of Hong Kong, China

2 School of Public Health and Primary Care, The Chinese University of Hong Kong, China

## References

[1] Joe, G. W, Lehman, W, & Simpson, D. D. Addict Death Rates during a Four-year Postreatment Follow-up. Am J Public Health (1982). , 72(7), 703-709.

[2] Klee, H, & Morris, J. Crime and Drug Misuse: Economic and Psychological Aspects of the Criminal Activities of Heroin and Amphetamine Injectors. Addict Res (1994). , 1(4), 377-386.

[3] Australia and NSWHeroin: An Assessment Current Situation, Trends, and Potential Risk for Australia and NSW. Office of Drug Policy, the Cabinet Office, NSW; (2002).

[4] Mcneece, C. A. DiNitto DM. Chemical Dependency, A System Approach. 3rd ed. Boston, MA: Pearson-Allyn & Bacon; (2003). , 45-62.

[5] Hong Kong Special Administration RegionPRC. Report on Review of Methadone Treatment Programme. Narcotics Division, Security Bureau; (2000).

[6] Cherry, A, Dillon, M. E, & Rugh, D. Substance Abuse: a Global View. London, Westport, Connecticut: Greenwood Press; (2002). , 1-20.

[7] American Psychiatric AssociationDiagnostic and Statistical Manual of Mental Disorders, Fourth Edition, Text Revision. Washington, DC: American Psychiatric Association; (2000). , 175-194.

[8] Gowing, L, Ali, R, & White, J. Opioid Antagonists with Minimal Sedation for Opioid Withdrawal. Cochrane Database Syst Rev (2002). CD002021.

[9] Seivewright, N. Community Treatment of Drug Misuse: more than Methadone. London: Cambridge University Press; (2000).

[10] Higgins JPTGreen S, editors. Cochrane Handbook for Systematic Reviews of Interventions version 5.1.0 [updated March (2011). http://www.cochrane-handbook.orgaccessed 8 August 2012).

[11] Guo, S, Jiang, Z. N, Wang, Y. D, Hu, G. C, Wu, Y. M, & Huang, M. S. A Comparative Study of Chinese Herbal Medicine with Clonidine Hydrochloride on Opiate Withdrawal Syndrome. Chinese Bulletin of Drug Dependence (1995). , 4(4), 210-216.

[12] US Department of health & Human Services. Acupuncture. NIH Consensus Statement Online 1997 Nov 3-5; 15(5) 1-34.

[13] Xu, M. Lee DTS, Chen Q, Deng PX, Deng B, Chan YY, et al. Meta-analysis of Acupuncture Therapy in the Treatment of Heroin Dependence: a Systematic Review of Randomized Evidence. Beat Drugs Fund, Research Project Report, (2007). , 1-110.

[14] Montazeri, K, Farahnakian, M, & Saghaei, M. The Effect of Acupuncture on the Acute Withdrawal Symptoms from Rapid Opiate Detoxification. Acta Anaesthesiol Sin (2002). , 40(4), 173-177.

[15] Song, X. G, Zhang, H, & Wang, Z. H. Clinical Observation on Acupuncture Combined with Methodone for Improving Heroin Withdrawal Syndrom. Chinese Acupuncture & Moxibustion (2002). , 12(12), 795-797.

[16] Wang, Z. T, Yuan, Y. Q, Wang, J, & Luo, J. K. Observations on the Efficacy of Auricular-plaster Therapy plus Medicine for Heroin Adiction. Shanghai Journal Acupuncture and Moxibustion (2005). , 24(12), 6-7.

[17] Zong, L, Hu, J, Li, Y, Lu, Y, & Xin, Y. F. Comparison of the Breaking Effects of Acupuncture, Chinese Medicine and Their Combination on Heroin Addiction. Shanghai Journal Acupuncture and Moxibustion (2001). , 20(2), 1-3.

[18] Zeng, X. L, Lei, L. M, & Lu, Y. H. Clinically Controlled Study on Detoxification of Heroin Dependence by Acupuncture on Points of the Governor Vessel. Chinese Acupuncture and Moxibustion. (2004). , 24(6), 385-387.

[19] Wu, L. Z, Cui, C. L, & Hang, J. S. Reduction of Methadone Dosage and Relief of Depression and Anxiety by 2/100Hz TENS for Heroin Detoxification. Chinese Journal of Drug Dependence (2001). , 10(2), 124-126.

[20] Shu, R, Wen, X. Y, & Ru, L. Q. Channel Balance-inducing Treatment for Late Withdrawal Syndrome of Heroin Dependence. Chinese Acupuncture and Moxibustion (2003). , 23(6), 325-328.

[21] Zhu, Z. C, Ju, L. H, Hu, J, & Xu, P. Effect of Electro-acupuncture on Drug-seeking Behaviour of the Heroin Self-administrating Rat. Journal of Acupuncture and Tuina Science (2005). , 3(4), 12-16.

[22] Jia, G. The Essence Re-exploration of Governor Vessel, Bladder Meridian, Conception Vessel and Kideny-essence. Chinese Archives of Traditional Chinese Medicine (2003). , 21(11), 1807-1808.

[23] Guan, C. X, & Xi, H. X. Investigate the Relation between Brain and Governor Vessel. Henan Journal of Traditional Chinese Medicine and pharmacy (2001). , 16(2), 52-53.

[24] Mu, X, Duan, H. Q, Chen, W, Gao, L. Y, & Yang, Z. J. Physiological Study on the Relationship between the Essence of Acupuncture Point and the Microvasculum. China Journal of Basic Medicine in Traditional Chinese Medicine (2001). , 7(12), 47-52.

[25] Yuan, X. Y. Quantitative and Dynamic Studies of Acupoint Microcirculation Perfusion. Beijing Journal of traditional Chinese Medicine (1994).

[26] Wen, H. L, & Teo, S. W. Experience in the Treatment of Drug Addiction by Electro-acupuncture. Hong Kong Nursing Journal (1975).

[27] Wen, H. L. Clinical Experience and Mechanism of Acupuncture and Electrical Stimulation in the Treatment of Drug Abuse. Am J Chin Medicine (1980). , 8(4), 349-353.

[28] Lam, T. H, Abdullah, A. S, Chan, S. S, & Hedley, A. J. Adherence to Nicotine Replacement Therapy versus Quitting Smoking among Chinese Smokers: a preliminary investigation. Psychopharmacology (Berl) (2005). , 177(4), 400-408.

[29] Hong Kong Special Administration RegionPRC. Feature Articles: Pattern of smoking. Thematic Household Survey. Hong Kong Monthly Digest of Statistics June (2009). The Census and Statistics Department. http://www.statistics.gov.hk/pub/B10100022009MM06B0500.pdfaccessed 8 August 2012).

[30] Hong Kong Special Administration RegionPRC. The Smoking (Public Health) Ordinance (Cap. 371). http://www.tco.gov.hk/textonly/english/legislation/legislation_so.htmlaccessed 8 August, (2012).

[31] Lancaster, T, Stead, L, Silagy, C, & Sowden, A. Effectiveness of Interventions to Help People Stop Smoking: Findings from the Cochrane Library BMJ (2000). , 321(7257), 355-358.

[32] Cho, S. H, & Whang, W. W. Acupuncture for Alcohol Dependence: a Systematic Review. Alcohol Clin Exp Res (2009). , 33(8), 1305-1313.

[33] Gates, S, Smith, L. A, & Foxcroft, D. R. Auricular Acupuncture for Cocaine Dependence. Cochrane Database Syst Rev (2006). CD005192.

[34] White, A. R, Rampes, H, Liu, J. P, Stead, L. F, & Campbell, J. L. Acupuncture and Related Interventions for Smoking Cessation. Cochrane Database Syst Rev (2006). CD000009.

[35] Tian, Z. M, & Chu, Y. W. Treating Smoking Addiction with the Ear Point Seed Pressing Method. The Journal of Chinese Medicine (1996). , 52-5.

[36] Huang, C. L, Lin, H. H, & Wang, H. H. Psychometric Evaluation of the Chinese Version of the Fagerstrom Tolerance Questionnaire as a Measure of Cigarette Dependence. J Adv Nurs (2006). , 55(5), 596-603.

[37] Biener, L, & Abrams, D. B. The Contemplation Ladder: Validation of a Measure of Readiness to Consider Smoking Cessation. Health Psychol (1991). , 10(5), 360-365.

[38] Shiffman, S, West, R. J, & Gilbert, D. G. Recommendation for the Assessment of Tobacco Craving and Withdrawal in Smoking Cessation Trials. Nicotine Tob Res (2004). , 6(4), 599-614.

[39] West, R, & Hajek, P. Evaluation of the Mood and Physical Symptoms Scale to Assess Cigarette Withdrawal. Psychopharmacology (Berl) (2004).

[40] White, A. R, Moody, R. C, & Campbell, J. L. Acupressure for Smoking Cessation: a Pilot Study. BMC Complement Altern Med (2007).

[41] Jarvis, M. J, Russell, M. A, & Saloojee, Y. Expired Air Carbon Monoxide: a Simple Breath Test of Tobacco Smoke Intake. Br Med J (1980). , 281(6238), 484-485.

[42] Russell, M. A, Merriman, R, Stapleton, J, & Taylor, W. Effect of Nicotine Chewing Gum as an Adjunct to General Practitioner Advice against Smoking. Br Med J (1983). , 287(6407), 1782-1785.

[43] Soria, R, Legido, A, & Escolano, C. Lopez Yeste A, Montoya J. A Randomised Controlled Trial of Motivational Interviewing for Smoking Cessation. Br J Gen Pract (2006). , 56(531), 768-774.

[44] Lau, E, Chan, A, Lau, Y. K, Lam, C. W, Ma, H. K, Hedley, A. J, et al. Report 1: A New Smoking Cessation Health Centre in Hong Kong. First interim report on the characteristics of clients attending the Smoking Cessation Health Centre (SCHC). Hong Kong Council on Smoking and Health (2001). Jan.

[45] Lau, E, Chan, A, Lau, Y. K, Lam, C. W, Ma, H. K, Hedley, A. J, et al. Report 2: Impact of Smoking Cessation Services on Smokers in Hong Kong and Predictors of Successful quitting. Hong Kong Council on Smoking and Health (2001). Sep.

[46] Jatlow, P, Toll, B. A, Leary, V, Krishnan-sarin, S, & Malley, O. SS. Comparison of Expired Carbon Monoxide and Plasma Cotinine as Markers of Cigarette Abstinence. Drug Alcohol Depend (2008). , 98(3), 203-209.

[47] Maclaren, D. J, Conigrave, K. M, Robertson, J. A, Ivers, R. G, Eades, S, & Clough, A. R. Using Breath Carbon Monoxide to Validate Self-reported Tobacco Smoking in Remote Australian Indigenous Communities. Popul Health Metr (2010).

Chapter 15

# Immediate Effects of Microsystem Acupuncture in Patients with Oromyofacial Pain and Craniomandibular Disorders (CMD): A Double-Blind Placebo-Controlled Trial

Irmgard Simma, Jochen M. Gleditsch,
Leopold Simma and E. Piehslinger

Additional information is available at the end of the chapter

http://dx.doi.org/10.5772/55066

## 1. Introduction

Patients with craniomandibular disorders (CMD) frequently suffer from pain and dysfunction in the temporomandibular joint (TMJ) and the masticatory muscles, as well as headaches, disorders of the cervical spine, difficulty in opening the mouth, joint clicking [1, 2, 3, 4, 5, 6, 7, 8, 9] sinusitis, chronic neck pain, and reduced mobility of the cervical spine [10, 11]. This variety of pain symptoms is known in dentistry as well as many other medical specialties.

Acupuncture has been acknowledged for more than 200 years as an effective means of achieving pain relief (Traditional Chinese Medicine or TCM) [12]. The fact that not only pain, but also muscular dysfunction and tension, psychosomatic disorders, and dysregulation of the lymphatic and immune systems respond well to acupuncture treatment has been confirmed in numerous scientific studies [13, 14, 15, 16]. Trials using MRI revealed immediate signals in specific regions of the brain [17, 18].

Modern pain research has incidentally disclosed various effects of acupuncture while neurophysiological explanations for these phenomena have also been provided. Targeted needle stimulation at specific points in the skin or mucosa activates the organism's regulatory and modulation abilities. Modulation of pain is achieved in several ways. One of the remarkable results of pain research is the activation of endorphins and neurotransmitters when acupuncture stimuli are applied [19, 20].

In traditional acupuncture, points of analogous reflex relations are found in linear sequence (chains), also known as meridians. In microsystem acupuncture - which is a recently discovered subject - systematic point patterns are found in specific parts of the body such as the auricle, the oral cavity, and others These microsystems of acupuncture may be described as somatotopies representing a multitude of organs and their respective functions. Microsystem points can only be detected in a state of irritation. Activation of microsystem points results in increased sensitivity and pressure in the microsystemaereas (f.i. auricle mouth, skulp,….) which is a sign of functional disorders in the corresponding organ.

The stimulation of microsystem points has proved to be a very effective method of acupuncture. For optimum results the microsystem points are preferably detected and pricked by means of the 'very-point' technique [21].

In cases of pain in the stomatognathic system and dysfunction of the TMJ, remote points stimulation on the hands, auricles, at the sternum, and particularly in the enoral retromolar area of the lower jaw were found to be effective in open trials. Pain relief and alleviation of muscular tension was achieved immediately after the application of 'very-point' therapy[21]. Very Point therapy is the most sensitivity point in the point area.

## 2. Statement of the problem

The effects of acupuncture have been reported in many studies, but just a few of these provide data from placebo-controlled trials. We performed a randomized, double-blind placebo-controlled study to investigate the immediate effects of acupuncture in patients with myofacial pain and craniomandibular disorders (CMD).

## 3. Application area and methods

Twenty-three women aged 18 to 64 years, with dysfunction and pain in the stomatognathic system (particularly in the TMJ) and no previous therapy, were recruited for the trial from February 2002 to July 2003. Consecutive patients who reported at the outpatient unit of the department of prosthetic dentistry Medical University Vienna (Prof. Dr. E. Piehslinger) with dysfunction and pain in the stomatognathic system not attributable to any known underlying disease were eligible if they were women between 18 and 65 years of age. (we had no male patients at this time) All patients who were contacted agreed to participate in the study. Patients were randomized on the basis of a computer-generated random permutation list into two groups: one group was treated with acupuncture (n=11) while the other group received sham laser treatment (n=12) [22, 23, 24]. Randomization was performed after consent had been obtained before the date of therapy. The study protocol was approved by the ethics committee of the Medical University of Vienna. The treatment was scheduled to be administered two to seven days after enrolment at the department of dentistry, Medical University of Vienna.

Patients were unaware as to whether they were receiving verum or placebo treatment; this was disclosed after the final assessment. Patients who received placebo treatment were informed after their sham treatment that a different type of treatment might be more effective, and needle acupuncture was offered (because of ethical reasons). All patients in the placebo group consented and were treated with acupuncture after the sham procedure and the actual necessarity

The physician who palpated the different muscles and registered the patients' pain scores was blinded to their verum or placebo status. Patients were assessed immediately before and after treatment.

The patients' subjective perception of pain was evaluated on a visual analog scale (VAS).

Muscle palpation included the following muscles and regions: atlanto-occipital region, anterior temporal muscle, medial temporal muscle, posterior temporal muscle, muscles of the cranio-mandibular junction, pterygoid muscles, masseter muscles, digastric muscle, and sternocleidomastoid muscle, on both sides.

Pain on muscle palpation was rated on a four-point scale in ascending intensity from 0 to 3.

Classical acupuncture points according to TCM, microsystem points, and special points that corresponded to the disorders in question were palpated. Table 1 shows the acupuncture points that were positive on palpation and those that were used in therapy.

| Acupuncture point | Palpation | Therapy |
|---|---|---|
| Upper jaw retromolar | 11 | 9 |
| Lower jaw retromolar | 8 | 4 |
| Upper jaw vestibule | 4 | 1 |
| Lower jaw vestibule | 4 | 0 |
| Large bowel 4 | 9 | 1 |
| Small bowel 3, 2 | 6 | 7 |
| Auricle | 9 | 9 |
| Sternum | 8 | 5 |
| Adler-Langer points | 8 | 0 |
| Others | 5 | 5 |

**Table 1.** Acupuncture points positive on palpation and used for acupuncture therapy (n=11).

In microsystem acupuncture, points that demonstrate a high degree of irritation have proved to be more suitable for therapy. These points were given preference. Adler points are para-cervical pressure points were used for diagnostic purposes as well as for assessment of therapy. [25]

For precise identification of points and subsequent insertion of needles we used the 'very-point' technique. The latter permits acupuncture points to be spotted and pricked with maximum accuracy. Points were detected on the skin in the oral cavity, and very fine and sharp needles were inserted here. First, the area surrounding the suspected enoral point was palpated manually. As the next step, the region in which the patient reported maximum sensitivity was tapped gently and tangentially with the therapy needle itself, preferably at an angle of about 45°. The point of greatest sensitivity and tenderness, the 'very point', is usually at the center of the region of irritation. The patient reacts accordingly by mimic expression and/or verbal affirmation. (only the verum group received this type of treatment.

Treatment was performed in a double-blind manner; neither the patient nor the person performing the evaluation was aware of the non-functioning laser pen. The sham laser instrument was an inactivated soft laser pen that emitted an ordinary red light. To enhance the credibility of the sham procedure, the emission of red light was accompanied by visual and acoustic signals.

The same point selection criteria were used in both groups. Every point was 'sham irradiated' for about two minutes. The laser pen did not touch the skin but was held at a distance of about 0.5 to 1 cm.

### 3.1. Statistical methods

The sample size was determined on the basis of data obtained from a preliminary open trial. Assuming a difference of one standard deviation with respect to the primary endpoint between groups, an alpha level of 5% and a power goal of 80%, each group was required to consist of 10 patients. The primary endpoint was the patient's subjective assessment of pain on a visual analog scale. Secondary endpoints were the intensities of pain on palpation of various muscles and muscle groups. The latter were summed up to obtain pain ratings for all muscles and muscle groups. Medians and quartile ranges were computed as estimates for central tendency and dispersion. Before/after treatment differences in VAS ratings and the sum score of pain on palpation were compared between groups by Mann-Whitney tests. For the primary endpoint, the alpha error was set to 0.05. Exploratory tests were performed for secondary endpoints, and uncorrected p-values are reported.

## 4. Results

Figure 1 shows results for muscles and muscle groups that were initially painful on palpation in at least 20% of verum or placebo patients. Pain reduction as assessed by palpation was more pronounced in the acupuncture group than in the sham laser group. Of 14 muscles or groups of muscles that were examined, nine were initially scored painful on palpation in 20% or more of patients. Pain on palpation was most commonly observed in the pterygoid and masseter muscles (up to 96% of patients). Acupuncture resulted in greater reduction of pain (average 40%) than placebo treatment (average 8%). A large number of patients had initially experienced pain in the shoulder and neck (91% in the acupuncture group and 58% in the placebo group). In the acupuncture group 64% of patients reported a reduction on the pain scale, while 20% had no pain at all on palpation after the treatment. In contrast, no patient in the placebo group was free of pain after sham treatment. Fifty percent of acupuncture patients who had initially experienced pain on palpation of the digastric muscle recovered after treatment. In more than 50% of placebo-treated patients, however, pain on palpation of the same muscle persisted after therapy. In the temporal muscles, acupuncture achieved a reduction in nearly all patients while no reduction in pain was observed after placebo treatment. Placebo treatment had no effect on the sternocleidomastoid muscle, whereas 64% of patients with verum acupuncture about 9% reduction in pain. Pain on palpation of the hyoid muscles was rare and resolved after acupuncture in most cases. A summary of pain ratings on palpation is given in Table 2.

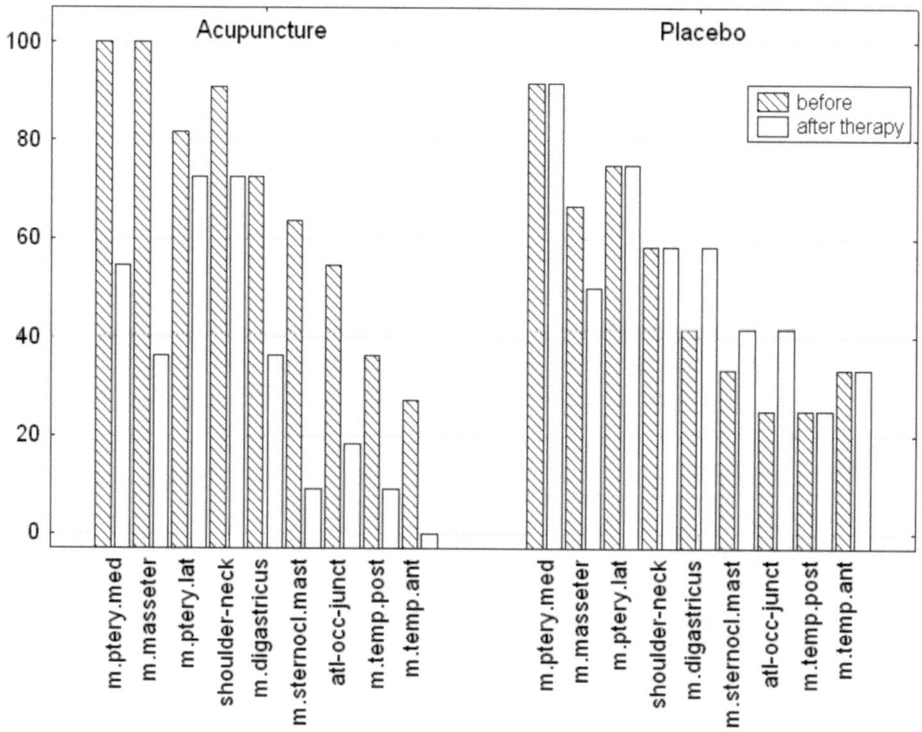


**Figure 1.** Percentage of patients in the acupuncture and placebo groups with pain on palpation of various muscles or groups of muscles before and after treatment

| | Treatment | | |
|---|---|---|---|
| | before | after | p-value* |
| Acupuncture | 22.5 ( 7.8) | 8.0 (10.0) | <0.001 |
| Sham | 19.0 (15.0) | 16.0 (20.0) | |

* Mann-Whitney test for before/after differences

**Table 2.** Median (quartile range) of the sum of pain ratings (0-3) assessed by palpation of 14 muscles.

The results of overall pain ratings on a visual analog scale (VAS) are summarized in Table 3. VAS scores were reduced after acupuncture as well as sham treatment, but the reduction was much more significant after acupuncture (p=0.031).

| | Treatment | | |
|---|---|---|---|
| | **before** | **after** | **p-value*** |
| Acupuncture | 40.5 (34.0) | 16.5 (33.0) | 0.031 |
| Sham | 41.0 (34.0) | 30.0 (28.5) | |

* Mann-Whitney test for differences before/after

**Table 3.** Median (quartile range) of visual analog (VAS) ratings of pain.

## 5. Discussion

In a previous trial comparing a single session of acupuncture with no treatment, a significant improvement in cervical mobility was reported in patients with chronic neck pain. This was in line with data reported by other authors [26, 27, 28]. The present study was designed to test the immediate effects of acupuncture on oromyofacial pain refractory to previous conventional therapy. Our results indicate that acupuncture therapy using remote points – either traditional points or corresponding microsystem points found in a state of irritation – has an immediate effect on motion-related pain as well as pain at rest in patients with CMD, TMJ and cervical spine mobility disorders.

Although the results in the control group indicate a certain placebo effect, it should be noted that these patients were also palpated and palpation and relaxation as such might have reduced pain. Pain in placebo-treated patients was reduced in one muscle (masseter), but increased in three others (digastric and sternocleidomastoid muscles, and atlanto-occipital region).

The absence of local therapy is especially important when patients are sensitive to treatment. Consequently, the frequency of a placebo effect may be higher. Moreover, the study demonstrates the importance of specific point selection performed by finger palpation, needle detection, and subsequent needle insertion at punctual sites of maximum sensitivity in a suspected point area. This 'very-point' method can be applied to the skin as well as mucous membranes.

In the mouth, a system of highly effective points is found in the mucous membranes. These points may serve as reflex points in modern pain therapy as well as acupuncture. Points in the mucous membrane, in a state of irritation, are highly sensitive to pressure during palpation. In these cases, reflex therapy of specific points is highly effective. The topography of the points determines the direction of potential therapeutic effects. Immediate relaxation and release of tension in the upper and lower jaw can be achieved especially in the retromolar area. The reflex action from the retromolar area primarily affects the cervical muscles, including the deep muscles of the receptor field of the neck. Although the immediate effects of enoral treatment

http://dx.doi.org/10.5772/55066

do not guarantee a permanent outcome, instant relief from muscular tension and pain is still an important and strong motivating factor for the patient. Once such initial relief and improvement has been achieved, the patient is more receptive to further treatment.

Specific traditional points on the sternum (Renmai), and the cervical Adler-Langer points were used to diagnose conditions as well as monitor the progress of patients.

Local pain points, also known as trigger points, were not treated locally in this study. Treatment was administered via remote points and superior systems in order to refrain from evoking memories of pain and avoid local pain during initial therapy.

One feature of microsystem acupuncture is that specific points serve as points of input for the organism's regulatory systems. Microsystem points are categorized as remote points, distant from the site of pain. This fact is greatly appreciated by patients who experience severe local pain. A very small number of patients did not respond to the treatment used in the study. These patients could be classified as non-responders to treatment via the regulatory system. The vast majority of patients, however, experienced immediate pain relief without the need to touch the affected area, and were therefore motivated to undergo subsequent therapy.

A single acupuncture session may provide immediate pain relief, alleviate muscle tension, enhance mobility, and improve the interplay between the TMJ and the cervical spine. This demonstrates the close interrelationship between the TMJ and the cervical region, craniomandibular dysfunction, and symptoms in the neck and shoulder. Such disorders have become very common and are relevant for a number of medical disciplines, amongst which dentistry plays a key role because occlusion of the teeth, muscles, the TMJ, and the cervical spine constitute a functional unit [29, 30, 31].

## 6. Conclusion

Pain reduction measured on VAS was significantly more pronounced after acupuncture than after placebo treatment ($p=0.031$). The sum of pain scores across 14 muscles was also reduced to a markedly greater extent after acupuncture than after sham laser treatment. Acupuncture may bring immediate pain relief in patients with oromyofacial disorders.

## Author details

Irmgard Simma[1], Jochen M. Gleditsch[1], Leopold Simma[1] and E. Piehslinger[2]

1 ÖGZMK-CAM (Complementary and Alternative Medicine in Dentistry) Society, Bregenz, Austria

2 University Clinic of Dentistry, Medical University of Vienna, Austria

## References

[1] Gelb, H.: Clinical management of head and TMJ pain and dysfunction. Saunders, Philadelphia 1977

[2] Wanman, A.; Longitudinal course of symptoms of craniomandibular disorders in men and women. A 10-year follow-up study of an epidemiologic sample. ActaOdontolScand 1996; 54:337-342

[3] Freesmeyer, W. B.: Funktionelle Befunde im orofacialen System und deren Wechselwirkung. Hanser, München 1987

[4] Slavicek, R.: Clinical and instrumental function analysis for diagnosis and treatment planning. Part 7 computer-aided axiography. JCO 1988; 22; 776-787

[5] Solberg, W. K.: Temporomandibular disorders: physical tests in diagnosis. Dr Dent J 160: 273-277, 1986

[6] Krogh-Poulsen, W.G.: Occlusaldisharmonie and dysfunction of the stomatognathic system. Dent Clin N Am 10, 627-635 (1966)

[7] Rauhala K., Oikarinen KS RaustiaAM (1999) Role of temporomandibular disorders (TCM) in facial pain: occlusion, muscle and TMJ pain. Cranio 17/4: 254-61

[8] Gsellmann B., M. Schmid-Schwap, E. Piehslinger, R. Slavicek: Anamnestic Findings in Patients with Temporomandibular Joint Disease, in: J Gnathol. 1995, Vol. 14, No.1: 41-46

[9] Hieber, G.: Kiefergelenksbeschwerden, in Dt. ZeitschriftfürAkupunktur 4/1999 S. 216-222

[10] Costen J.B.: A syndrom of ear and sinus symptoms dependant upon distrurbed function of the temporomandibular joint. Ann OtolRhinolLaryngol 43: 1-15; 1934,

[11] Travell, J.: TMJ pain referred from muscles of the head and neck. J Prosthet Dent 1960; 10:745-763

[12] WHO indication list for acupuncture, 1970

[13] Irnich, D., Behrens, Molzen, H., König, A., N., Gleditsch, J., et all.:Randomised trial acupuncture compared with conventional massage and „sham" laser acupuncture for treatment of chronic neck pain. Brit.Med.journal 322 (2001) S.1574-1577

[14] Irnich, D., Behrens, N., Gleditsch, J., et al.: Immediate effects of dry needling and adupuncture at distant points in chronic neck pain. Pain 99 (2002) S. 83-89

[15] Rosted, P.; (2001) Practical recommentations for the use of acupuncture in the treatment of temporomandibular disorders based on the outcome of published controlled studies. Oral Dis 7/2: 109-15

[16] Bossy, J.; Immune Systems Defense Mechanisms and Acupuncture Fundamental and Practical Aspects. Am. Jours. Acup. 18 (1990) 219-232

[17] HUI K.K.S; Liu, J., Chen. A. J. W. et al.: Acupunture modulates the limbic system and subcortical structures of the human brain, in: Neuroimage 7 (1998) 441

[18] Pert, A.; et all.: Alterations in rat central nervous system endorphins following trans-auricularelectroacupuncture, in: Brain Research 224 (1981) 83-93

[19] Chapmann, C.R.; Mechanisms of Pain an analgetic Compounds, New Work 1979

[20] Sandkühler, J.; The organsisation and function of endogenous antiocieptive systems, in: Prog. Neurobiol. 1 (1996) 49-81

[21] Gleditsch, J.M.: The „Very Point" Technique: a Needle Based Point Detection Method – Acupuncture in Medicine XIII (1995)

[22] Irnich, D., Behrens, Molzen, H., König, A., N., Gleditsch, J., et all.:Randomised trial acupuncture compared with conventional massage and „sham" laser acupuncture for treatment of chronic neck pain. Brit.Med.journal 322 (2001) S. 1574-1577

[23] Streitberger, K.; Kleinhenz, J.; Introducing a placebo needle into acupuncture research. Lancet 1998:352:364-365

[24] Vincent, C.; Lewith, G.;: Placebo controls für acupuncture studies. J. Royal Soc Med 1995; 88:199-202

[25] Adler, E.;Störfeld und Herd im Trigeminusbereich. GGM Heidelberg 2005;

[26] Löhnert et al; Akupunktur bei Zervikalsyndromen, in: Manuelle Medizin, 34 (1996) 269-274

[27] Gleditsch, J.M.: Oral Acupuncture, in: Acupuncture in Medicine, Journal of the BMAS 13 (1995) 15-19

[28] Melzack, R.; Trigger points and acupuncture points for pain: Correlations and implications, in: Pain 3 (1977) S. 3-23

[29] Rauhala, K., Oikarinen, K.S.; Raustia AM. (1999) Role of temporomandibular disorders (TMD) in facial pain: occlusion, muscle an TMJ pain. Cranio 17/4: 254-61

[30] Rosted: Practical recommendations fort he use of acupuncture in the treatment of temporarmandibular disorders based on the outcome of published controlled studies

[31] Lu, D.P.; Lu, G.P; Kleinmann, L.; (2001) Acupuncture and clinical hypnosis for facial and head and neck pain: a single crossover comparison. Am J ClinHypn 44/2: 141-8

Chapter 16

# Acupuncture in Military Medicine

Alexandra M. York, Kevin G. Berry, Rick C. Welton,
Joan A. G. Walter, Richard C. Niemtzow and
Wayne B. Jonas

Additional information is available at the end of the chapter

http://dx.doi.org/10.5772/55146

## 1. Introduction

Pain treatment and management remains one of the biggest challenges to modern medicine today. A recent Centers for Disease Control and Prevention (CDC) report found that 25 percent of U.S. adults reported experiencing a full day of pain within the past 30 days and one in 10 said their pain lasted one year or more. The most common complaints were low back pain followed by migraine or severe headache and joint pain[1].

Current research efforts to understand pain mechanisms have revealed a complex picture in which the biological mechanisms of pain reach beyond the nervous system to other areas and systems associated with depression, anxiety, and sleep, areas of the mind and psyche. A recent nationwide survey found that one in five Americans say their pain has resulted in major lifestyle changes in employment, residence, or personal freedom and mobility. Participants viewed the medical community as being only partially successful in helping patients manage their pain[2].

New, multi-disciplinary approaches to pain management have been developed and many therapies exist, however the dominant component of these approaches continues to be prescription and over-the-counter medications. While the use of medications is necessary and often effective, it does present the risk of overreliance, misuse, and abuse. Over the last decade there have been a number of reviews highlighting not only a significant rise in prescription medication, but also a sharp climb in abuse particularly for those between the ages of 18-25[3].

Military medicine is faced with similar challenges to successful pain management and treatment. However, many factors such as work cycles, organizational structure, mission and patient population of the military generate unique issues when formulating a strategy for pain management[4]. While the adequate and appropriate management of pain is a daunting issue for the military, recent engagements have put the issue of pain front and center.

The Global War on Terrorism and the wars in Iraq and Afghanistan have produced an increasing number of combat veterans returning with complex multi-trauma. Most of these injuries are caused by roadside, vehicle-mounted, and variously concealed improvised explosive devices (IEDs) that cause extensive direct and indirect concussive, blunt and projectile-induced damage. Due to significant improvements in individual body and vehicle armor, more sophisticated and responsive emergency medical and surgical care, and advanced air evacuation system capabilities, these injuries have become more survivable. In some cases, the very body armor that saves lives may contribute to head, neck, and extremity injuries, which in turn often progress to long-term disability and/or pain. Added to the physical wounds of war are the psychological and emotional sequelae associated with civilian and guerilla warfare, mass casualties and asymmetric warfare. As a result, large numbers of combat veterans experience a trauma spectrum response that includes pain, sleep and other somatic disorders, anxiety, post-traumatic stress, and other symptoms.

Due to the stigma associated with being taken out of the fight and away from their battle team, it is common for U.S. combatants to delay seeking medical help unless the injuries are significantly debilitating. It is variously reported that 15 to 20 percent of combat veterans returning without obvious physical injury have some degree of persistent mild traumatic brain injury and post-traumatic stress disorder. For others being treated for life-threatening injuries due to combat trauma, the sometimes hidden symptoms of repetitive concussive injury and combat stress are also present. These multiple overlapping injuries typically lead to chronic, more severe multi-system disorders well after the crisis of initial injury subsides. In many cases, the primary presenting problem is "depression, anxiety, or chronic pain" without other obvious physical manifestations. But upon further investigation, a profile of Wounded Warriors has been identified. These soldiers have had one or more concussive, blunt or projectile- induced injury, seek help several months to years after that injury, and describe persistent, multi-system symptoms of varying degrees and severities. This is reminiscent of "Gulf War Syndrome" or "Chronic Multi-symptom Illness" defined in the first gulf war.

All levels of the U.S. military medical departments and the Department of Defense engaged in a strategic reassessment of how to best respond to the needs of these Wounded Warriors in a way that also helped alleviate delayed deployments due to ongoing medical problems, the rising costs of medical care with fewer positive outcomes, and increasingly adverse and costly effects of drug and procedure-oriented solutions to treatment.

## 2. The pain experience in the military

To more fully understand the complexity inherent in addressing the pain caused by poly-trauma it is necessary to consider how the expression of pain is dictated by a number of factors in addition to direct tissue injury. Those who have experienced pain of any kind would attest

http://dx.doi.org/10.5772/55146

it is not a pleasant experience and one they would happily do without. However from an ontogeny perspective, pain serves a preservation purpose.

The primary role of pain is aptly summarized by Nikola Grahek in his book titled "Feeling Pain and Being in Pain":

---

*The capacity to feel pain upon harmful external stimulation or upon internal bodily damage is certainly the most precious gift bestowed on us by Mother Nature for self-protective purposes. However,...when in pain, we dislike it very much, and will do anything to get rid of it or at least alleviate it, especially if the pain is intrusive or severe5. (p.7)*

---

Grahek further explains that the pain system, at its fundamental level, can be viewed as serving two purposes – as a system of avoidance and as a system that promotes restoration or repair. As an avoidance system, pain warns us to stay clear of dangerous stimuli by assisting us in detecting the danger before any serious bodily damage befalls us. Its genius is in its preventative capacity which serves to protect and maintain survival. In instances in which damage has already occurred, the restorative system that promotes healing is facilitated by movement-limiting pain.

While typically functioning as it should – prevention and repair – the pain system has the potential to be overwhelmed. Instead of being triggered by painful stimuli, the system becomes overly sensitive to non-harmful stimuli (allodynia) or it may register an increased sensitivity to stimuli (hyperesthesia) or register pain sensation in non-damaged tissue (hyperalgesia). When this occurs, the perceived pain is no longer directly tied to the injury, and is thus maladaptive.

Recent scientific research indicates that a patient's psychological state may significantly influence their experienced pain, and that the perception of pain involves multiple factors beyond the direct physiological injury. Such factors contribute to the persistence of pain experience even after an injury has healed, and to the sensation of pain in an area devoid of any injury. Pain is now understood as a bio-psycho-social phenomenon rather than a strictly physiological one[6]. [See Gatchel for a more complete summary of the changing theories of pain]

The interplay of psycho-social factors and biology is strikingly on display in poly-trauma injuries. The persistent and chronic nature of pain associated with traumatic injuries has been well documented[7]. Additionally, there is a high incidence of concurrent Post-Traumatic Stress Disorder (PTSD), depression, and anxiety with these injuries. The overlapping and multi-component nature of traumatic injuries, both psychological and physical, has been recently characterized by Jonas et al. as war-related, trauma spectrum response (wrTSR). They propose mind-brain/body injuries, such as traumatic brain injury (TBI), are more appropriately addressed by a constellation (whole systems) view of the impact of that injury[8]:

---

*Triggered by combined mind-brain/body injuries (MBIs), the various manifestations of wrTSR share many common pathophysiological and recovery mechanisms....environmental and/or psychosocial insult can induce a core constellation of common symptoms that includes: (1) psychological and emotional distress (e.g., depression, anxiety, or anger); (2) cognitive impairment; (3) chronic and often refractory pain of organic and psychosomatic origins; (4) drug/opioid desensitization (with abuse potential); and (5) somatic (sleep, appetite, sexual, and energy) dysfunction.8*

---

The assessment of these components in complex interaction with each other and not as separate problems provides a more comprehensive picture of traumatic injury, and one that is more in line with the actual bio-psycho-social experience of the pain caused by the injury. To the extent that this is true, combat related pain has the potential to be exacerbated by the psychological aspects of war fighting. Addressing this constellation with approaches that impact them collectively will provide a more logical and likely efficient and effective framework than isolating them as "co-morbidities" each with their own specific treatments.

Combined physical, psychological, and social injury is not limited to injuries that are a result of a blast or combat. The majority of injuries from Operation Iraqi Freedom (OIF), Operation Enduring Freedom (OEF), and Operation New Dawn (OND) are not directly related to battle injuries. An evaluation of medical evacuations over the course of the nine years of OIF/OEF/OND found that most medical evacuations were not directly related to battle injuries. Instead, musculoskeletal disorders and mental disorders accounted for more than half[9]. This data is also supported by another evaluation that found non-battle injuries as the single largest category responsible for medical evacuations (approximately 36 percent) with fracture, inflammation/pain, and dislocation as the leading diagnosis. The leading body regions where the injury occurred were back, knee, and wrist/hand[10].

There is evidence suggesting that injury severity and functional recovery are similar across all groups – combat injury related to a blast exposure, injury due to combat, and injury in a noncombat zone. Not surprisingly blast exposure is associated with broader physical injuries, use of oral analgesics, and higher rates of PTSD and other psychiatric diagnoses when compared to non-blast injuries[11]. Whether blast related, combat related, or non-combat related, the majority of injuries resulting from OIF/OEF/OND are associated with psychological and social injuries that further complicate the successful management of pain regardless of its etiology.

Most clinicians and investigators find that pain, when viewed as a constellation of traumatic physical, psychological, and social injury, is quite different from that of multi-system trauma sustained in civilian circumstances and unrelated to combat operations. The additional significant family, relationship, and community factors are also aggravated as a result of the increased operational tempo of multiple combat-related deployments. The stress of repetitive deployments and rigorous training schedules even in the absence of combat-related trauma takes service members away from the family, and the family away from their normal support systems.

Initiated by combined "mind-brain-body" injury the array of wrTSR manifestations and behaviors probably share common pathophysiological and recovery mechanisms. One would therefore expect the need for an integrated, patient and family-centered, multi-disciplinary (body, mind, spirit, social, professional, and community), co-located team approach to evaluation, collaborative problem prioritization, intervention, monitoring, reconditioning, and reintegration back to military duty or to a productive civilian lifestyle.

http://dx.doi.org/10.5772/55146

However, the traditional approach to helping service members and their families recover and reintegrate into functional and meaningful military or civilian lifestyles is focused on pathology, disease and illness identification. Treatment is sought at separate medical departments and clinics (medical, mental health, and surgical specialties), military installations, and community programs. Each program independently evaluates and treats individuals (usually service and family members separately) in an asynchronous, non-integrated process. And, each typically deconstructs each separate problem affecting a particular body part or system in isolation, and prescribes a particular medication or procedure for that specific problem. Frequently these various and separately prescribed treatments interact and cause additional adverse effects. Even when chronic pain is managed as the primary problem, traditional measures focus on poly-pharmacy and localized procedures.

Although physical therapy, ultrasound, cold and heat applications, electrical stimulation, and chiropractic adjustment are applied, these modalities are usually added to a traditionally heavy medication load. This adds to the complexity of management and further increases risks of adverse or counterproductive interactions. When employed, psychological evaluations and counseling occur separately, and may add other drugs and treatments to the load.

Pharmacological agents go a long way in addressing acute pain and, when properly used, potentially preventing the development of chronic pain[12]. However, the use of pain medication comes at a high cost to the patient[13]. Recent studies and media reports have documented the risks (drug addiction, abuse, and overuse) associated with addressing the bio-psycho-social manifestations of pain with a poly-pharmacological approach[14],[15]. A 2008 Department of Defense (DoD) survey of health-related behaviors among active duty personnel revealed approximately 25 percent reported abusing prescribed medications within 12 months prior to the survey. Pain relievers were reported to be the most abused medication. The report also highlighted that prescription drug abuse within the military is significantly higher than among civilians[16].

The military has recently begun to recognize the limitations and risks associated with a primarily pharmacological approach to pain and psychological injury.

---

*"When the kids leave for school in the morning, Dad's on the couch. The pain is controlled, victory for us and medicine – we did a good job. But when the kids come home from school in the afternoon, Dad's still on the couch. Medicine is still saying it's doing its job because the pain is controlled, but this person's quality of life is probably not what they want it to be, definitely not what the spouse wants it to be, [and] not what their family wants it to be." 17*

COL Galloway, Chief of Staff, U.S. Army's Pain Management Task Force

---

Spurred by the challenges of treating complex, overlapping physical and psychological injuries the military has begun to open the door to non-traditional approaches to pain management particularly acupuncture.

## 3. A Holistic approach to pain

Complementary and integrative (CI) therapies have existed for centuries albeit more so among consumers than the medical community. However, the shift of CI therapies from the periphery to a more mainstream position in conventional medicine began in the U.S. in the 1960s and 1970s and has continued ever since[18]. Spurred by compelling effectiveness evidence and documentation of its popularity among the public[19] CI therapies have increasingly become integrated into traditional medical care. More than other CI therapies, acupuncture has undergone a significant integration particularly as a complement to traditional pain management approaches.

The preferred use of acupuncture for pain can be explained by a number of factors including its underlying theory, evidence base, and delivery. The theory and approach of acupuncture is guided by a different underlying assumption than conventional medicine. In conventional medicine it is assumed the expression of symptoms such as pain is directly tied to a disease or dysfunction in the physiological system. However in acupuncture, all aspects of a patient – physical, psychological, symptoms, and other characteristics – are understood to contribute to a pattern of imbalance[20]:

---

*The Chinese method is based on the idea that no single part can be understood except in its relation to the whole. A symptom, therefore, is not traced back to a cause, but is looked at as a part of a totality. If a person has a complaint or symptom, Chinese medicine wants to know how the symptom fits into the patient's entire being and behavior. Illness is situated in the context of a person's life and biography20 (p.7)*

---

The theories that guide acupuncture are precisely what make it an ideal complement to the bio-psycho-social model of pain management. The resolution offered in an acupuncture treatment not only acknowledges the interplay of the internal and external factors involved in the manifestation of pain in the patient, but it utilizes those factors to generate a holistic, healing approach that goes beyond symptom management. Note, however, that this holistic framework means that simply adding acupuncture as another add-on, asynchronous modality in the same manner other isolated treatments are provided may not optimize its effectiveness for the entire spectrum of illness in wrTSR.

The underlying theory of acupuncture makes it an ideal candidate for inclusion into an integrative approach to pain management and the current effectiveness evidence goes even further in strengthening the justification of its integration. Over the past decade and a half there has been a significant increase in both the quantity and quality of acupuncture studies. A number of significant findings and consensus statements have confirmed and further elucidated the effectiveness of acupuncture and its mechanistic underpinnings[21],[22].

More recently a number of reviews summarizing and evaluating the evidence of acupuncture for chronic pain conditions have been conducted. A systematic review evaluating 51 randomized controlled trials (RCT) for varying pain conditions found that the majority of high-quality studies that produced positive findings involved musculoskeletal pain[23]. A meta-analysis, examining systematic reviews of acupuncture for chronic pain from 2005-2008, found acupuncture to be effective for chronic osteoarthritis of the knee and headache. Improvement was maintained for both short term (defined as less than three months after randomization) and long term (three months or longer). Consistent with previous literature, the results for back pain were mixed – true acupuncture was superior to sham in the short term, but the evidence for the long term was mixed[24]. Further, a review evaluating and summarizing Cochrane reviews of acupuncture for chronic pain conditions found that four reviews concluded acupuncture was effective for neck disorders, tension-type headaches, and peripheral joint osteoarthritis[25].

While the current evidence of acupuncture for depression and anxiety remains mixed due to many factors[26] it is still regarded as a promising therapy. A number of RCTs evaluating acupuncture for generalized anxiety disorder or anxiety neurosis have demonstrated positive results[27]. Additionally acupuncture, particularly ear acupuncture, has shown benefit in addressing peri-operative anxiety[27]. Regarding depression, a recent systematic review concluded that while the quality of studies examining acupuncture for depression had improved, there was still insufficient evidence to draw a firm conclusion either in support for or against acupuncture[28]. Although the research evaluating acupuncture for PTSD is still in its infancy, the evidence so far indicates acupuncture could be very effective. In 2007 a three-arm RCT comparing acupuncture to cognitive behavioral therapy (CBT) to a wait-list control found that acupuncture provided treatment effects similar to CBT that were maintained three months post-treatment. Additional studies are needed to confirm these initial findings.

A discussion of acupuncture effectiveness would not be complete without mention of the non-specific effects of acupuncture. Much attention has been given to the fact that in many cases the effectiveness of true acupuncture has been found to be no greater than sham or placebo acupuncture. While often viewed in a negative light, this observation only serves to further illuminate the effects of acupuncture. From a reductionist, disease treatment framework, non-specific effects are to be isolated and minimized in favor of specific effects. However from a more holistic and healing oriented framework being suggested here, they become core mechanisms to enhance and maximize – facilitating the self-healing mechanisms not associated with a single disease or illness syndrome. Acupuncture is more than the act of needle insertion. It is embedded in a ritual that includes a narrative interaction and trusting relationship between the patient and acupuncturist. This interaction and relationship have been shown to activate immune markers and specific neurotransmitters associated with symptom improvement[29]. In many cases, especially for patients with a wide spectrum of problems, as in wrTSR, these effects may be just what are needed.

Taken together, the underlying theory of acupuncture and the current evidence of its effectiveness support its inclusion into an integrative pain management strategy and the adoption of a holistic model similar to one on which it is based. The U.S. military has come to a similar determination and through a number of recent initiatives has made significant strides in integrating acupuncture into its pain management paradigms.

## 4. Military medicine initiatives — Creating a path for integration

Each of the United States Armed Forces provides the manpower, equipment, and facilities to organize and sustain required capabilities, including health readiness, in order to maintain a ready force across a range of military operations. By doctrine the Army, Navy and Air Force are responsible for the force health protection, health service delivery, and health systems support in alignment with Department of Defense policy and guidance.[30] The Navy is the primary health readiness provider for the Marine Corps. The U.S. Coast Guard under the Department of Homeland Security is the fifth armed service and, when directed by the appropriate authority, deploys with the U.S. military. The uniformed U.S. Public Health Service supports the Coast Guard for health readiness and it receives additional support from other branches of the Department of Defense when deployed with them.

Traditionally the United States Army, Navy/Marine Corps, Air Force and Coast Guard (when assigned to the Department of Defense) have approached health readiness somewhat differently because of differences in mission capabilities, practices, and culture. In 2007 the medical departments of the armed forces, under the purview of the Assistant Secretary of Defense for Health Affairs, developed the Joint Force Health Protection Concept of Operations to improve joint war fighting capabilities.[31] This was the first time the health and medical requirements for U.S. troops irrespective of branch of service were codified.

The Department of Defense revised this policy in 2010 and 2011 expanding Joint Force Health Protection into a hierarchy of health and medical requirements documents. At the topmost level was the new overarching Health Readiness Concept of Operations policy that spelled out the optimal health service that would go "anytime, anywhere" in support of military operations consistent with the then newly expanded Military Health System Strategic Plan composed of four mission elements: casualty care and humanitarian assistance/disaster response; fit, healthy, and protected force; healthy and resilient individuals, families, and communities; education, research, and performance improvement.[30] While some capabilities critical for military medical operations are explicitly delineated, complementary and alternative medicine (CAM), integrated medicine and acupuncture are not mentioned.

In the United States and on permanent overseas bases and stations, in-garrison medical and preventive health services are generally provided to service members by their own military medical department. Under United States Code, Title 10, Chapter 55, family members, retirees, and in special cases others are entitled to receive a broad-based healthcare benefit that is part of the Defense Health Program under the policy direction of the Assistant Secretary of Defense for Health Affairs in the Military Healthcare System.

In 2011 the Department of Defense provided a medical benefit to 9.7 million people for a total cost of $52 billion. The vast majority of the money covered the cost of actual care. In 2011, 17,476 active duty medical personnel medically supported 321,751 service members deployed overseas, and medically evacuated 6,943 casualties including 221 amputees. "TRICARE" is the military medical system for the health care of its active and retired service members and families. The Department of Defense Health Service Delivery Concept of Operations describes an ability "to build healthy communities by managing and delivering the health benefit, through the use of military treatment facilities, and the TRICARE network of healthcare providers."[32]

The former Army Surgeon General, LTG Eric B. Schoomaker, chartered the Army Pain Management Task Force in August 2009 to develop and recommend strategies for "comprehensive pain management that is holistic, multidisciplinary, and multimodal in its approach, utilizes state of the art/science modalities and technologies, and provides optimal quality of life for Soldiers and other patients with acute and chronic pain." The Task Force included a variety of medical specialties and disciplines predominantly from the Army but included representatives from the Navy, Air Force, TRICARE Management Activity, and Veterans Health Administration (VHA) as well.

The Task Force reviewed pain management in the United States, concluding that variability is common depending on provider and medical care delivery system factors. The report found that pain can be effectively managed by over the counter and prescription medications but that there are unintended consequences to the overreliance on them, with abuse highest in the 18-25 year old age demographic that encompasses many war casualties. The report acknowledged patients' interest in treatments other than or in addition to medication, with CAM a popular option.

Many of the Military Health System's (MHS) challenges with pain management are very similar to those faced by other medical systems, but the MHS also faces some unique issues because of its distinctive mission, structure and patient population. For example:

- The nation expects the MHS to provide the highest level of care to those carrying war's heaviest burdens.
- The transient nature of the military population, including patients and providers, makes continuity of care a challenge for military medicine.
- Pain management challenges associated with combat polytrauma patients require integrated approaches to clinical care that cross traditional medical specialties, not all of which are universally available across the MHS.

[The Army Medical Command] and MHS lack a comprehensive pain management strategy that addresses current deficiencies. As a result, pain management initiatives are fragmented - often driven by local champions and subject to retirements, changes of command, and annual budget priorities for their continued existence.[33] (page E-2)

The Army Pain Management Task Force concluded that "improving pain management across the DoD will require a significant reorganization, education, and training effort that will be most effective if pursued as a part of a DoD and [Veterans Health Affairs] partnership." Additional pain medicine specialists would be needed as would support teams. The teams would manage pain employing a biopsychosocial model of care evolving the standard of care pain management to one not excessively rely on medication and creates a collaborative interdisciplinary approach among providers from differing specialties.

The Task Force encouraged the DoD to responsibly explore safe and effective use of advanced and non-traditional approaches to pain management and to "support efforts to make these modalities covered benefits once they prove safe, effective and cost efficient." [5] (page E-2)

The Army urged DoD to "establish pain as a priority, with an urgency that leads to practice changes" with attention of prevention, prompt and appropriate treatment to relieve acute pain and eliminate progression to chronic pain when possible. Cooperation between the DoD and VHA would lead to shared common educational materials, venues, protocols, and formularies providing "a standardized DoD and VHA vision and approach to pain management to optimize the care for Warriors and their Families."[5] (page E-3)

In the body of the Task Force Report, acupuncture is specifically identified among 109 recommendations. The recommendation for standardized minimum training, skill attainment and credentials includes acupuncture, spinal manipulation and an expansion of treatment modalities to include CAM and integrative medicine. [5] (page 19). Training, skills and credentials are necessary preconditions to a holistic integrative multi-modal patient-centered care plan. Acupuncture, Yoga/Yoga Nidra, non-allopathic chiropractic care, therapeutic massage, biofeedback, and the mind-body techniques of meditation and mindfulness, combined active and passive modalities, are recommended Tier 1 modalities: the highest level of supporting scientific evidence. [5] (page 44).

The Army Medical Command issued a directive to the Army direct medical care system to engage in a comprehensive pain management campaign plan. The issuance took the format of an Army operational order.[34] The campaign plan included acupuncture and yoga as modalities to reduce overreliance on medication. The operational order provided the mechanism and authority to make acupuncture available in Army military treatment facilities, for credentialing acupuncturists and or other providers to add acupuncture as a privilege when trained and skilled.

In a June 2011 meeting to discuss improving pain management for Warriors and Veterans through the use of integrative medicine General Schoomaker remarked, "This is a unique, historic moment to capitalize on what we know works to effectively treat pain. It marks the beginning of a cultural shift in how health care is practiced in the military."[35]

The Army Surgeon General's establishment of the Pain Management Task Force coincided with the U.S. Congress' passage of the National Defense Authorization Act for 2010. The final version of that bill, signed into law by the President, included Section 711, which required the Secretary of Defense to develop and implement a comprehensive pain management policy for the Military Health System and to report on its progress to Congress.

While each service has introduced integrative medicine therapies into their pain management paradigm, the U.S. Army Medical Command currently has the strongest mandate for integration with unequivocal support in terms of policy, procedures and resources for acupuncture, yoga, and other alternative pain management modalities that have an adequate base of evidence. The goals of the Army campaign are to meet patient demand for complementary and alternative medicine that is integrated holistically into the lives of Soldiers and family members, and to reduce excessive use, or supplement judicious use of pain medications. The

Army Task Force recommended changing the paradigm of pain management to include patient activities in addition to therapy delivered passively by a provider.

The military health benefit continues to evolve, and is based on evidence of efficacy and cost effectiveness. Traditional Chinese Medicine and acupuncture are not yet covered benefits of the TRICARE military health system, but acupuncture in one form or another is available to some beneficiaries on a limited basis within some military treatment facilities. The challenge for proponents of acupuncture and those who seek its benefits is that access is dependent on local factors: i.e., acceptability of the practice in the eyes of local military medical leaders, local credentials and privileging policies, referral mechanisms, and most importantly the availability of acupuncture practitioners.

The challenge of access to acupuncture services is also a challenge of training. Increasing the number of providers trained in acupuncture will in turn increase the availability of acupuncture. Within the last decade, the U.S. Air Force has committed a number of resources to increasing acupuncture availability and training.

The impetus for increased acupuncture availability began with establishment of the first ever, full-time, medical acupuncture clinic at Andrews Air Force Base, Maryland in 2002. Through the efforts of two medical acupuncturists Col (Ret) Richard Niemtzow, MD, PhD, MPH and Col (Ret) Stephen M. Burns, MD the clinic offered acupuncture treatments aimed at addressing pain in a more holistic way. The clinic, due to growing demand for acupuncture and reported benefits [36] recently transitioned into an Acupuncture Center (AC).

In addition to the direct offering of acupuncture through the AC, and because of the success of the AC, the Air Force in 2009 sponsored the training of 44 active duty military physicians in medical acupuncture. Representatives from all three services – Army, Navy, Air Force, and a variety of medical specialties participated in the training. The Navy's Bureau of Medicine and Surgery offered a similar training program in 2009-2010 to Navy participants [37].

These training programs generated a cadre of military physicians now capable of offering acupuncture services. However the time constraints of current clinical practice (approximately 10 to 20 minutes per patient) presents a challenge to physicians offering a more traditional acupuncture treatment that includes a comprehensive diagnostic evaluation and treatment [37]. Additionally, military physicians practice in a number of austere training and combat-operational environments that are not always conducive to a traditional acupuncture treatment; and the frequent deployments and military household moves render a transitory nature to patients, making follow-up more difficult. In response to these clinical challenges, a number of simple, standardized acupuncture protocols have been developed [37]. While these approaches may not take advantage of the complete holistic models needed, they do offer new, non-drug and non-stigmatizing options for pain and are scalable to a large population. The Samueli Institute is currently testing the effectiveness of this standardized approach compared to a more holistic acupuncture model and conventional care on pain in service members with TBI. This research will help determine the "dose" and framework needed for delivery of acupuncture in the most efficient manner.

In addition, the military is using other acupuncture approach models. These include the Helms Medical Institute auricular trauma protocol (ATP) [38] which is an ear acupuncture protocol in which needles are administered sequentially to the following points: hypothalamus, amygdala, hippocampus, Master Cerebral, and Point Zero. The needles are typically left in for 30-120 minutes. The rationale for this protocol is based on the concept that the three affected neurological structures in traumatic stress – amygdala, hippocampus, and prefrontal cortex – are correlated with somatotopic reflex zones found on the ears. The "Koffman Cocktail" is a bilateral, 4-point acupuncture protocol developed by U.S. Navy Capt Robert L. Koffman, MD which has been suggested to be a calming and centering treatment [37]. The best known of these standardized protocols is battlefield acupuncture (BFA). BFA is a bilateral, 5-point ear acupuncture protocol aimed at addressing a number of pain conditions [39]. The following acupuncture points are sequentially administrated: Cingulate Gyrus, Thalamus point, Omega 2, Point Zero, and Shen Men. Either the left or right ear is chosen for the placement of the needles, or the needles are administered bilaterally until pain attenuation is reached. BFA was developed by Dr. Niemtzow and has demonstrated preliminary success for a number of refractory pain conditions [40], and has been associated with improved quality of life [36].

The additional expressed appeal of these simple, standardized acupuncture protocols lies in the ability to teach a variety of providers who have no formal acupuncture training. The Air Force Medical Service, through the Acupuncture Center, has begun to teach "mini-courses" in BFA. The course is conducted by medical acupuncturists who have been trained in BFA and have used it extensively in their own practice. The BFA course is typically conducted over a one or two day time period and instruction includes background on the mechanistic theory of BFA and a supervised clinical practice [37].

While these initiatives represent a profound change in military medicine in terms of approach and delivery, how they are affecting acupuncture availability and utilization across the military is unclear. Currently there has been no formal analysis of acupuncture availability or utilization. However a number of media reports have documented the availability and use of acupuncture throughout the military. These reports detail stories of both the front line and state side use of acupuncture for PTSD, mild TBI, and pain.

On the front line, acupuncture has been used to treat PTSD and mild TBI at the Concussion Restoration Care Center (CRCC), Camp Leatherneck, Afghanistan. The CRCC is part of a joint Navy-Marine Corps effort, Operation Stress Control and Readiness Program, in which psychiatrists and psychologists are placed within combat teams to provide mental health care to troops in Afghanistan[41]. The former director of CRCC reported that, of the troops he personally treated, a majority of them experienced improvements in sleep and decreases in anxiety levels and frequency of headaches. Another story details acupuncture being used by a military physical therapist to treat service members at the Courage Clinic, Camp Victory, Iraq[42]. More recently acupuncture has begun to be offered to patients and crewmembers aboard the Military Sealift Command hospital ship USNS Mercy in Vietnam for pain and associated ailments[43]. Acupuncture was also used for pain management and stress relief aboard the hospital ship USNS Comfort as part of a humanitarian and civic assistance mission[44].

In the U.S. acupuncture has been used at a number of military treatment facilities (MTFs) as a part of holistic, multi-disciplinary programs. As mentioned earlier, the Acupuncture Center at Joint Andrews Base has utilized acupuncture for a number of pain conditions, sleep, and psychological issues[36]. At Walter Reed National Naval Medical Center (WRNNMC) acupuncture has been used for phantom limb pain and it is used in the Specialized Care Program (SCP) at the Deployment Health Clinical Center. The SCP is a three-week, multidisciplinary, therapy program for service members with post-deployment health concerns[45]. At the National Intrepid Center of Excellence in Bethesda, Maryland acupuncture is used for treating stress and psychological disorders such as TBI and post-traumatic stress[46]. In Texas acupuncture is part of the medical care offered to the Warrior Transition Brigade at Ft. Hood for pain management and stress relief[47] and it is part of the Integrative Medicine Center (IMC) at Ft. Bliss. The IMC was the first physical health and integrative medicine clinic in the Department of Defense when it opened its doors approximately six years ago[48]. Also, the Naval Medical Center San Diego (NMCSD) has been offering acupuncture since 1999 for the treatment and management of pain[49] and just this year acupuncture was reported to be one of the complementary therapies offered in the Wounded Warrior Program at Naval Hospital Camp Pendleton[50].

An unpublished paper[51] examining the differences in the amount of services utilized between non-acupuncture and acupuncture patients for the same diagnosis within the DoD provides information, albeit preliminary and limited, on acupuncture availability and impact on cost from the perspective of a military treatment facility (MTF). The paper reports that in 2008 the DoD had more than 40 licensed acupuncturists and that acupuncture was offered at 40 different MTFs. Data on acupuncture utilization revealed that in 2008 there were 12,209 clinical encounters that received an acupuncture code (Common Procedural Terminology (CPT code). The majority of this patient population was between the ages of 20 and 49 and active duty personnel. The top three diagnoses accompanying acupuncture codes were for low back pain, fibromyalgia (myalgia), and neck pain. The author highlighted possible reasons for the increased encounters by patients receiving acupuncture: 1) those who receive acupuncture usually do so as part of a program of other therapies that would result in more encounters and 2) patients who elect to utilize acupuncture usually tend to do so as a last resort therefore their conditions are usually more difficult to treat and are associated with increased encounters.

The paper concluded that patients who received acupuncture had more encounters resulting in an increase of "revenue" for MTFs of approximately $2 million as calculated in the study[51]. The fact that the study did not address per patient per year government costs or opportunity cost for the MTF prevents definitive conclusions to be drawn. While the limited analysis reported in this paper sheds some preliminary light on the cost impact of acupuncture on the military health system, there has yet to be a rigorous, comprehensive assessment of cost analyses of acupuncture across the DoD. Recent economic analyses of acupuncture within civilian health care systems have found it to be cost-effective for chronic pain[51], low back pain[52],[53], headache[54], and neck pain[55].

The integration of any new therapy into an existing system of care requires continued evaluation and assessment. While there has been a considerable amount research examining the effectiveness of acupuncture conducted in the civilian population, there has been a paucity of acupuncture research conducted in the military population. A review conducted to assess the quantity and quality of acupuncture research within the military and veteran populations found a total of only two RCTs, two observational studies, and four descriptive studies[56]. The mixed quality of these studies did not allow the authors to draw any definitive conclusions regarding the effect of acupuncture. However the review did note that there are indicators pointing to an increase in acupuncture research within these populations. A quick search of the clinicaltrials.gov database (a database that provides the public with information about current ongoing clinical research studies) found approximately a dozen trials examining the effectiveness of acupuncture for a wide range of conditions including sleep, quality of life, sore throat, gastro-esophageal reflux disease (GERD), Gulf War Illness, and acute pain.

Additionally the review highlighted a select number of completed or ongoing studies that examined acupuncture for pain and stress disorders. Studies included an observational trial conducted in 2005 evaluating the benefits of acupuncture offered through the Acupuncture Center at the Joint Andrews Base for acute and chronic pain in active duty military personnel, dependents, and retirees. Significant reductions in pain and improved quality of life scores were reported[36]. A number of studies have been completed however the results have yet to be published. They include a pilot study evaluating the feasibility of integrating BFA into the aeromedical evacuation system from Ramstien Air Base, Germany to Joint Andrews Base and another pilot study examining acupuncture for phantom limb pain that yielded promising preliminary data. In 2006 a RCT evaluated acupuncture for PTSD in a cohort of service members and the results were presented at a symposium in 2008. Finally the review mentioned an exploratory, randomized study to examine the effectiveness of acupuncture for TBI related headache in an active duty population at Walter Reed National Naval Medical Center that began in 2011[56]. Of particular interest is the design of this study which will compare a standardized ear acupuncture technique (developed by a medical acupuncturist) to an individualized, semi-standard acupuncture protocol (developed by a licensed acupuncturist and psychiatrist)[57]. While headache is the primary outcome of this study additional secondary measures examining sleep, stress, depression, and anxiety will be collected.

While these reports of current and ongoing research will add valuable information in terms of acupuncture effectiveness, a significant gap remains between how acupuncture is being utilized and the amount of acupuncture research that has been conducted in military populations. An increase in research efforts will be required to determine if these military initiatives are successfully being translated into improved health outcomes and cost savings.

## 5. Conclusion

The initiatives discussed in this chapter represent recognition by the military health system that successful pain management requires a more comprehensive, holistic approach. They also represent a clear commitment by the military to augment the current health care system to allow for the inclusion of these therapies as complements to conventional pharmacological and multi-disciplinary approaches.

http://dx.doi.org/10.5772/55146

As it has been noted here and elsewhere [58] many barriers still exist and will need to be addressed before full integration is realized. They include increasing the availability of acupuncture through changes in credentialing and privileging polices for those already trained and increasing acupuncture training opportunities; developing curricula to educate medical students and current providers in integrative therapies; and to develop assessment tools that capture effectiveness outcomes and impact outcomes (utilization and cost/benefit analyses). As of August 2012 evidence-based complementary modalities are not yet a TRICARE (health care program for Uniformed Service members, retirees and their families worldwide) benefit.

## Acknowledgements

The authors would like to thank Doug Cavarocchi for his assistance in the preparation of this manuscript. This work is supported by the U.S. Army Medical Research and Materiel Command under Award No. W81XWH-06-1-0279 to Samueli Institute. The views, opinions and/or findings contained in this work are those of the author(s) and should not be construed as an official Department of the Army position, policy or decision unless so designated by other documentation.

## Author details

Alexandra M. York[1], Kevin G. Berry[1], Rick C. Welton[1], Joan A. G. Walter[1], Richard C. Niemtzow[2] and Wayne B. Jonas[1]

1 Samueli Institute, USA

2 United States Air Force Acupuncture Center, Joint Base Andrews, USA

## References

[1] CDC National Center for Health Statistics Press OfficeNew Report Finds Pain Affects Millions of Americans. (2006). http://www.cdc.gov/nchs/pressroom/06facts/hus06.htmAccessed August 8, 2012.

[2] Peter, D. Hart Research Associates. Americans Talk About Pain. (2003). http://www.researchamerica.org/uploads/poll2003pain.pdf.Accessed August 8, 2012.

[3] Sehgal, N, Manchikanti, L, & Smith, H. S. Prescription opioid abuse in chronic pain: a review of opioid abuse predictors and strategies to curb opioid abuse. *Pain Physician.* Jul (2012). Suppl):ES, 67-92.

[4] Office of The Army Surgeon General. (2010). *Report to Surgeon General: Pain management Task Force Report: Providing a standardized DoD and VHA vision and approach to pain management to optimize the care for warriors and their families.*

[5] Grahek, N. *Feeling Pain and Being in Pain.* 2nd ed: MIT Press; (2007).

[6] Gatchel, R. J. Perspectives on pain: a historical overview. In: R.J. Gatchel DCT, ed. *Psychosocial Factors in Pain: Cretical Perspectives.* New York, NY: Guilford Press; (1999)., 1999, 3-17.

[7] Turk, D, & Okifuji, A. Psychological factors in chronic pain: evolution and revolution. *J Consult Clin Psychol.* (2002)., 70, 678-690.

[8] Jonas, W, Walter, J, Fritts, F, & Niemtzow, R. Acupuncture for the Trauma Spectrum Response: Scientific Foundations, Challenges to Implementation. *Medical Acupuncture.* (2011)., 23(4), 249-262.

[9] Armed Forces Health Surveillance Center*Causes of medical evacuations from Operations Iraqi Freedom (OIF), New Dawn (OND) and Enduring Freedom (OEF), active and reserve components, U.S. Armed Forces, October 2001September 2010.* Washington, D.C.February, (2011).

[10] Hauret, K. G, Taylor, B. J, Clemmons, N. S, Block, S. R, & Jones, B. H. Frequency and causes of nonbattle injuries air evacuated from operations iraqi freedom and enduring freedom, u.s. Army, *Am J Prev Med.* Jan (2010). Suppl):S94-107., 2001-2006.

[11] Clark, M. E, Walker, R. L, Gironda, R. J, & Scholten, J. D. Comparison of pain and emotional symptoms in soldiers with polytrauma: unique aspects of blast exposure. *Pain Med.* Apr (2009)., 10(3), 447-455.

[12] Black, I. H, & Mcmanus, J. Pain management in current combat operations. *Prehosp Emerg Care.* Apr-Jun (2009)., 13(2), 223-227.

[13] Nicholas, M. K, Molloy, A. R, & Brooker, C. Using opioids with persisting noncancer pain: a biopsychosocial perspective. *Clin J Pain.* Feb (2006)., 22(2), 137-146.

[14] Becker, W. C, Fiellin, D. A, Gallagher, R. M, Barth, K. S, Ross, J. T, & Oslin, D. W. The association between chronic pain and prescription drug abuse in Veterans. *Pain Med.* Apr (2009)., 10(3), 531-536.

[15] Doa, J, Carey, B, & Frosch, D. For Some Troops, Powerful Drug Cocktails Have Deadly Results. *New York Times*(2011). A1.

[16] Bray, R. M, Pemberton, M. R, Lane, M. E, Hourani, L. L, Mattiko, M. J, & Babeu, L. A. Substance Use and Mental Health Trends Among U.S. Military Active Duty Personnel: Key Findings From the 2008 DoD Health Behavior Survey. *Military Medicine.* (2010)., 175(6), 390-399.

[17] Garamone, J. Military Medicine Works on Managing Pain. (2011). http://www.defense.gov/news/newsarticle.aspx?id=65812Accessed August 8, 2012.

[18] Whorton, J. C. *Nature Cures: The History of Alternative Medicine in America*: Oxford University Press; (2004).

[19] Eisenberg, D. M, Davis, R. B, Ettner, S. L, et al. Trends in alternative medicine use in the United States, 1990-1997: results of a follow-up national survey. *JAMA.* Nov 11 (1998). , 280(18), 1569-1575.

[20] Kaptchuk, T. J. *The Web That Has No Weaver*: McGraw-Hill; (2000).

[21] Park, J, Linde, K, Manheimer, E, et al. The status and future of acupuncture clinical research. *J Altern Complement Med.* Sep (2008). , 14(7), 871-881.

[22] Schnyer, R, Lao, L, Hammerschlag, R, et al. Society for Acupuncture Research: 2007 conference report: "The status and future of acupuncture research: 10 years post-NIH Consensus Conference". *J Altern Complement Med.* Sep (2008). , 14(7), 859-860.

[23] Ezzo, J, Berman, B, Hadhazy, V. A, Jadad, A. R, Lao, L, & Singh, B. B. Is acupuncture effective for the treatment of chronic pain? A systematic review. *Pain.* Jun (2000). , 86(3), 217-225.

[24] Hopton, A. MacPherson H. Acupuncture for chronic pain: is acupuncture more than an effective placebo? A systematic review of pooled data from meta-analyses. *Pain Pract.* Mar-Apr (2010). , 10(2), 94-102.

[25] Lee, M. S, & Ernst, E. Acupuncture for pain: an overview of Cochrane reviews. *Chin J Integr Med.* Mar (2011). , 17(3), 187-189.

[26] Pilkington, K, Kirkwood, G, Rampes, H, Cummings, M, & Richardson, J. Acupuncture for anxiety and anxiety disorders--a systematic literature review. *Acupunct Med.* Jun (2007).

[27] Pilkington, K, Kirkwood, G, Rampes, H, Cummings, M, & Richardson, J. Acupuncture for anxiety and anxiety disorders- A systematic literature review. *Acupuncture in Medicine.* (2007).

[28] Smith, C. A, Hay, P. P, & Macpherson, H. Acupuncture for depression. *Cochrane database of systematic reviews (Online).* (2010). CD004046.

[29] Kaptchuk, T. J. Placebo studies and ritual theory: a comparative analysis of Navajo, acupuncture and biomedical healing. *Philos Trans R Soc Lond B Biol Sci.* Jun 27 (2011). , 366(1572), 1849-1858.

[30] Woodson, J. Health Readiness Concept of Operation (CONOPS). Washington, DC: Office of Stratgic Management Office of Assistant Secretary of Defense (Health Affairs); (2010).

[31] Smith, D, & Timberlake, G. Joint Force Health Protection Concept of Operations. Washington, DC: Joint Staff J4 Health Services Support Division; (2007).

[32] Woodson, J. Health Service Delivery Concept of Operations (CONOPS). Washington, DC: Office of Strategic Managment Office of the Assistant Secretary of Defense (Health Affairs); (2011).

[33] Thomas, R. Pain Managment Task Force: Final Report May 2010. Washington, DC: Army Medical Command; (2010).

[34] Jones, D. J. OPERATION ORDER 10-76 (USAMEDCOM COMPREHENSIVE PAIN MANAGEMENT CAMPAIGN PLAN). Washington, DC: US Army Medical Command; (2010).

[35] Military to Implement Integrative Medicine for Comprehensive Pain Management*The Bravewell Collaborative* (2010). http://www.bravewell.org/current_projects/military_medicine/.Accessed August 5, 2012, 2012.

[36] Niemtzow, R. C, Burns, S. M, Cooper, J, Libretto, S, Walter, J, & Baxter, J. Acupuncture clinical pain trial in a military medical center: Outcomes. *Medical Acupuncture.* (2008). , 20(4), 255-261.

[37] Pock, A. R. Acupuncture in the U.S. Armed Forces: A Brief History and Review of Current Educational Approaches. *Medical Acupuncture.* December 20, (2011). , 23(4), 205-208.

[38] Helms, J. M, Walkowski, S. A, Elkiss, M, Pittman, D, Kouchis, N. S, & Lawrence, B. HMI Auricular Trauma Protocol: An Acupuncture Approach for Trauma Spectrum Symptoms. *Medical Acupuncture.* December 20, (2011). , 23(4), 209-213.

[39] Niemtzow, R. C, Litscher, G, Burns, S. M, & Helms, J. M. Battelfield Acupuncture: Update. *Medical Acupuncture.* (2009). , 21(1), 43-46.

[40] Goertz, C. M, Niemtzow, R, Burns, S. M, Fritts, M. J, Crawford, C. C, & Jonas, W. B. Auricular acupuncture in the treatment of acute pain syndromes: A pilot study. *Mil Med.* Oct (2006). , 171(10), 1010-1014.

[41] Voorhees, C. Acupuncture Makes Strides in Treatment of Brain Injuries, PTSD. *Armed with Science* (2011). http://science.dodlive.mil/2011/06/20/acupuncture-makes-strides-in-treatment-of-brain-injuries-ptsd-video/Accessed August 6, 2012.

[42] Bradford, L. Holistic healing offers new alternative to medicine. (2010). http://www.army.mil/article/34359/Accessed August 6, 2012.

[43] Feddersen, M. Acupuncturist Re-Visits his Ancient Craft. (2012). http://www.navy.mil/submit/display.asp?story_id=68373.Accessed August 6, 2012.

[44] Grannan, D. Unique Pain Relief Offered to Dominicans on Comfort. (2009). http://www.navy.mil/submit/display.asp?story_id=44716.Accessed August 6, 2012.

[45] DCoE Strategic CommunicationsWounded Warriors Share their Views on Acupuncture. In: Defense Ceners of Excellence, ed. *The DCoE Blog.* , 20122010

[46] Gantz, S. Navy psychiatrist uses acupuncture to open veterans to healing body and mind. (2011). http://www.gazette.net/article/20110706/NEWS/707069991/&template=gazette.Accessed August 8, 2012.

[47] Montgomery, G. Warrior care year-round commitment to Fort Hood's WTB. (2011). http://www.army.mil/article/69918/Warrior_care_year_round_commitment_to_Fort_Hood_s_WTB/.Accessed August 8, 2012.

[48] Kennemer, J. Fort Bliss Soldiers have integrative medicine options. (2010). http://www.army.mil/article/35942/fort-bliss-soldiers-have-integrative-medicine-options/ Accessed August 8, 2012.

[49] Puscian, A. NMCSD Provides an Alternative Medicine. (2009). http://www.med.navy.mil/sites/nmcsd/Pages/Did%20You%20Know/dyk-201002.aspx.Accessed August 8, 2012.

[50] Calestini, M. Wounded Warrior care at Camp Pendleton is team effort. In: U.S. Navy and Marine Corps Health Care, ed. *Navy Medicine Live.* , 20122012

[51] Ambrosio, E. M, Bloor, K, & Macpherson, H. Costs and consequences of acupuncture as a treatment for chronic pain: A systematic review of economic evaluations conducted alongside randomised controlled trials. *Complement Ther Med.* Oct (2012). , 20(5), 364-374.

[52] Moritz, S, Liu, M. F, Rickhi, B, Xu, T. J, Paccagnan, P, & Quan, H. Reduced health resource use after acupuncture for low-back pain. *J Altern Complement Med.* Nov (2011). , 17(11), 1015-1019.

[53] Thomas, K. J. MacPherson H, Ratcliffe J, et al. Longer term clinical and economic benefits of offering acupuncture care to patients with chronic low back pain. *Health Technol Assess.* Aug (2005). iii-iv, ix-x, , 1-109.

[54] Witt, C. M, Reinhold, T, Jena, S, Brinkhaus, B, & Willich, S. N. Cost-effectiveness of acupuncture treatment in patients with headache. *Cephalalgia.* Apr (2008). , 28(4), 334-345.

[55] Willich, S. N, Reinhold, T, Selim, D, Jena, S, Brinkhaus, B, & Witt, C. M. Cost-effectiveness of acupuncture treatment in patients with chronic neck pain. *Pain.* Nov (2006).

[56] York, A, Crawford, C, Walter, A, Walter, J, Jonas, W, & Coeytaux, R. Acupuncture research in military and veteran populations: A Rapid Evidence Assessment of the Literature. *Medical Acupuncture.* (2011). , 23(4), 229-236.

[57] Lee, C, Wallerstedt, D, Duncan, A, et al. Design and rationale of a comparative effectiveness study to evaluate two acupuncture methods for the treatment of headaches associated with traumatic brain injury. *Medical Acupuncture.* (2011). , 23(4), 237-247.

[58] Hickey, A. H. Military Medical Acupuncture and CAM: Next Steps. *Medical Acupuncture*. December 20, (2011). , 23(4), 281-285.

Section 4

# Assessment and Accessibility in Acupuncture Therapy

Chapter 17

# The Evolution of Patient-Based Outcome Assessment Instruments in Acupuncture Research: Choosing Patient-Based Outcomes

Raheleh Khorsan, Alexandra York, Ian D. Coulter,
Remy R. Coeytaux, Rachel Wurzman,
Joan A. G. Walter and Kevin Berry

Additional information is available at the end of the chapter

http://dx.doi.org/10.5772/55265

## 1. Introduction

In this chapter, we present the patient-based outcome assessment (PBOA) instruments that have been used to determine outcomes in acupuncture clinical research, and highlight measures that are feasible, practical, economical, reliable, valid, and responsive to clinical change. The material in this chapter has been previously published in the Journal of Alternative and Complementary Medicine (See Footnote[*1]). This chapter has been edited to reflect and enhance, in particular, recent discussions on measures that cover issues of specific concern to the patient (i.e. health and wellbeing). It must be noted that often patient reported outcomes are measured by questionnaires that cover issues of specific concern to the patient. However, patient reported outcomes should be distinguished from PBOAs. Patient reported outcomes connotes patient-provided (rather than clinician observed) information; however, the information sought may or may not be focused on what the patients consider the most important health-related outcomes. An example of a patient-reported outcome is a sleep diary, in which patients track and report hours of sleep during a trial of a sleep medication. On the other hand, patient based outcomes explore the patient's health from her own perspective, and include

1 *. Material in this chapter is republished from a journal article in the Journal of alternative and complementary medicine (New York, N.Y.): Khorsan R, York A, Coulter ID, Wurzman R, Walter JA, Coeytaux RR. Patient-based outcome assessment instruments in acupuncture research. J Altern Complement Med. 2010 Jan;16(1):27-35. Reprint permission was granted via email correspondence on July 09, 2012 5:05 PM

measures of health that may lie outside of traditional medical surveys. An example of a PBOA related to a sleep medication trial is a self-report sleep diary in which the patient rates how refreshed she feels following medication-induced sleep. For the purposes of this chapter we define PBOA as any questionnaire, interview schedule and other related method or that assesses the *patient's* health, illness and benefits of health care interventions from the *patient's* perspective.

As health care costs continue to escalate in the U.S, especially in the military, there is renewed pressure on both payers and providers to demonstrate that the services provided by all clinicians are cost effective. There is also an emphasis on quality of patient care, manifested through an increasing demand for evidence based medicine demonstrated through performance measurement. Health care clinicians, patient advocates, regulatory authorities, administrators and policy makers are increasingly recognizing that patient focused outcome research, as captured by PBOA, is an important component of current quality based initiatives, and the evaluation of health care services.

Outcome instruments can provide information on the effectiveness of interventions and inform "real life" clinical practice. There is a range of outcome instruments available for acupuncture research and clinical practice, yet choosing the best outcome instrument is difficult due to numerous factors. [1,2]. Some of the important features of outcome measurements include that the instrument should: "(1) be valid, i.e. must measure what it sets out to test; (2) be reliable and consistent, i.e. it should give reproducible results on different occasions or with comparable groups; [3] (3) be responsive to clinical change; (4) be economical, (5) be feasible to administer; and (6) make it possible to compare findings to other studies, populations, or standard norms, etc. (p.356) [4] In addition to these considerations, the patient health status must also be considered, and it should be particularly suited to measure those aspects of health that the intervention of interest is likely to affect. Selecting suitable outcome instruments can be time consuming and challenging. There are hundreds of outcome measure and instruments available. Instruments can be patient-completed (self- administered) questionnaires, physiological tests, clinician-completed observation scales, task-specific activities/tests and impairment tests.

Assessing health outcomes associated with acupuncture is particularly challenging. [5] Acupuncture has been claimed as an effective treatment for certain chronic pain conditions. [6,7] According to the National Institutes of Health (NIH) Consensus Development Conference Statement there is "clear evidence for acupuncture's efficacy for treating postoperative and chemotherapy nausea and vomiting, [8,9] the nausea of pregnancy, [10] and postoperative dental pain." [11] Acupuncture has also been claimed effective for other various pain conditions such as migraines, [12-14] back pain, [14] tennis elbow, [15,16] menstrual cramps, [17] fibromyalgia, [18] and carpal tunnel syndrome. [19]

However, acupuncture, like many Complementary and Alternative Medicine (CAM) therapies, often does not involve a standardized protocol but rather is tailored to meet the patient's unique clinical presentation, needs or desires. In addition, previous studies have found that acupuncture may result in subtle improvements in a general sense of well-being in ways that may not be measured by standardized instruments. [5] Therefore using PBOAs to assess the benefits of acupuncture can be particularly meaningful, since they are customized to address patients' unique clinical needs and therapeutic goals. There still remains the challenge "to define *a priori* a single set of clinical outcomes to assess." [5]

### 1.1. The review

The objectives of the original review were to: 1) assess the available literature and identify the most common pain, disability, and quality-of-life PBOA instruments used in acupuncture research; 2) describe a framework for identifying appropriate sets of instruments; and 3) address the challenges associated with these instruments that are relevant to acupuncture. This chapter reassesses the available literature and identifies the most common PBOA instruments used in the original review. Also, this chapter enhances and builds on the discussion concerning the frameworks, in identifying appropriate sets of instruments and some of the challenges associated with the use of these instruments to measure acupuncture's effects.

## 2. Methods

We conducted our original search in 2009. At that time, our search included all published clinical trial abstracts in the PubMed database from inception to Feb 2009. We performed another search in August 2012. This secondary search included all abstracts for clinical studies published in PubMed from Feb 2009 to August 2012.

Our original search in 2009 was conducted in two phases. Initially, a broad systematic search was performed to identify existing instruments for measuring pain, disability, general health status and well-being found in acupuncture therapy studies. To be included in this phase of the review, an instrument had to be used in at least 3 separate studies that met our search criteria. Patient outcome instruments were included if they were found cited in the abstract of a paper reporting research related to acupuncture. We used the same methodology for our search from Feb 2009 to August 2012.

We categorized the type of patient outcome instruments into two categories: physiological or patient-based. We used our definition of PBOA to sort and review those articles in full that included PBOA and acupuncture. Because of time limitations, we did not pull the full text articles for our secondary search from Feb 2009 to August 2012. Therefore we cannot discuss whether a recent study (Feb 2009-August 2012) has a PBOA instrument as a primary or secondary measure (See table 1).

For each instrument that was included, a second search was conducted to identify papers reporting research on its psychometric properties. This second phase of searching was not confined to studies of acupuncture. Data on the psychometric properties of identified instruments were subsequently extracted and compared (See table 2).

| | Included studies (Inception - April 2009) | | Studies with No PBOA (Inception - April 2009) | | Included studies (April 2009 - Aug 2012) | |
|---|---|---|---|---|---|---|
| | n | % | n | % | n | % |
| Total number of studies | 258 | | 112 | | 206 | |
| **Study design** | | | | | | |
| RCT | 182 | 70.543% | 39 | 34.821% | 203 | 98.544% |
| CCT | 28 | 10.853% | 23 | 20.536% | 38 | 18.447% |
| CO | 8 | 3.101% | 0 | 0.000% | 9 | 4.369% |
| Mixed Design | 2 | 0.775% | 11 | 9.821% | 9 | 4.369% |
| Pilot | 25 | 9.690% | 9 | 8.036% | 40 | 19.417% |
| CT | 8 | 3.101% | 0 | 0.000% | 0 | 0.000% |
| SR | 5 | 1.938% | 11 | 9.821% | 7 | 3.398% |
| Other | 0 | 0.000% | 19 | 16.964% | 0 | 0.000% |
| **General Topic** | | | | | | |
| musculoskeletal | 86 | 33.333% | 24 | 21.429% | 1 | 0.485% |
| women's Health | 25 | 9.689% | 10 | 8.929% | 6 | 2.913% |
| headache | 24 | 9.302% | 7 | 6.250% | 1 | 0.485% |
| other type of conditions | 21 | 8.139% | 23 | 20.536% | 18 | 8.738% |
| neurologic condition | 20 | 7.751% | 7 | 6.250% | 7 | 3.398% |
| mental health | 18 | 6.976% | 5 | 4.464% | 5 | 2.427% |
| gastrointestinal disorders | 14 | 5.426% | 3 | 2.679% | 12 | 5.825% |
| addiction | 11 | 4.263% | 3 | 2.679% | 7 | 3.398% |
| autoimmune condition | 8 | 3.1% | 11 | 9.821% | 27 | 13.107% |
| cardiovascular condition | 8 | 3.1% | 8 | 7.143% | 2 | 0.971% |
| cancer and treatment related symptoms | 7 | 2.713% | 3 | 2.679% | 91 | 44.175% |
| pulmonary disorder | 5 | 1.937% | 2 | 1.786% | 3 | 1.456% |
| allergy | 4 | 1.55% | 1 | 0.893% | 16 | 7.767% |
| urological disorder | 4 | 1.55% | 5 | 4.464% | 1 | 0.485% |
| sleep disorder | 3 | 1.162% | 0 | 0.000% | 45 | 21.845% |
| PBOA Instrument is primary | 192 | 74.418 | NA | NA | U | U |
| PBOA Instrument is secondary | 21 | 8.139 | NA | NA | U | U |
| PBOA Instrument is valid and reliable | 223 | | NA | | U | U |

PBOA, patient-based outcome assessment; CO, cohort study; CCT, controlled clinical trial; CT=other clinical trial; Pilot, pilot study; RCT, randomized control trial; SR, systematic review.

**Table 1.** Study Characteristics

http://dx.doi.org/10.5772/55265

| | *Assessing* | *Validity* | *Reliability* | *Clinical Responsiveness* | *Cost* | *Feasibility* | *Comparability* |
|---|---|---|---|---|---|---|---|
| Visual Analog Scale (VAS) | General Pain Intensity (Acute or Chronic) | X | X | X | Training: None Equipment: None Cost: Copying Permission: U | Self-administered, 1 min | X |
| Numerical Pain Rating Scale (NRS) | General Pain Intensity (Acute or Chronic) | X | X | X | Training: None Equipment: None Cost: Copying Permission: U | Self-administered, 1 min | X |
| McGill Present Pain Index (MPI or MPQ) (Including: the McGill Short Form Pain Questionnaire) | General Pain Intensity (Acute or Chronic) | X | X | X | Training: None Equipment: None Cost: Copying Permission: U | Self-administered, 5-10min | X |
| Oswestry Pain Disability Index (ODI) (Including: revised versions 1.0, 2.0, AAOS/MODEMS, "revised ODI") | Functional Disability & Back Pain (Acute or Chronic) | X | X | X | Training: None Equipment: None Cost: Copying Permission: Needed[a] | Self-administered, 5 min | X |
| Roland Morris Disability/Activity Questionnaire (Including: revised versions RM-23, RM-18) | Functional Disability & Back Pain (Acute & Subacute) | X | X | X | Training: None Equipment: None Cost: Copying Permission: None[a] | Self-administered, 5 min | X |
| SF-36 (Including modified versions) | Health Related Quality of Life | X | X | X | Training: None Equipment: Possibly Cost: Varies Permission: Needed, co-copyright holders[b] | Self-administered, 5 min | X |
| Nottingham Health Profile (NHP) | Health Related Quality of Life | X | X | X | Training: None Equipment: None Cost: Copying Permission: None | Self-administered, 7-10 min | X |
| Western Ontario and McMaster Universities (WOMAC) Osteoarthritis Index | Functional Disability & Arthritis Pain (Acute or Chronic) | X | X | X | Training: None Equipment: None Cost: Copying Permission: U | Self-administered, 5-10min | X |

| | *Assessing* | *Validity* | *Reliability* | *Clinical Responsiveness* | *Cost* | *Feasibility* | *Compara bility* |
|---|---|---|---|---|---|---|---|
| Pain Disability Index | Functional Disability & Pain (Acute & Subacute) | X | X | X | Training: None Equipment: None Cost: Copying Permission: U | Self-admin-istered, 5-10min | X |
| Beck Depression Inventory (BDI) | Depression | X | X | X | Training: None Equipment: None Cost: Copying Permission: U | Self-admin-istered, 5-10min | X |
| Hamilton depression scale (HAMD) | Depression | X | X | X | Training: None Equipment: None Cost: Copying Permission: U | Self-admin-istered, 5-10min | X |
| Measure Yourself Medical Outcome Profile (MYMOP) | Primary Care Setting | X | X | X | Training: None Equipment: None Cost: Copying Permission: Needed: Register as a user[c] | Self-admin-istered, 7-10min | X |
| Hospital Anxiety & Depression Scale (HADS) | Hospital General Medical Outpatient | X | X | X | Training: None Equipment: None Cost: Copying Permission: Needed[d] | Self-admin-istered, 5-10min | X |

[a] The instruments (RM-24 & ODI version 2.0) are include in Roland and Fairbank (2000) appendixes (Roland M, Fairbank J. The Roland-Morris Disability Questionnaire and the Oswestry Disability

Questionnaire. Spine 2000; 25: 3115–3124). When used in the forms reproduced in the appendixes (Roland and Fairbank 2000), no permission is required from the authors or from Spine.

[b] RAND Health, a research division of the RAND corporation, the Medical Outcomes Trust (MOT), Health Assessment Lab (HAL), and QualityMetric Incorporated are co-copyright holders of the

Short Form Health Surveys.

[c] User registration is required at www.pms.ac.uk=mymop=index.php?c¼contact&s¼register.

[d] For purchase of questionnaire contact GL Assessments.

X, Available; U, unavailable.

**Table 2.** Common Pain, Disability, Depression, Health Status, and Well Being Measures use in clinical acupuncture research (Total n= 464)

### 2.1. Inclusion and exclusion criteria

Originally the studies eligible for inclusion in the review included peer reviewed clinical trials, case reports, and randomized controlled trials for which a full abstract was available. A sensitive search was originally conducted for key search terms for 'acupuncture', 'pain', 'disability', 'well-being' and 'outcome measures'. Search terms for 'acupuncture' and 'pain' were limited to the title or abstract to constrain the magnitude of the review yield to a manageable size. For example search terms included: Acupuncture, Acupuncture Therapy, Acupuncture, Ear, Acupuncture Points, Acupuncture Analgesia, patient, outcome, measure, assessment and derivatives of each.

Acupuncture was defined according to the National Institutes of Health (NIH) National Center for Complementary and Alternative Medicine (NCCAM). [11]
The search restrictions were human, clinical trial, editorial, letter, meta-analysis, practice guideline, randomized controlled trial, and review for which a full abstract was available. Full length manuscripts were pulled whenever possible. This review also obtained full length manuscripts that reported the psychometric properties of the PBOA instruments. Hard copies were obtained of the instruments of interest that were reported in included papers. All abstract reviewed were in English. The search was restricted to instruments targeted towards adults (i.e. 16 years or older). No upper age limit was set.

Of the 520 abstracts reviewed 111 abstracts were case reports. Nearly always, a case report is written after the fact (after something of interest was noted in a given person). Therefore, a research-oriented outcome measure would not be expected to have been administered in a case report. For the purposes of this review, we exclude case reports from the final analysis.

We instead expanded our search to include all acupuncture clinical studies including but not limited to pain (see figure 2). This systematic review excluded studies on laser acupuncture, TENS, dry needling, audits, surveys, literature reviews, commentaries and proceedings.

The complete search strategy is illustrated in Figures 1 and 2. The database searched was PubMed. All papers were screened for pain, disability, general health status and well-being instruments that were reported in the title, abstract, and full article.

## 3. Results

The original search initially identified 582 articles. After screening of title/abstract, 212 articles were excluded. From the remaining 370 citations, 258 manuscripts identified explicit PBOA, while 112 abstracts did not include any PBOA (Fig. 1). A total of 258 manuscripts were extracted and reviewed (Table 1). When we conducted our secondary search for new papers (2009-2012) we found an additional 242 abstracts. Of the 242 article abstracts, 206 manuscript abstracts identified explicit PBOA, while 12 abstracts did not include any PBOA (Fig. 2). We excluded the 12 articles that did not include any PBOA from our discussion section and tables; therefore, this chapter discusses the results of an aggregate total 464 articles with PBOA instruments.

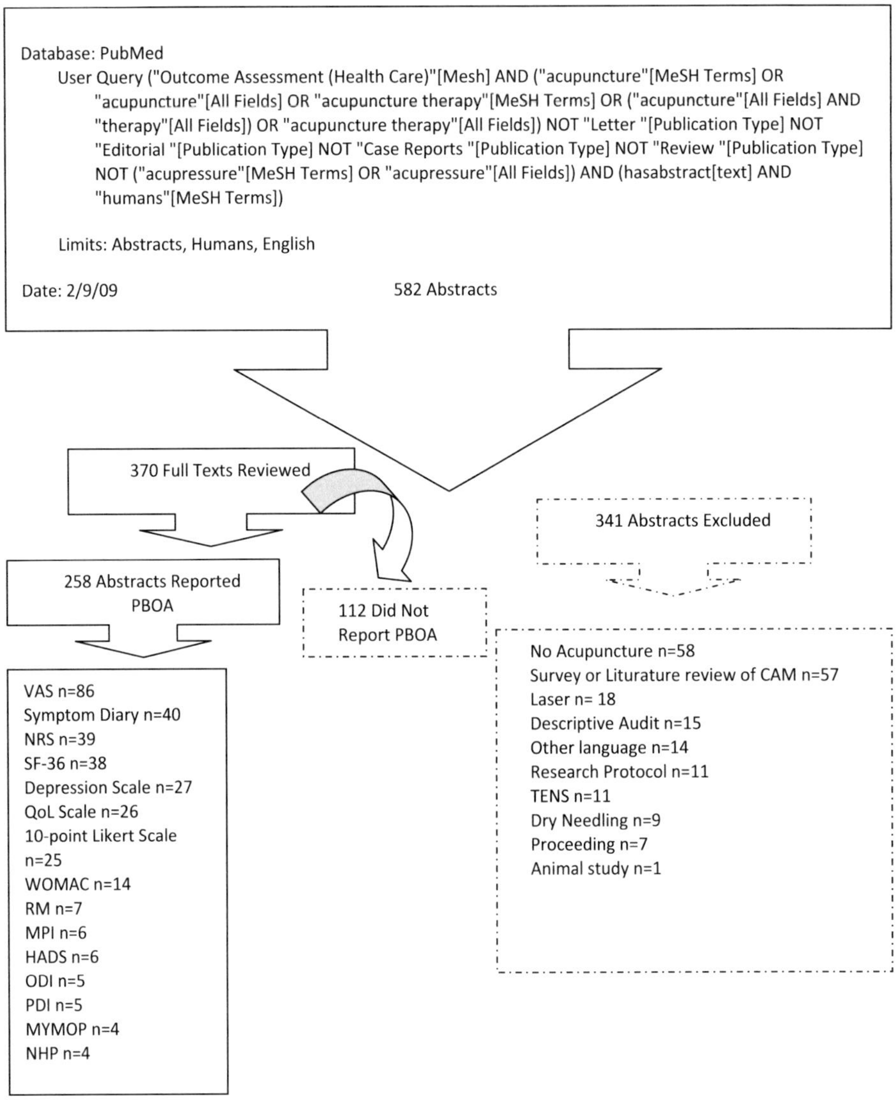


**Figure 1.** Primary search inclusion / exclusion flow chart

The original (inception) and secondary searches (2009-2012) both found that randomized control trials (RCTs) were the most common design for clinical acupuncture studies that met the criteria for inclusion in this discussion. In addition, musculoskeletal disorders were the most the most common condition researched in the included acupuncture studies. Of those instruments reviewed, the Visual Analog Scale (VAS) was

http://dx.doi.org/10.5772/55265

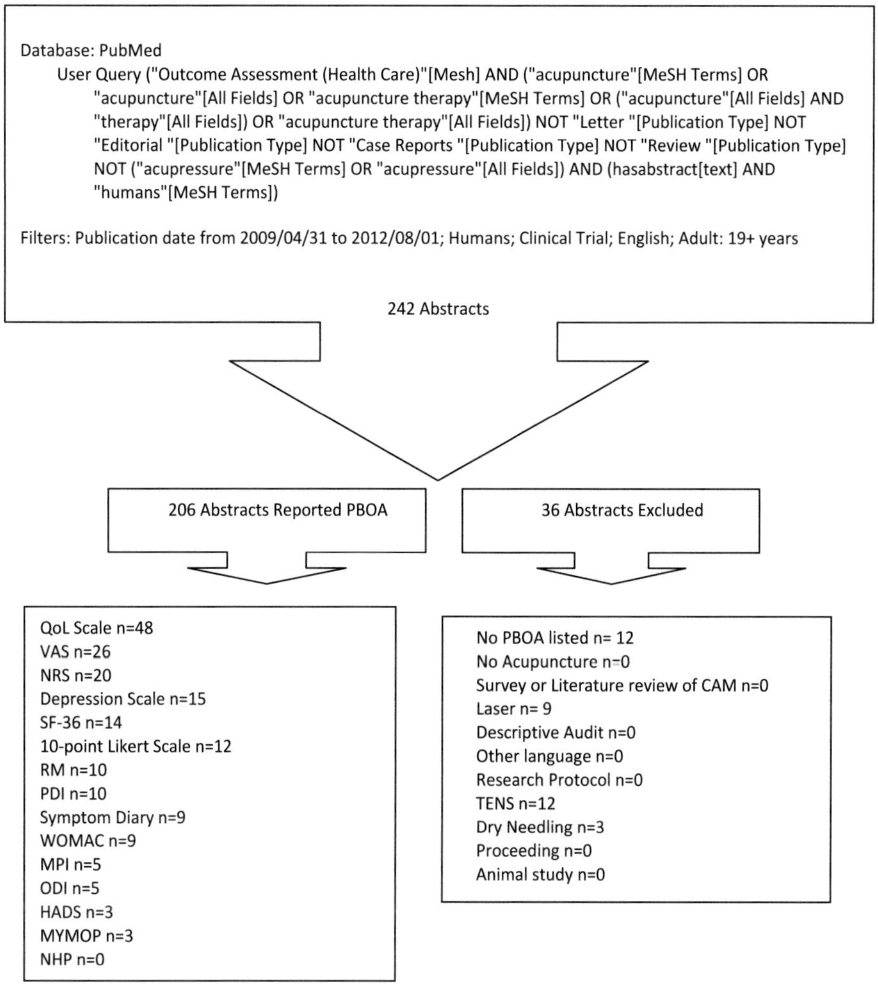


**Figure 2.** Secondary search inclusion / exclusion flow chart

the most common PBOA measure identified. Furthermore, we found that the VAS and the Numerical Pain Rating Scales (NRS) are the most common scales used to measure pain intensity. [20] The most commonly used health status and well being instrument was the SF-36. The vast majority of studies included PBOA instruments as their primary measure (~70%).

When we conducted our search in 2009, we found that the most common instruments used in acupuncture studies were single dimensional pain scales such as the VAS (n=86) and NRS (n=39). Also in 2009, we found that about 60% of all acupuncture studies in this review used some sort of Quality-of-Life (QoL) measure.

In 2012, of those instruments reviewed during our secondary search, the Quality of Life Scale (QoL) was the most common PBOA measure identified. The Medical Outcomes Study Short Form-36 (SF-36) was the most common QoL instrument used across all study designs and conditions. Similar to our original search in 2009, the VAS and the Numerical Pain Rating Scales (NRS) were the most common scales used to measure pain intensity.

The most common multi-dimensional pain scales used in acupuncture pain studies were the McGill pain questionnaire (MPQ), the Oswestry Pain Disability Index (ODI), the Roland Morris Disability/Activity Questionnaire (RM), and the Western Ontario and McMaster Universites (WOMAC) Osteoarthritis Index. Table 1 provides a summary and characteristics of the studies included. Data on the psychometric properties of identified instruments were subsequently extracted and compared (See Table 2).

The number of study participants in the original search included studies ranged from 5 to 14,161 subjects. There were 11 studies that included 1,000 or more subject participants. The vast majority of the studies identified in this review employed a battery of instruments rather than a single instrument. Most study abstracts included a number of different PBOA instruments as well as including both patient and clinician reported instruments.

Our review found that identifying the main outcome of interest, i.e. pain as the primary outcome measure, was common is acupuncture studies. This was especially true for our most recent review of the literature (2009-2012). However, we also found that the types of existing PBOA instruments used in acupuncture clinical studies varied widely in their length and content from study to study. Some studies lacked standardized protocols for choosing PBOA instrument (~20%).

## 4. Discussion

There seems to be an increase in studies from Feb 2009 to Aug 2012 that incorporate PBOA. In 2009 we found that 582 clinical trial abstracts for acupuncture that reported PBOA. On Aug 1, 2012 we found 242 clinical trial abstracts that incorporate PBOA. This large increase, in a short time span, in clinical acupuncture studies that incorporate PBOA may reveal the considerable maturation of the field of acupuncture research. Langevin et al. [21] published white paper, identifies gaps in knowledge underlying the paradoxes and proposes strategies for their resolution through translational research. The authors recommend that acupuncture treatments should be studied (1) “top down” as multi-component “whole-system” interventions and (2) “bottom up” as mechanistic studies that focus on understanding how individual treatment components interact and translate into clinical and physiological outcomes. They state that, "the complexity of acupuncture interventions makes it unlikely that even a battery of standardized outcomes will adequately capture the richness of practitioners' experiences, which may inform optimal study design." Langevin et al. recommend that, qualitative methods be used "to explore the meaning that patients ascribe to an intervention, the process and context by which healing occurs, outcomes that are relevant and meaningful to patients, and how interventions fit within everyday lives [22]." [21] We discuss these challenges in more detail in below sections.

### 4.1. Challenges and psychometric properties associated with PBOA instruments and acupuncture

The goal of this section is to provide the reader with a rich outline of the important aspects of the PBOA instruments examined in this review, rather than to discuss all the published works relating to the PBOA instruments. Toward that effort, we will briefly discuss some of the studies that highlight important aspects of a PBOA instrument (i.e., validity) that are significant when considering its use as an outcome measure in acupuncture research or clinical care.

The VAS is a patient completed analogue instrument that evaluates pain intensity and function, typically on a 100-mm-long horizontal or vertical line anchored at each end with a statement representing the extremes of the dimension being measured. The patient places a mark on the appropriate position on the line to represent his pain level. Generally, the NRS styles also include a horizontal line, but unlike the VAS, the NRS uses whole numbers (typically 0-10) to measure pain severity.

Both instruments provide pain intensity estimates relatively quickly, are highly patient-centered, have the most value when looking at change within individuals and are of less value for comparing across a group of individuals at one time point. Also both instruments are quick and simple to administer, [23] easy to translate into other languages, inexpensive, [24] and readily available. [25]

The single dimensional pain intensity scales (i.e. the VAS and NRS) have been criticized for their lack of sensitivity, oversimplifying the patient's experience of pain, and their single dimension of pain (e.g. intensity). [26] Also the VAS and NRS may not be an effective PBOA instrument for patients who have cognitive or motor problems, and in young children and elderly patients. [27]

Both in 2009 and 2012, we found that many (~60% or more) of all acupuncture studies in this review used some sort of Quality-of-Life (QoL) measure. QOL is a broad multidimensional concept that usually includes subjective evaluations of both positive and negative aspects of life. [28]

As stated, the Medical Outcomes Study Short Form-36 (SF-36) was the most common QoL instrument used across all study designs and conditions. The SF-36, often referred to as the MOS SF-36 [29], and the RAND 36-Item Health Survey 1.0 (distributed by RAND Corporation) are identical scales with 36-item general health. In 2012, we found that the majority of acupuncture clinical studies included QoL measures. For acupuncture and other CAM studies, QoL instruments such as the Centers for Disease Control and Prevention's (CDC) health-related quality of life (HRQOL) defines health as a multidimensional construct that includes physical, mental, and social domains. This broad multidimensional aspect of QoL measure may also be presented as a challenge since the term "quality of life" has meaning for nearly everyone and every academic discipline, individuals and groups can define it differently. Although health is one of the important domains of overall quality of life, there are other domains as well—for instance, jobs, housing, schools, the neighborhood. Aspects of Culture, values, and spirituality are also key aspects of overall quality of life that add to the complexity of its measurement." [30] Nevertheless, it seems that a many acupuncture studies use QoL as a measure of health surveillance and intervention outcome. There are substantial reliability and validity data for Qol measures such as the SF-36. [31-34] Other QoL measures used were the NIH-Chronic Prostatitis Symptom Index (NIH-CPSI), the Nottingham Health Profile (NHP), and the EuroQol 5-Dimension form (EQ-5D).

For pain related studies such as headache, musculoskeletal, cancer,and treatment related symptoms the most common scales used in acupuncture clinical research included the VAS, NRS, 10-point Likert scale on subjective experience and global wellbeing (n=25), and symptom diary (n=40). However, most studies did not include citations for the use of the 10-point Likert scale on subjective experience and global wellbeing and symptom diary. Therefore it is unknown if there are any validity or reliability issues associated with these instruments. The Symptom Diary was also commonly used among acupuncture studies of pulmonary, sleep, and urological disorders. We were unable to determine whether the Symptom Diaries used in acupuncture research were structured, meaning that the research participants recorded particular information related to a specific health event or a particular research question; or unstructured (i.e., journals, used to explore a patient's spontaneous thoughts and feelings in relationship to a particular event). [35] No study in this review cited a standardized and validated Symptom Diary. While there are validated Symptom Diaries available (i.e., the Diagnostic Headache Diary), [36] it may be that most researchers are unable to find in the published literature a specific diary that meets their particular research question and therefore each research team devises its own diary. [37]

Aside from brief or predictable procedure related pain, more comprehensive pain assessment requires the determination of other characteristics of the pain, such as location and quality, and its effect on mood and function. Multidimensional pain assessment tools have been developed to quantitate these aspects of pain.

Our results found that the most common multi-dimensional pain scales used in acupuncture pain studies were the McGill pain questionnaire (MPQ), the Oswestry Pain Disability Index (ODI), the Roland Morris Disability/Activity Questionnaire (RM), and the Western Ontario and McMaster Universities (WOMAC) Osteoarthritis Index.

McGill pain questionnaire (MPQ), also known as the Melzack pain questionnaire, was developed by Ronald Melzack of McGill University in 1975. This original questionnaire attempted to specify pain experience using 78 pain descriptors on 4 dimensions; I) sensory (items 1-10), II) affective (items 11-15), III) evaluative (items 16) and; IV) an additional miscellaneous descriptor (items 17–20). [38] In 1980, Melzack noted that the MPQ was too long and complex for use in most clinical trials, and a short form of the MPQ (SF-MPQ) was derived from commonly used sensory and affective descriptors in the clinical studies Melzack conducted up to that time.

The ODI, like the MPQ, is a self-report questionnaire designed for assessing the degree of functional limitation in patients seeking secondary care for low-back pain, while the RM is designed for assessing the degree of functional limitation in patients with low-back pain in primary care. [39] The development, testing, and properties of both measures have been extensively examined and adequately reviewed (Table 2). Both instruments have been translated into many languages and used to evaluate outcome in a range of populations, settings, and interventions.

The WOMAC is a disease specific, self administered questionnaire that evaluates three dimensions: pain (5 questions), stiffness (2 questions), and physical function (17 questions). [40] The WOMAC was constructed to evaluate patients' experience of osteoarthritis (OA) of the knee and hip. It was designed in the late eighties in response to the lack of a multidimensional instrument that could measure clinically important, patient-relevant symptoms of OA in the knee and hip. [41]

The reliability and validity of the WOMAC has been demonstrated in a number of studies. [40-45] Overall the WOMAC has been compared to many instruments [46-55] with mixed results depending on which subscales (physical function, pain, and stiffness) were being evaluated or on what specific condition was being evaluated (total hip arthroplasty, total knee arthroplasty, OA of knee, OA of hip, rheumatoid).

Disability and depression scales were mainly used in acupuncture studies on mental health, neurologic conditions, addiction, autoimmune condition and musculoskeletal disorders. The most common disability and depression scales were the Pain Disability Index (PDI), and Beck Depression Inventory (BDI).

The PDI is a patient-completed, condition-specific functional status questionnaire. [56] The PDI rates the level of disability on a numerical rating scale (0=no disability and 10=maximum disability) assessing 7 broad categories of activity including items on recreation, personal care, activities related to home and family, work, frequency and quality of sex life, social activity and general life-support functions (e.g. eating, sleeping, and breathing). [57-59]

The BDI [60-62] is a multiple-choice self-report inventory among the most widely used instruments for measuring the severity of depression and related mental health. Both instruments were created to measure the intensity, severity, and depth of depression. There are several versions of both instruments.

The PDI and the BDI have been translated into many languages and used to evaluate outcome in a range of populations, settings, and interventions.

### 4.2. Measures for acupuncture in primary care settings and hospitals

The Measure Yourself Medical Outcome Profile (MYMOP), and the Hospital Anxiety and Depression Scale (HADS) [63,64] were used in several acupuncture clinical studies, including acupuncture for chronic pain management and in the elderly (Fig. 1). MYMOP is an outcome measure originally developed to measure aspects and symptoms that a patient determines are most important to her or him, and their effects. It is a sensitive measure of within-person change over time, is applicable to the whole spectrum of illness seen in primary care, is capable of measuring the effects of a wide variety of care, and enables the patient to score the chosen variables. [65] The HADS consists of 14 questions, 7 for anxiety and 7 for depression. Although it was originally designed for hospital general medical outpatients, it has been extensively used for other populations such as in primary care. [63, 64]

The psychometric properties for the HADS have been extensively evaluated and validated across a range of populations, settings, and interventions.

### 4.3. PBOA instruments in acupuncture versus conventional therapy research

In 2006, Hull et al., [5] researched the various methods of assessing clinically meaningful change associated with a course of acupuncture treatments. They reported that assessing outcomes associated with acupuncture is particularly challenging compared to other therapies because "acupuncture may result in subtle improvements in a general sense of well-being in ways that may not be measured by standardized instruments, and acupuncture treatments often are customized to meet individual patients' unique clinical needs and therapeutic goals, thereby making it difficult to define a priori a single set of clinical outcomes to assess" (p. 247). [5] We believe that Hull et al. correctly assert that the effects of acupuncture cannot be easily quantified by commonly examined clinical outcomes due to its whole systems construct.

CAM therapies are often based on whole medical systems that are built upon complete systems of theory and practice, as is true for acupuncture. [66] Most research on acupuncture effects and application remains inconclusive among contemporary biomedical researchers and clinicians because the acupuncture research does not generally involve a standardized protocol. Acupuncturists generally tailor the treatments and therapeutic objectives to meet the individual patient's unique clinical presentation, needs, or desires. In addition, Hull et al. state that, "such individualized treatment approaches and therapeutic objectives may limit the ability of standardized instruments to assess meaningful clinical change among groups of patients" (p. 248). [5]

### 4.4. Next steps: The need for more comparative research

The allopathic medical model limits treatment modalities to medications alone or in combination with, procedures, surgery and physical therapy. A more whole person integrative approach opens the therapeutic window to other options that can provide healing benefits.

The gold standard double blind placebo controlled drug trial has an honored place in modern science-based medicine but this method of study does not provide information about the patient as a person across the full spectrum of their health goals, expectations and needs. Regardless of the mechanisms by which acupuncture might provide benefit or harm patient-based outcome assessments must be developed that can be trusted, provide meaning and point the way toward their impacts.

Many patients suffer from chronic conditions for which standard diagnostics and treatments do not result in understanding, cure or satisfactory strategies to achieve better health with disease. In these cases other systems of medicine suggest approaches that may offer hope, relief, facilitate healing, and result in a greater degree of health. Additionally, for some people a surgical, molecular and biological cure may result in unnecessary disability because the barriers to whole-person healing and thriving were not removed. Each person can be responsible for some determinants of their own health and well-being and some whole-person alternative medical models better assure personal involvement and activation in the promotion of health and healing. Maturing our understanding of patient-based outcomes assessments can facilitate personalized, precision and participatory health behaviors and activities. Acupuncture and other non-pharmacological means to address acute, chronic and syndromic conditions should be addressed by comparative research to reveal optimal healing effective and safe strategies.

### 4.5. Finding more information on PBOA instruments

There are electronic databases established as sources of information on PBOA instruments for clinical and research use. Some can be accessed free of charge, whereas others require membership or fees. Khorsan *et al* discuss many common electronic databases and translated version of PBOA instruments available for researchers and clinicians [4]. One such source is the Patient-Reported Outcomes Measurement Information System (PROMIS). [67] PROMIS was originally developed as an NIH Roadmap network project intended to develop, validate, and standardize item banks to measure patient-reported outcomes relevant across common medical conditions. [68]The PROMIS is a publicly available system that can be added to and modified periodically, and which allows clinical researchers to access a common repository of items and computerized adaptive tests. The PROMIS is also a network for researchers and clinicians to collaborate on the collection of self-reported data from diverse populations with a variety of chronic diseases, using agreed-upon methods, models, and questionnaires.

### 4.6. Limitation

This study does not review all the measures found. It reviews the most frequently used measures. It therefore isn't a review of all the 'pain disability' measures. The aims of this review are to assess the common measures available and used, to identify the PBOA, and to describe a framework for identifying appropriate sets of measures, while addressing the unique challenges associated with use of these measures to assess acupuncture. A limitation of our review was that the outcome instrument had to appear in at least 3 publications in order to be included.

## 5. Conclusion

In conclusion, acupuncture researchers, like all clinical researchers, should assess the appropriateness of their treatment approach defined and measured by clinically significant change and determine patient satisfaction with the intervention. We found in this review that acupuncture research includes a combination of validated instruments, such as common standardized questionnaires that assess functional status or health-related QoL before and after the administration of a therapeutic intervention for a specific condition. Examples include the VAS, NRS, and SF-36 and disease specific QoL instrument such as the WOMAC, BDI, and RM used to quantify change over time. However, acupuncture research also included a wide variety of unvalidated instruments like the 10-point Likert scale on subjective experience and global well-being and Symptom Diary. Both types of measures were used to capture particular health and wellbeing information from the study participants in relationship to a specific health event or an experience based on a particular research question that no single instrument and no combination of validated scales alone could achieve. The large number of unvalidated PBOA instruments in acupuncture research may be associated with the paradigm of whole systems medicine [5]. Therefore, instruments such as MYMOP may be most useful for assessing clinical change in patients who present for acupuncture treatment with a variety of symptoms, clinical conditions, and therapeutic objectives.[5] Further research is needed to determine whether these results apply across other whole medical system therapies compared more so than to conventional therapy research.

## Acknowledgements

No conflict of interest exists for any of the authors of this study. The views, opinions and/or findings contained in this report are those of the author(s) and should not be construed as an official Department of the Army position, policy, or decision unless so designated by others. This work is supported by the US Army Medical Research and Materiel Command under Award No. W81XWH-06-1-0279 through the Samueli Institute.

## Author details

Raheleh Khorsan[1*], Alexandra York[2], Ian D. Coulter[3,4,5], Remy R. Coeytaux[6,7], Rachel Wurzman[8], Joan A. G. Walter[2] and Kevin Berry[1]

*Address all correspondence to: rkhorsan@siib.org

1 Military Medical Research and Integrative Medicine, Samueli Institute, Corona del Mar, CA, U.S.A.

2 Military Medical Research, Samueli Institute, Alexandria, VA, U.S.A.

3 University of California Los Angeles, Los Angeles, CA, U.S.A.

4 RAND/Samueli Chair for Integrative Medicine and Senior Health Policy Researcher, RAND Corp., Santa Monica, CA, U.S.A.

5 Research Faculty, Southern California University of Health Sciences, Whittier, CA, U.S.A.

6 Center for Clinical Health Policy Research, Duke University, U.S.A.

7 Department of Community and Family Medicine, Duke University, U.S.A.

8 Georgetown University Medical Center, Interdisciplinary Program in Neuroscience, Washington DC, U.S.A.

## References

[1] Ware, J. E. Jr., Brook RH, Davies AR, Lohr KN. Choosing measures of health status for individuals in general populations. *Am J Public Health.* Jun (1981). , 71(6), 620-625.

[2] Wollersheim, H, Hermens, R, Hulscher, M, et al. Clinical indicators: development and applications. *Neth J Med.* Jan (2007). , 65(1), 15-22.

[3] Prady, S. L, Thomas, K, Esmonde, L, & Crouch, S. MacPherson H. The natural history of back pain after a randomised controlled trial of acupuncture vs usual care--long term outcomes. Acupunct Med. (2007). Dec;, 25(4), 121-9.

[4] Khorsan, R, Coulter, I. D, Hawk, C, & Choate, C. G. Measures in chiropractic research: choosing patient-based outcome assessments. J Manipulative Physiol Ther. (2008). Jun;, 31(5), 355-75.

[5] Hull, S. K, Page, C. P, Skinner, B. D, Linville, J. C, & Coeytaux, R. R. Exploring outcomes associated with acupuncture. J Altern Complement Med. (2006). Apr;, 12(3), 247-54.

[6] Ernst, E, Pittler, M. H, Wider, B, & Boddy, K. Acupuncture: its evidence-base is changing. *Am J Chin Med.* (2007). , 35(1), 21-25.

[7] Wang, S. M, Kain, Z. N, & White, P. F. Acupuncture analgesia: II. Clinical considerations. *Anesth Analg.* Feb (2008). table of contents., 106(2), 611-621.

[8] Dibble, S. L, Luce, J, Cooper, B. A, et al. Acupressure for chemotherapy-induced nausea and vomiting: a randomized clinical trial. *Oncol Nurs Forum.* Jul (2007). , 34(4), 813-820.

[9] Lee, A, & Done, M. L. Stimulation of the wrist acupuncture point 6 for preventing postoperative nausea and vomiting. *Cochrane Database Syst Rev.* (2004). CD003281.

[10] Einarson, A, Maltepe, C, Boskovic, R, & Koren, G. Treatment of nausea and vomiting in pregnancy: an updated algorithm. *Can Fam Physician.* Dec (2007). , 53(12), 2109-2111.

[11] National Center for Complementary and Alternative Medicine (NCCAM)An Introduction to Acupuncture. July 28, (2008). http://nccam.nih.gov/health/acupuncture/.Accessed Aug 26, 2008.

[12] Endres, H. G, Diener, H. C, & Molsberger, A. Role of acupuncture in the treatment of migraine. Expert Rev Neurother. (2007). Sep;, 7(9), 1121-34.

[13] Linde, K, Allais, G, Brinkhaus, B, Manheimer, E, Vickers, A, & White, A. R. Acupuncture for migraine prophylaxis. Cochrane Database Syst Rev. (2009). Jan 21; (1):CD001218.

[14] Vickers, A. J, Cronin, A. M, Maschino, A. C, Lewith, G, Macpherson, H, Victor, N, Sherman, K. J, & Witt, C. Linde K; Acupuncture Trialists' Collaboration. Individual patient data meta-analysis of acupuncture for chronic pain: protocol of the Acupuncture Trialists' Collaboration. Trials. (2010). Sep 28;11:90.

[15] Bjordal, J. M, Lopes-martins, R. A, Joensen, J, Couppe, C, Ljunggren, A. E, Stergioulas, A, & Johnson, M. I. A systematic review with procedural assessments and meta-analysis of low level laser therapy in lateral elbow tendinopathy (tennis elbow). BMC Musculoskelet Disord. (2008). May 29;9:75.

[16] Chang, W. D, Wu, J. H, Yang, W. J, & Jiang, J. A. Therapeutic effects of low-level laser on lateral epicondylitis from differential interventions of Chinese-Western medicine: systematic review. Photomed Laser Surg. (2010). Jun;, 28(3), 327-36.

[17] Smith, C. A, Zhu, X, He, L, & Song, J. Acupuncture for primary dysmenorrhoea. Cochrane Database Syst Rev. (2011). Jan 19;(1):CD007854.

[18] Cao, H, Liu, J, & Lewith, G. T. Traditional Chinese Medicine for treatment of fibromyalgia: a systematic review of randomized controlled trials. J Altern Complement Med. (2010). Apr;, 16(4), 397-409.

[19] Kumnerddee, W, & Kaewtong, A. Efficacy of acupuncture versus night splinting for carpal tunnel syndrome: a randomized clinical trial. J Med Assoc Thai. (2010). Dec;, 93(12), 1463-9.

[20] Hjermstad, M. J, Fayers, P. M, Haugen, D. F, Caraceni, A, Hanks, G. W, Loge, J. H, Fainsinger, R, & Aass, N. Kaasa S; European Palliative Care Research Collaborative (EPCRC). Studies comparing Numerical Rating Scales, Verbal Rating Scales, and Visual Analogue Scales for assessment of pain intensity in adults: a systematic literature review. J Pain Symptom Manage. (2011). Jun;, 41(6), 1073-93.

[21] Langevin, H. M, Wayne, P. M, Macpherson, H, Schnyer, R, Milley, R. M, Napadow, V, Lao, L, Park, J, Harris, R. E, Cohen, M, Sherman, K. J, Haramati, A, & Hammers-

chlag, R. Paradoxes in acupuncture research: strategies for moving forward. Evid Based Complement Alternat Med. (2011). Epub 2010 Oct 11.

[22] Verhoef, M. J, Casebeer, A. L, & Hilsden, R. J. Assessing efficacy of complementary medicine: adding qualitative research methods to the "Gold Standard". J Altern Complement Med. (2002). Jun;, 8(3), 275-81.

[23] Jensen, M. P, Karoly, P, & Braver, S. The measurement of clinical pain intensity: a comparison of six methods. *Pain.* Oct (1986)., 27(1), 117-126.

[24] Mccaffery, M, & Pasero, C. Assessment tools. *Pain: clinical manual.* 2 ed. St. Louis: Mosby, Inc.; (1999)., 1999, 58-88.

[25] Scott, J, & Huskisson, E. C. Graphic representation of pain. *Pain.* Jun (1976)., 2(2), 175-184.

[26] Flaherty, S. A. Pain measurement tools for clinical practice and research. *AANA J.* Apr (1996)., 64(2), 133-140.

[27] Reich, A, Heisig, M, Phan, N. Q, Taneda, K, Takamori, K, Takeuchi, S, Furue, M, Blome, C, Augustin, M, Ständer, S, & Szepietowski, J. C. Visual Analogue Scale: Evaluation of the Instrument for the Assess-ment of Pruritus. Acta Derm Venereol. (2011). Nov 21. doi:, 00015555-1265.

[28] The WHOQOL GroupThe World Health Organization Quality of Life Assessment (WHOQOL). Development and psychometric properties. Soc Sci Med (1998)., 46, 1569-1585.

[29] Ware, J. E. Jr., Sherbourne CD. The MOS 36-item short-form health survey (SF-36). I. Conceptual framework and item selection. *Med Care.* Jun (1992). National Center for Chronic, 30(6), 473-483.

[30] Disease Prevention and Health PromotionHealth-Related Quality of Life (HRQOL):HRQOL Concepts. http://www.cdc.gov/hrqol/concept.htm.Accessed: August 1, (2012). Page last reviewed: March 15, 2011; Page last updated: March 17, 2011

[31] Ware, J. E. Jr. The SF-36 health survey. In: Spilker B, ed. *Quality of life and pharmacoeconomics.* 2nd ed. Philadelphia, PA: Lippincott-Raven; (1996)., 1996, 337-345.

[32] Ware, J. E. Jr., Gandek B. Overview of the SF-36 Health Survey and the International Quality of Life Assessment (IQOLA) Project. *J Clin Epidemiol.* Nov (1998)., 51(11), 903-912.

[33] Ware, J. E. Jr., Kosinski M, Bayliss MS, McHorney CA, Rogers WH, Raczek A. Comparison of methods for the scoring and statistical analysis of SF-36 health profile and summary measures: summary of results from the Medical Outcomes Study. *Med Care.* Apr (1995). Suppl):AS, 264-279.

[34] Ware, J. E. Jr. The status of health assessment (1994). *Annu Rev Public Health.* 1995;, 16, 327-354.

[35] Ross, M. M, Rideout, E. M, & Carson, M. M. The use of the diary as a data collection technique. West J Nurs Res (1994). , 16, 414-425.

[36] Russell, M. B, Rasmussen, B. K, Brennum, J, et al. Presentation of a new instrument: The diagnostic headache diary. Cephalalgia (1992). , 12, 369-374.

[37] Coeytaux, R. R, Frasier, P. Y, & Reid, A. Patient-centered outcomes for frequent headaches. Headache (2007). , 47, 480-485.

[38] Melzack, R. The McGill Pain Questionnaire: major properties and scoring methods. *Pain.* Sep (1975). , 1(3), 277-299.

[39] Peat, G. *PPA recommendations for low back pain-related functional limitation outcome measures.* London: The Chartered Society of Physiotherapy; July (2004).

[40] Mcconnell, S, Kolopack, P, & Davis, A. M. The Western Ontario and McMaster Universities Osteoarthritis Index (WOMAC): a review of its utility and measurement properties. *Arthritis Rheum.* Oct (2001). , 45(5), 453-461.

[41] Bellamy, N. Pain assessment in osteoarthritis: experience with the WOMAC osteoarthritis index. *Semin Arthritis Rheum.* May (1989). Suppl 2):14-17.

[42] Martin, D. P, Engelberg, R, Agel, J, & Swiontkowski, M. F. Comparison of the Musculoskeletal Function Assessment questionnaire with the Short Form-36, the Western Ontario and McMaster Universities Osteoarthritis Index, and the Sickness Impact Profile health-status measures. *J Bone Joint Surg Am.* Sep (1997). , 79(9), 1323-1335.

[43] Finch, E, Walsh, M, Thomas, S. G, & Woodhouse, L. J. Functional ability perceived by individuals following total knee arthroplasty compared to age-matched individuals without knee disability. *J Orthop Sports Phys Ther.* Apr (1998). , 27(4), 255-263.

[44] Bellamy, N, & Womac, a. year experiential review of a patient-centered self-reported health status questionnaire. *J Rheumatol.* Dec (2002). , 29(12), 2473-2476.

[45] Wright, J. G, & Young, N. L. A comparison of different indices of responsiveness. *J Clin Epidemiol.* Mar (1997). , 50(3), 239-246.

[46] Bruce, B, & Fries, J. Longitudinal comparison of the Health Assessment Questionnaire (HAQ) and the Western Ontario and McMaster Universities Osteoarthritis Index (WOMAC). *Arthritis Rheum.* Oct 15 (2004). , 51(5), 730-737.

[47] Stratford, P. W, Kennedy, D. M, & Hanna, S. E. Condition-specific Western Ontario McMaster Osteoarthritis Index was not superior to region-specific Lower Extremity Functional Scale at detecting change. *J Clin Epidemiol.* Oct (2004). , 57(10), 1025-1032.

[48] Wolfe, F, Michaud, K, Kahler, K, & Omar, M. The Short Arthritis Assessment Scale: a brief assessment questionnaire for rapid evaluation of arthritis severity in research and clinical practice. *J Rheumatol.* Dec (2004). , 31(12), 2472-2479.

[49] Salaffi, F, Carotti, M, & Grassi, W. Health-related quality of life in patients with hip or knee osteoarthritis: comparison of generic and disease-specific instruments. *Clin Rheumatol.* Feb (2005). , 24(1), 29-37.

[50] Escobar, A, Quintana, J. M, Bilbao, A, Arostegui, I, Lafuente, I, & Vidaurreta, I. Responsiveness and clinically important differences for the WOMAC and SF-36 after total knee replacement. *Osteoarthritis Cartilage.* Mar (2007). , 15(3), 273-280.

[51] Rosemann, T, Joos, S, Koerner, T, Szecsenyi, J, & Laux, G. Comparison of AIMSSF, WOMAC, x-ray and a global physician assessment in order to approach quality of life in patients suffering from osteoarthritis. *BMC Musculoskelet Disord.* (2006). , 2.

[52] Whitfield, K, Buchbinder, R, Segal, L, & Osborne, R. H. Parsimonious and efficient assessment of health-related quality of life in osteoarthritis research: validation of the Assessment of Quality of Life (AQoL) instrument. *Health Qual Life Outcomes.* (2006).

[53] Garbuz, D. S, Xu, M, & Sayre, E. C. Patients' outcome after total hip arthroplasty: a comparison between the Western Ontario and McMaster Universities index and the Oxford 12-item hip score. *J Arthroplasty.* Oct (2006). , 21(7), 998-1004.

[54] Quintana, J. M, Escobar, A, Bilbao, A, Arostegui, I, Lafuente, I, & Vidaurreta, I. Responsiveness and clinically important differences for the WOMAC and SF-36 after hip joint replacement. *Osteoarthritis Cartilage.* Dec (2005). , 13(12), 1076-1083.

[55] Soohoo, N. F, Vyas, R. M, Samimi, D. B, Molina, R, & Lieberman, J. R. Comparison of the responsiveness of the SF-36 and WOMAC in patients undergoing total hip arthroplasty. *J Arthroplasty.* Dec (2007). , 22(8), 1168-1173.

[56] Tait, R. C, Chibnall, J. T, & Krause, S. The Pain Disability Index: psychometric properties. *Pain.* Feb (1990). , 40(2), 171-182.

[57] Pollard, C. A. Preliminary validity study of the pain disability index. Percept Mot Skills. (1984). Dec;59(3):974. PubMed PMID: 6240632.

[58] Tait, R. C, Chibnall, J. T, & Krause, S. The Pain Disability Index: psychometric properties. Pain. (1990). Feb;PubMed PMID: 2308763., 40(2), 171-82.

[59] Jerome, A, & Gross, R. T. Pain disability index: construct and discriminant validity. Arch Phys Med Rehabil. (1991). Oct;, 72(11), 920-2.

[60] Johnson, D. A, & Heather, B. B. The sensitivity of the Beck depression inventory to changes of symptomatology. Br J Psychiatry. (1974). Aug;, 125(0), 184-5.

[61] Salkind, M. R. Beck depression inventory in general practice. J R Coll Gen Pract. (1969). Nov;, 18(88), 267-71.

[62] Schwab, J, Bialow, M, Clemmons, R, Martin, P, & Holzer, C. The Beck depression inventory with medical inpatients. Acta Psychiatr Scand. (1967). , 43(3), 255-66.

[63] Bjelland, I, Dahl, A. A, Haug, T. T, & Neckelmann, D. The validity of the Hospital Anxiety and Depression Scale: An updated literature review. J Psychosom Res (2002). , 52, 69-77.

[64] Tang, W. K, Wong, E, Chiu, H. F, et al. Examining item bias in the anxiety subscale of the Hospital Anxiety and Depression Scale in patients with chronic obstructive pulmonary disease. Int J Methods Psychiatr Res (2008). , 17, 104-110.

[65] Paterson, C. Measuring outcomes in primary care: A patient generated measure, MYMOP, compared with the SF-36 health survey. BMJ (1996). , 312, 1016-1020.

[66] Boon, H, Macpherson, H, Fleishman, S, et al. Evaluating complex healthcare systems: A critique of four approaches. Evid Based Complement Altern Med (2007). , 4, 279-285.

[67] Fries, J. F, Bruce, B, & Cella, D. The promise of PROMIS: Using item response theory to improve assessment of patient reported outcomes. Clin Exp Rheumatol (2005). suppl 39):SS57., 53.

[68] Cella, D, Yount, S, Rothrock, N, et al. The Patient-Reported Outcomes Measurement Information System (PROMIS): Progress of an NIH Roadmap cooperative group during its first two years. Med Care (2007). suppl 1):SS11., 3.

Chapter 18

# Evaluating the Geography and the Visibility Tendencies of Acupuncture Treatment Locations in Metropolitan Toronto

Stephen P. Meyer

Additional information is available at the end of the chapter

http://dx.doi.org/10.5772/54599

## 1. Introduction

Acupuncture treatment can be delivered from the offices of health care professionals. Acupuncture is most commonly practiced by individuals working within the complementary and alternative medicine (CAM) sector; such as those self-identifying as 'primary' acupuncture practitioners, and chiropractors, massage therapists and naturopaths will often administer acupuncture treatment as part of their holistic approach to medicine. On the conventional medicine (CM) side, some dentists use acupuncture to help patients deal with anxiety [1], pain [2] and to control the gag reflux through 'hypnopuncture' [3] and 'integrative' family doctors and physiotherapists may suggest or administer acupuncture treatment for chronic pain issues [4].

Generally speaking, health care professionals and medical facilities are not located equally over geographic area. The spatial disparities in health care accessibility that these supply configurations create for citizens within various jurisdictions continues to be an important concern of medical geographers, policymakers and the like. Researchers examining the geography of health care supply in countries such as Canada have, more often than not, assessed the CM sector with analysis on the distribution of, and accessibility patterns to, family doctors, specialists and/or hospitals [5-13]. Analysis on the spatial properties of CAM is emerging at a more modest rate (for reviews of the literature see [14-18]) and there are examples of empirical geographic research on specific CAM health care such as chiropractors and naturopaths [19-26]. Although acupuncture research continues to expand within a number of fields [27], there is need for geographic study [28] which, aside from contributions from Meyer [18,29], remains underdeveloped.

In Canada, many practitioners that administer health services are small business owners functioning in competitive markets. This is certainly true of CAM operators (such as acupuncture practitioners, chiropractors and naturopaths), but also dentists. The economic success of a small health care establishment is undoubtedly dependent on favorable patient outcomes, but profitability may also be a function of visibility as most consumer services need to be 'seen' to be accessible to new patrons. Indeed, visibility has strong geographic connotations. "What we see is that which lies within our field of vision, where the boundaries of this field are shaped by the spatial and temporal properties of the here and now" [30]. A business's ability to be 'within our field of vision' may be enhanced in a number of ways; such as by being strategically situated in a high traffic/ high volume location or by placing advertisements in various media. Visibility requirements will vary with the operator; a well-respected health care provider may, with time, rely less on being visible and more on an excellent reputation. Nevertheless, understanding where health care providers are located, in light of visibility characteristics, is the first step in appreciating the magnitude of these possible advantages. As such, this study focuses on the specific case of acupuncture services in the Toronto census metropolitan area (CMA), located within the Canadian province of Ontario.

## 2. Methodology

Four types of health care providers that offer acupuncture services are considered: primary acupuncture practitioners, chiropractors, naturopaths and dentists. Primary acupuncture offices represent locations where acupuncture treatments are definitely offered; whereas chiropractor and naturopath offices are locations with likely acupuncture services and dentist offices are locations with possible acupuncture options. Therefore, a number of 2012 datasets, purchased from InfoCanada [31], were utilized for the Toronto metropolitan area:

1. The locations, characteristics (sales, employment and the like) and advertising habits (such as yellow pages, website ads and overall advertising expenditure) of 306 offices for which acupuncture is the primary medical service;
2. The locations, characteristics and advertising habits of 848 chiropractic and 149 naturopathic proprietors (for a total of 997); and
3. The locations, characteristics and advertising habits of 2,942 dentist offices.

All of these offices were placed on a road network layer [32] using the ArcGIS (version 10.0) 'address locator' geocoding function. Within the geographic information system (GIS) environment, these points were compared with respect to visibility advantages. More specifically, each office point was evaluated in terms of being within or beyond 'high visibility areas' and if each office participated in a high or low 'visibility approach'.

High visibility areas are comprised of two components: high visibility polygons and high visibility arcs (lines). By extracting blocks from an Ontario land use map [33], a layer of high visibility polygons was created by isolating commercial land use blocks and blocks adjacent to commercial areas. In a similar fashion, highways and major roads were taken from an Ontario road network layer [32] and saved as a specific high visibility arc (road) layer. Logically, offices in and around commercial zones and/or on well-travelled streets will feature high traffic volume and thus are high visibility areas. Conversely, low visibility areas are those that are not near commercial zones and not along a major road or highway. Acupuncture, chiropractor/naturopath and dentist office points were, hence, denoted as being located in high or low visibility areas. A high visibility approach was defined in this study as an office that utilizes a display ad in the yellow pages and/or has an above average advertising to sales ratio. A low visibility approach means the office does not have a listing in the yellow pages or only a regular listing (no display ad) and an advertising to sales ratio that is below average (as measured for all offices within the given category in metropolitan Toronto). Therefore, the three health care categories were further stratified by visibility approach (high or low). Online advertising was not specifically integrated into the visibility approach measure due to so few practitioners with a website listing in this database, but general observations are made nevertheless.

Based on these visibility 'area' and 'approach' stipulations, a series of layers/maps were derived in the GIS environment and important geographic patterns concerning the visibility tendencies of those offering, or potentially offering, acupuncture services were realized. Essentially, points were allocated into four groups: 1) high visibility area with a high visibility approach, 2) high visibility area with a low visibility approach, 3) low visibility area with a high visibility approach and 4) low visibility area with a low visibility approach.

The point distributions of these four visibility categories, for each of the three health care categories, were analyzed further to understand within metropolitan Toronto patterns. Specifically, a nearest neighbor analysis of the point patterns was employed using the application within ArcGIS. The nearest neighbor significance test indicates if an observed pattern of points deviates from a theoretical (random) distribution sufficiently enough to be considered significantly clustered or dispersed in space [34]. A nearest neighbor ratio (or index) is derived and this allows for point distributions, within the same sample area, to be compared directly in terms of the degree of clustering and/or dispersion. The ratio/index values were calculated using the Manhattan city block method (right angle distance computations) with the actual metropolitan Toronto area (5,905.71 kilometers square). The nearest neighbor analysis provided more elucidation into the visibility tendencies of the health care providers and corroborated the patterns displayed in the maps. Also, to more precisely assess municipality differences within metropolitan Toronto, a census subdivision (CSD) layer [35] and Census of Canada 2011 population and population change variables were used [36]. See Figure 1 for the location of each municipality.

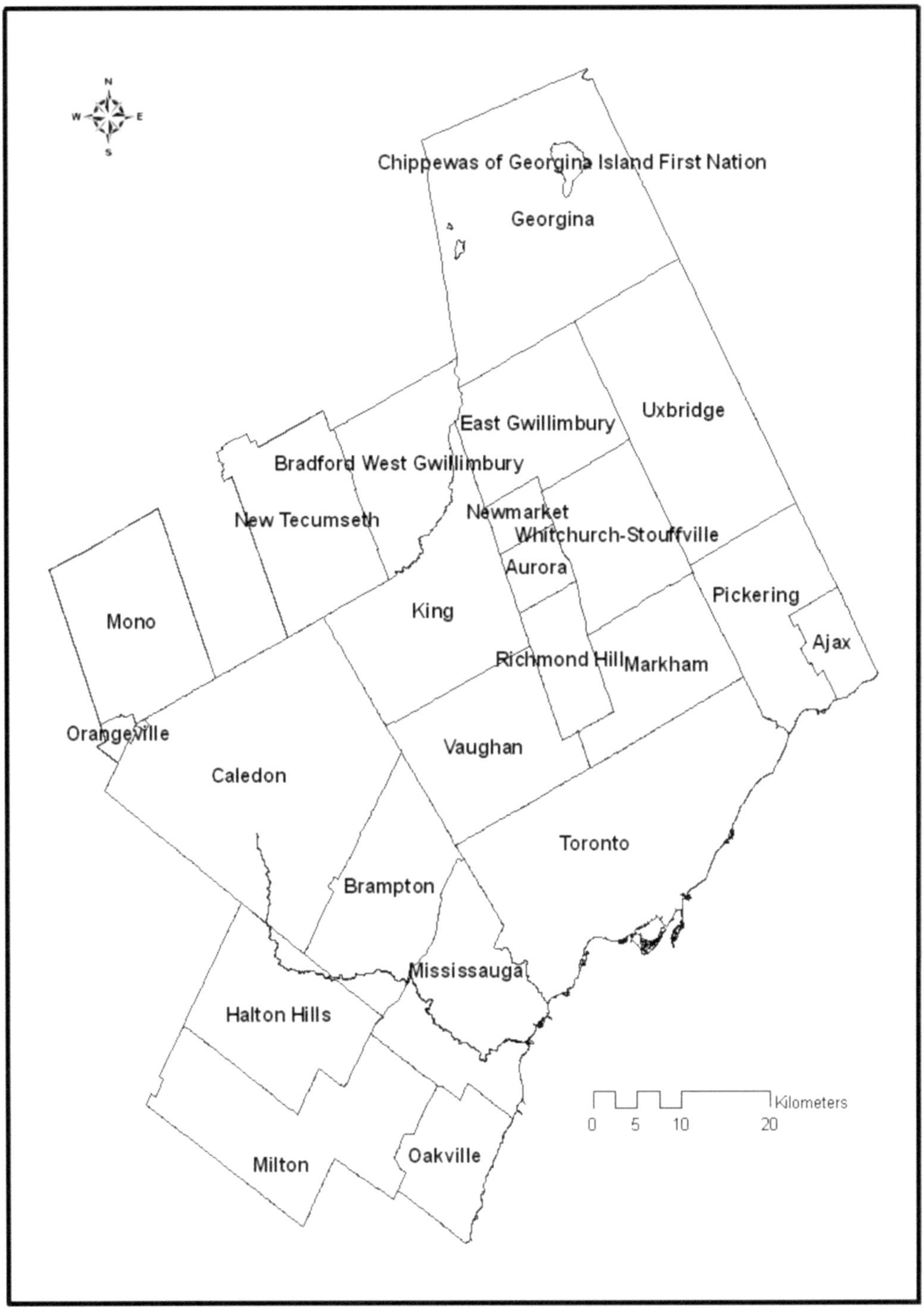


**Figure 1.** Municipalities in metropolitan Toronto

http://dx.doi.org/10.5772/54599

## 3. Observing the overall trends

Primary acupuncture, chiropractor/naturopath and dentist office enumerations follow general population trends with disproportionate tallies in the most populous municipalities such as, particularly, the City of Toronto, but also Mississauga and other CSDs in excess of 100,000 people (see Table 1 and the point configurations on Figure 2, 3 and 4). However, other important, but more subtle, differences are detectable. For instance, of the 306 acupuncture offices in metropolitan Toronto, the City of Toronto contains 60.46% of the cases and the addition of Mississauga, Brampton, Markham and Vaughan brings the proportion to 83%. Dentist office percentages are not as high for the City of Toronto (54.49%), but when the five municipalities, with more 200,000 in population, are combined, the percentage is similar (81.64%). In contrast, the chiropractor/naturopath category in the City of Toronto and the top five most populated municipality proportions are lower by comparison (49.85% and 74.02% respectively). Although general correspondence between office frequencies and CSD population is apparent, the same is not true of population change. For example, only modest office tallies occur in some of the less populated yet fast growing CSDs (such as Whitchurch-Stouffville, Bradford-West Gwillimbury and Milton) and a disproportionately high number of office points occur in Toronto and Mississauga in spite of below average population growth in these municipalities. Perhaps a stronger association between health care office numbers and population change will emerge in time and larger municipalities with very high growth rates, such as Brampton, Vaughan, Ajax and Milton, may be particularly worthy of investigation in the future.

As shown on the maps, considerable portions of metropolitan Toronto have few office points and other parts show quite high densities. This suggests a concentrated pattern and the degree of 'clustering' varies with health care type. The nearest neighbor indices for acupuncture, chiropractor/naturopath and dentist health care types were 0.576, 0.509 and 0.349, respectively, and all were statistically significantly clustered at a confidence interval of 99%. Acupuncture offices are less clustered and this may seem counterintuitive given that there are large areas within the Toronto CMA completely void of primary acupuncture practitioners whereas the chiropractor/naturopath and dentist points appear to 'fill in' the maps to a greater extent. Yet, even in the south-central, where all three categories have considerable proportions, the distribution varies. Dentist offices almost continuously cover the City of Toronto and into adjacent Mississauga, southern parts of Vaughan, Richmond Hill and Markham.

| Census subdivision (CSD) | Pop 2011 | Acu. | Chi. or nat. | Den. | Pop change 2006-11 (%) |
|---|---|---|---|---|---|
| Toronto | 2,615,060 | 185 | 497 | 1,603 | 4.5 |
| Mississauga | 713,443 | 33 | 108 | 340 | 6.7 |
| Brampton | 523,911 | 8 | 31 | 174 | 20.8 |

| Census subdivision (CSD) | Pop 2011 | Acu. | Chi. or nat. | Den. | Pop change 2006-11 (%) |
|---|---|---|---|---|---|
| Markham | 301,709 | 17 | 47 | 133 | 15.3 |
| Vaughan | 288,301 | 11 | 55 | 152 | 20.7 |
| Richmond Hill | 185,541 | 19 | 42 | 98 | 14.0 |
| Oakville | 182,520 | 7 | 51 | 110 | 10.2 |
| Ajax | 109,600 | 6 | 15 | 43 | 21.6 |
| Pickering | 88,721 | 3 | 14 | 38 | 1.0 |
| Milton | 84,362 | 3 | 19 | 40 | 56.5 |
| Newmarket | 79,978 | 7 | 30 | 51 | 7.6 |
| Caledon | 59,460 | 1 | 9 | 19 | 4.2 |
| Halton Hills | 59,008 | 2 | 13 | 26 | 6.7 |
| Aurora | 53,203 | 0 | 16 | 36 | 11.7 |
| Georgina | 43,517 | 1 | 6 | 11 | 2.8 |
| Whitchurch-Stouffville | 37,628 | 0 | 5 | 13 | 54.3 |
| New Tecumseth | 30,234 | 0 | 11 | 12 | 9.1 |
| Bradford–West Gwillimbury | 28,077 | 0 | 3 | 11 | 16.8 |
| Orangeville | 27,975 | 1 | 8 | 14 | 3.9 |
| East Gwillimbury | 22,473 | 0 | 4 | 3 | 6.7 |
| Uxbridge | 20,623 | 1 | 5 | 10 | 7.6 |
| King | 19,899 | 1 | 6 | 5 | 2.1 |
| Mono | 7,546 | 0 | 2 | 0 | 6.7 |
| Chippewas of Georgina | 275 | 0 | 0 | 0 | -22.1 |
| Toronto CMA | 5,583,064 | 306 | 997 | 2,942 | 9.2 |

**Table 1.** Acupuncture, chiropractor/naturopath and dentist offices, population and population change for municipalities of metropolitan Toronto

http://dx.doi.org/10.5772/54599

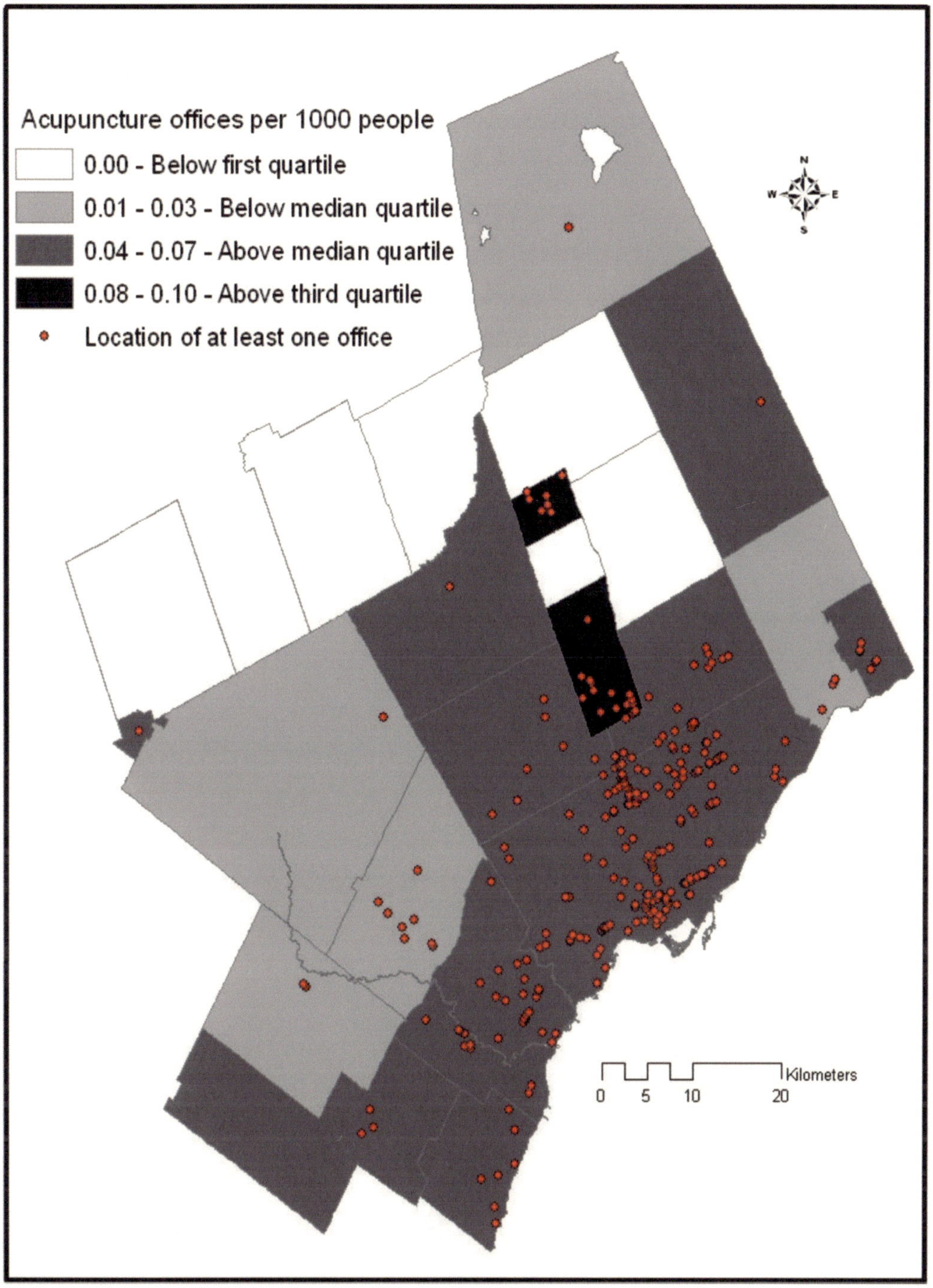


**Figure 2.** Location of acupuncture offices and acupuncture offices per 1000 people for municipalities in metropolitan Toronto

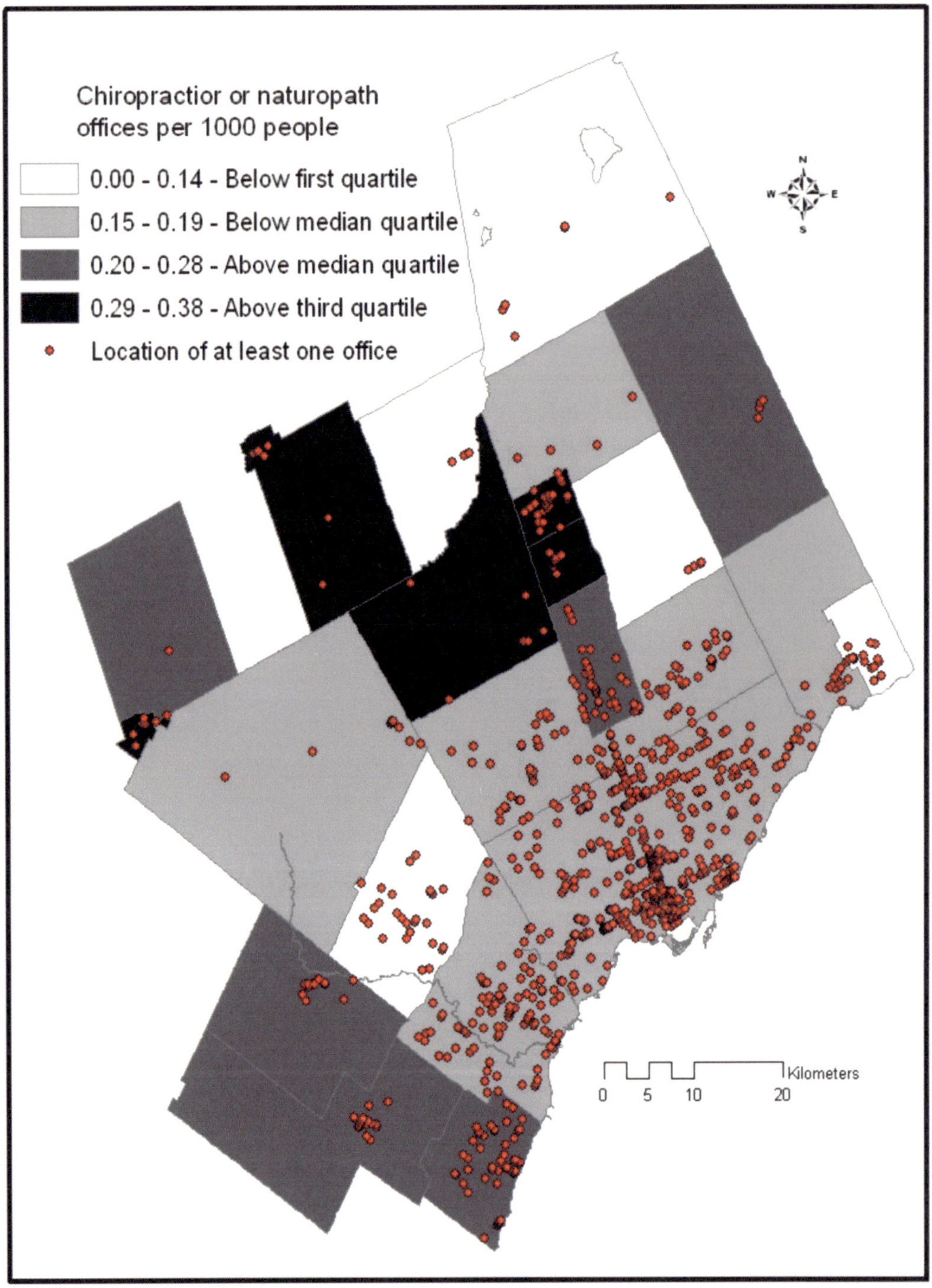


**Figure 3.** Location of chiropractor or naturopath offices and chiropractor or naturopath offices per 1000 people for municipalities in metropolitan Toronto

http://dx.doi.org/10.5772/54599

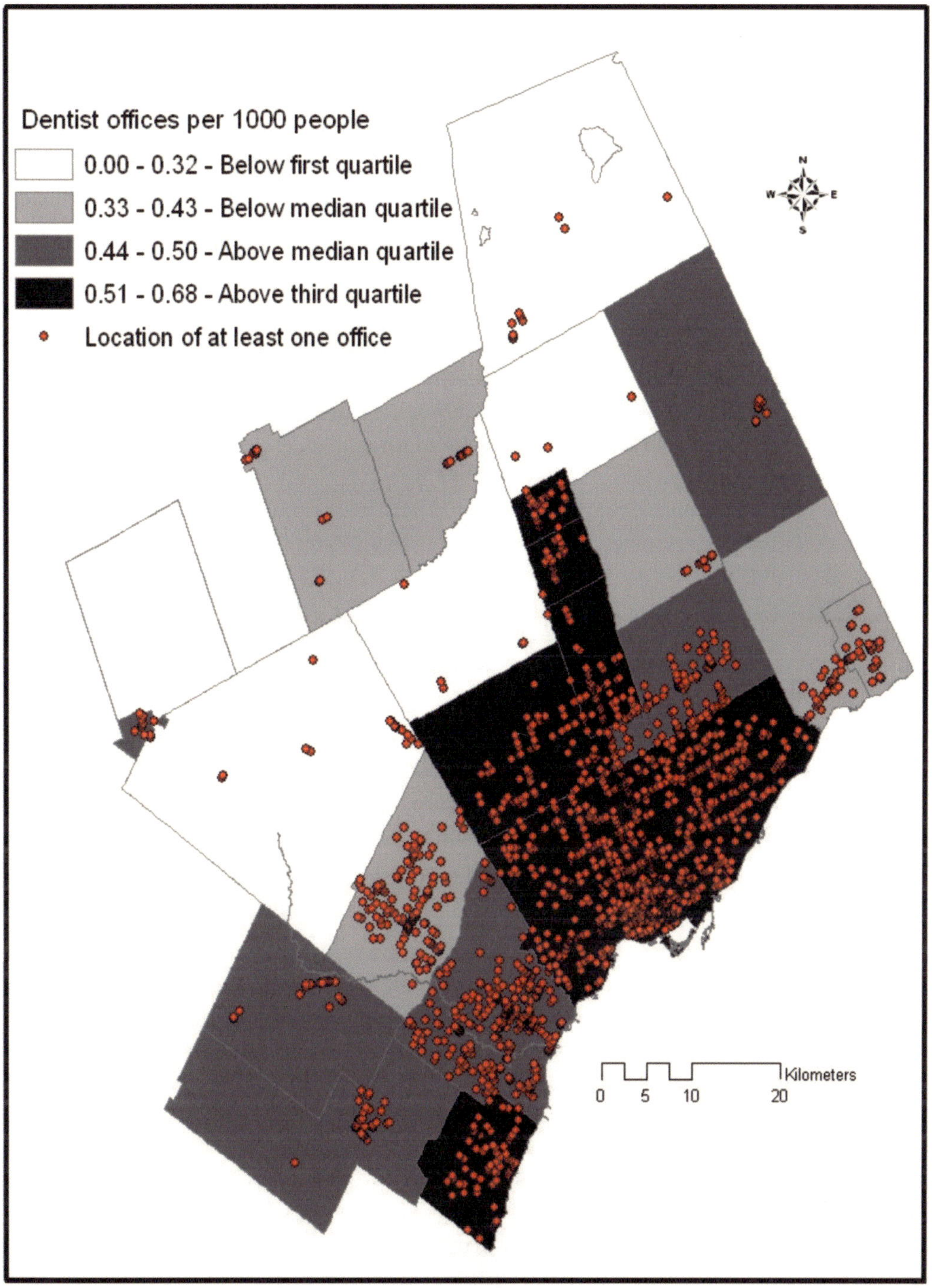


**Figure 4.** Location of dentist offices and dentist offices per 1000 people for municipalities in metropolitan Toronto

Southern Oakville and central Brampton are also substantially covered, which is certainly pushing the nearest neighbor index downward (more clustered). On the other hand, the chiropractor/naturopath and acupuncture categories show high concentrations in the southern municipalities as well, but the point patterns tend to be less regular and more prone to 'peaks and valleys' over space; moving the index towards random (1.00) by comparison. Subtle differences aside, all three health care point distributions are certainly not even close to 'dispersed'. A dispersed pattern would indicate more equal allocation throughout the study area. Thus, the clustered patterns illustrated on the maps and measured by the nearest neighbor analysis imply that patients/customers proximity to these offices varies by municipality.

By standardizing office tallies by population and the maps by quartile classification, the relative presence and absence of the three health care categories can be more plainly observed (see the polygons on Figures 2, 3 and 4). Acupuncture offices per 1,000 people, with values above the median quartile, show a spatially continuous pattern throughout the south-central and include the 'non-connected' municipalities of Orangeville, Uxbridge and Ajax. While several of these municipalities display relative presence, only two (Richmond Hill and Newmarket) are in the upper quartile. The spatial pattern of dentist offices per capita (Figure 4) is similar to the acupuncture office display, but with a greater number of CSDs in the upper quartile (the City of Toronto, Vaughan, Aurora and Oakville) and a comparatively more pronounced southwestern presence. In the case of both the acupuncture and dentist maps, the northern portions of most of the Toronto CMA exhibit below median offices per capita values and this suggests that dentists and acupuncture practitioners, in general, do not favor these areas. The chiropractor/naturopath map provides interesting contrast and is almost a 'negative mirror image' of the other two patterns. Only the relative importance of the extreme southwest, Newmarket, Richmond Hill, Uxbridge and Orangeville are common to all three health care types. Perhaps most striking is that most of southern metropolitan Toronto (including the City of Toronto) is below the median quartile for chiropractors and/or naturopaths in per capita terms. Conversely, northern CSDs such as King, New Tecumseth and Mono uniquely emphasize the chiropractor/naturopath classification.

Although the sheer numbers of offices and degree of clustering differ substantially, the office per capita spatial patterns for acupuncture practitioners and dentists are quite similar while the chiropractor/naturopath category more unique. It is intriguing that this spatial congruency between primary acupuncture practitioners and dentists occurs even though the former is most commonly associated with the CAM sector and the latter usually viewed as 'conventional' medicine. That chiropractors and/or naturopaths emphasize several areas not comparatively abundant in primary acupuncture practitioners or dentists (such as the northern parts of the metropolis) may suggest a 'substitution' situation; as chiropractors and naturopaths are likely to offer acupuncture services. As such, the maps may be indicating that areas within the Toronto CMA not comparatively rich in primary acupuncture practitioners per capita may still receive acupuncture and related therapies from other CAM providers, such as chiropractors and naturopaths. The geographic sameness of dentists and primary acupuncture offices per person does not necessarily indicate market overlap. These would be 'imperfect substitutes' in most cases, as dentists offering acupuncture are likely to do so in a more focused fashion, rather than

http://dx.doi.org/10.5772/54599

'full body' treatment options common to primary acupuncture specialists. Thus, there are some areas of metropolitan Toronto that display relatively high per capita values for all three types of health care, such as the extreme west, and other regions present more distinct health care biases. Yet, many of these overall trends do vary with office visibility characteristics.

## 4. Focusing on visibility tendencies

It is far more common for offices to be in high visibility areas, compared to low visibility areas, and the proportions of offices in high visibility areas are reasonably similar for the health care types: 76.47%, 76.03% and 80.86% for acupuncture, chiropractor/naturopath and dentist, correspondingly. Whereas, visibility approach varies much more by type; proportions in the high category are: 22.55% (acupuncture), 53.56% (chiropractor/naturopath) and 39.39% (dentist). Other complexities emerge when visibility area and visibility approaches are cross-compared (see Tables 2 and 3).

| Health care type and visibility characteristics | # of offices | Average sales ($) | Average employment |
|---|---|---|---|
| Acupuncture | | | |
| High visibility area with a high visibility approach | 51 | 555,392.16 | 4.37 |
| High visibility area with a low visibility approach | 183 | 480,692.13 | 2.92 |
| Low visibility area with a high visibility approach | 18 | 425,222.22 | 3.28 |
| Low visibility area with a low visibility approach | 54 | 487,113.21 | 3.06 |
| All acupuncture offices | 306 | 492,076.67 | 3.22 |
| Chiropractor/naturopath | | | |
| High visibility area with a high visibility approach | 409 | 770,668.30 | 4.65 |
| High visibility area with a low visibility approach | 349 | 786,870.69 | 4.65 |
| Low visibility area with a high visibility approach | 125 | 766,864.00 | 4.69 |
| Low visibility area with a low visibility approach | 114 | 684,000.00 | 3.68 |
| All chiropractor/naturopath offices | 997 | 766,150.75 | 4.55 |
| Dentist | | | |
| High visibility area with a high visibility approach | 930 | 1,434,896.77 | 7.44 |
| High visibility area with a low visibility approach | 1,449 | 1,054,632.85 | 5.40 |
| Low visibility area with a high visibility approach | 229 | 1,400,676.83 | 7.34 |
| Low visibility area with a low visibility approach | 328 | 1,003,161.59 | 5.11 |
| All dentist offices | 2,942 | 1,195,570.70 | 6.16 |

**Table 2.** Health care type and visibility characteristics in metropolitan Toronto compared by number of offices, average sales and average employment estimates

### 4.1. The 'high visibility area with a high visibility approach' group

Offices located in high visibility areas (along major roads and/or near or within commercial blocks) and employing a high visibility approach (above average advertising to sales ratio and/ or a display ad in the yellow pages) tend to be the largest operations and/or the most 'successful'. Sales and employment values are the highest (acupuncture and dentist) or at least above average (chiropractors/naturopaths) in each of the groupings. Given that there is comparatively high cost involved in simultaneously pursuing above average advertising and maintaining a high traffic location, it is perhaps not surprising that more modestly-sized offices would choose, or be forced into, a different visibility approach.

The high visibility area/approach subset does show variability by health care type in terms of proportional location preferences. As shown on Table 3, acupuncture offices in this category are far less likely to be in the core of metropolitan Toronto (the City of Toronto) in comparison to chiropractors/naturopaths and dentists. Given that acupuncture offices are much smaller, the higher rents of these highly visible areas of Toronto (in addition to the costs associated with above average advertising) may dampen their numbers in these locations. High visibility area/approach acupuncture practitioners more frequently practice in the inner band (Mississauga, Brampton, Vaughan, Markham and Pickering) and the outer band (the remaining municipalities) areas. In contrast, more than 40% of chiropractors/naturopaths and dentists choose the City of Toronto. The nearest neighbor indices indicate significant clustering, but acupuncture practitioners are comparably the least concentrated: 0.639 (acupuncture), 0.572 (dentist) and 0.449 (chiropractor/naturopath). Since chiropractors/naturopaths and dentists emphasize the high visibility 'core' areas more than the acupuncture category, it is predictable that these nearest neighbor values would be further away from random (1.00).

Offices in this category are utilizing what might be termed the optimal visibility strategy. It is illuminating that it is only with chiropractor and/or naturopaths in which this visibility type is most frequent. Perhaps this implies that chiropractors and/or naturopaths are in more competitive markets compared to dentists and primary acupuncture practitioners. This may also point to strong business acumen. It is not uncommon for students in chiropractic and naturopathic schools to be exposed to small business workshops in which the attributes of being 'visible' are predictably illustrated.

### 4.2. The 'high visibility area with a low visibility approach' group

Almost 60% of acupuncture offices (59.80%) and a sizable proportion of dentists (49.25%), chiropractors and/or naturopaths (35.01%) fall into this category making it the overall most common visibility outcome. These are offices that locate in high traffic areas, but pursue comparatively less aggressive advertising approaches and tend to be in the intermediate to high range in sales and employment. Strikingly, this visibility group clearly favors the core; almost three-quarters of acupuncture offices and two-thirds of chiropractors/naturopaths and dentists are in the City of Toronto. The configuration of points are the most clustered of any other visibility designation for acupuncture and dentist (with nearest neighbor index values of 0.557 and 0.349, respectively) and comparatively concentrated for chiropractor/naturopath (0.557).

http://dx.doi.org/10.5772/54599

| Health care type and visibility characteristics | Core | Inner band | Outer band |
|---|---|---|---|
| Acupuncture | | | |
| High visibility area with a high visibility approach | 21.57 | 47.06 | 31.37 |
| High visibility area with a low visibility approach | 74.86 | 15.85 | 9.30 |
| Low visibility area with a high visibility approach | 22.22 | 38.89 | 38.89 |
| Low visibility area with a low visibility approach | 61.11 | 22.22 | 16.67 |
| All acupuncture offices | 60.46 | 23.53 | 16.01 |
| Chiropractor/naturopath | | | |
| High visibility area with a high visibility approach | 42.78 | 27.38 | 29.83 |
| High visibility area with a low visibility approach | 63.04 | 21.78 | 15.19 |
| Low visibility area with a high visibility approach | 38.40 | 28.80 | 32.80 |
| Low visibility area with a low visibility approach | 47.37 | 27.19 | 25.44 |
| All chiropractor/naturopath offices | 49.85 | 25.58 | 24.57 |
| Dentist | | | |
| High visibility area with a high visibility approach | 44.52 | 32.15 | 23.33 |
| High visibility area with a low visibility approach | 65.08 | 23.33 | 11.59 |
| Low visibility area with a high visibility approach | 32.75 | 37.12 | 30.13 |
| Low visibility area with a low visibility approach | 50.61 | 34.76 | 14.63 |
| All dentist offices | 54.49 | 28.45 | 17.06 |
| Offices of all three types | 53.83 | 27.42 | 18.75 |

Note: The 'core' area is the City of Toronto; the 'inner band' is comprised of Mississauga, Brampton, Vaughan, Markham and Pickering; the 'outer band' is the remaining municipalities.

**Table 3.** Health care type and visibility characteristics compared by 'core', 'inner band' and 'outer band' municipalities in metropolitan Toronto (shown in percentage)

Why does this visibility classification occur so frequently? Certainly this relates to the modest size of most of these offices, with acupuncture practitioner locations being the smallest. There might be limited funds available for advertising; and being 'clustered' in a high visibility location, and disproportionately in the high population density environment of the City of Toronto, might be necessary in these competitive markets. In effect, these are offices that have chosen a location with high traffic volume over 'eye catching' advertising in the yellow pages or websites. A key influence on this group is being proximate to vehicle and/or pedestrian traffic flow. This may also explain why so few offices of this visibility group are in the outer band of municipalities of metropolitan Toronto, where traffic volume opportunities would be comparatively reduced.

### 4.3. The 'low visibility area with a high visibility approach' group

This visibility group is rare, in terms of office frequency, and the point configurations are less clustered and distributed quite evenly across the Toronto CMA. The acupuncture and dentist classes have the lowest number of office tallies of any visibility group (5.88% and 7.78%, correspondingly) and chiropractors/naturopaths (12.54%) are below average. The nearest neighbor indices are well above the norm for each respective health care type: 0.811 compared to 0.576 for acupuncture, 0.792 vis-à-vis 0.509 for the chiropractor/naturopath category and 0.551 compared to 0.493 for dentists. In fact, the nearest neighbor index for acupuncture (0.811) was statistically insignificance (with 99% confidence) and thus random. The comparatively even distribution across the core, inner band and outer band spatial divisions echo the nearest neighbour results. Notice that the proportions all stay within the 20-40% range for each health care type (see Table 3); a result that does not occur for any other visibility group. This evenness is complemented with the highest proportions in the outer band; again, for all three health care categories.

The rareness of this visibility group is perhaps surprising. One might assume that if an office was not in a high volume location, it would have to compensate for this lack of physical visibility with virtual visibility, through ads in the yellow pages, websites and other creative means of promotion. Yet, the results show that if this strategy is being employed, it does not occur very often.

### 4.4. The 'low visibility area with a low visibility approach' group

This group is, for all intents and purposes, the most disadvantaged in terms of visibility; and is described as offices in low traffic areas with relatively limited propensity to advertise. This group is quite regularly found in the core (ranging from 47.37% to 61.11%) and is definitely below average in size. While more clustered than the 'low visibility area with a high visibility approach' assembly of points, these offices tend to be more spread out than the two 'high visibility area' groups. The nearest neighbor indices for this visibility group provide confirmation: acupuncture 0.790, chiropractor/naturopath 0.636 and dentist 0.493.

Given the small size (in terms of average sales and employment), limited advertising and propensity to be away from high volume areas, one might expect that many of these health care providers have their business and residence at the same address. If the lack of 'formal' advertising is by choice, perhaps this visibility type can also be described as professionals who rely chiefly on 'word of mouth' to capture new customers.

## 5. Conclusions and implications for acupuncture spatial accessibility

The visibility traits of health care providers that administer (or may administer) acupuncture services are complex. Nevertheless, this study did demonstrate that the visibility tendencies of various acupuncture treatment locations leave interesting and distinctive geographies and a greater appreciation of these patterns builds upon our knowledge regarding the motivations and potential profitability of small health care business owners. The majority of primary acupuncture (PA), chiropractor/naturopath and dentist offices are attracted to high visibility/high volume areas and some of these employ high visibility/more aggressive advertising approaches to attract new patrons. Many practitioners are in high visibility locations, but eschew aggressive advertising and on occasion the reverse occurs (offices in low visibility areas but with a high visibility approach). The former constitutes the most frequent 'visibility' classification' and implies the importance of strategic site choices, in which being in a highly visible location may be replacing the need to advertise lavishly on websites and yellow pages. The latter category may have motivations that follow similar logic: because these offices have fewer geographic advantages, the approach to advertising and self-promotion needs to be more aggressive to compensate. There is also a significant minority of cases that are in low visibility areas and also forego high visibility (advertising) approaches. These may describe professionals who stay in business, and perchance are very profitable, primarily on the strength of a sterling reputation. It is possible that for this one very select group of health care professionals, geography and promotion are irrelevant as patients find them regardless.

Studying acupuncture treatment locations, in a wider sense, enhances our understanding of the complex reasons for spatial disparities in health care accessibility and potentially aids policymakers concerned with more adequately equating health care opportunities amongst all citizens within a jurisdiction. For instance, there is quite striking spatial imbalances of PA offices throughout the Toronto metropolitan area which deviate only slightly by visibility approach. Many communities and municipalities in Greater Toronto do not have local PA services and/or are below the median in terms of offices per capita. The general trend is that people most 'come south' to patronize these particular offices, but this is unlikely to accurately demonstrate true accessibility disadvantages in the more peripheral areas. Chiropractors and naturopaths display a far greater presence in Toronto's peripheral/northern municipalities; and if acupuncture services are offered by these chiropractors and naturopaths, then accessibility disadvantages across metropolitan Toronto may not be as acute. It is less likely that dentists are playing the same role; although the very specialized acupuncture procedures carried out in some dentist's offices may create partial overlap with PA services in some areas. Admittedly, it remains uncertain how clearly most people differentiate the acupuncture services rendered from naturopaths, chiropractors, dentists and primary acupuncturists. Thus, from a business competitiveness standpoint, it is also not certain if PA offices should vigorously promote differences in acupuncture technique from other providers. More precisely evaluating commonalities and distinctions should be investigated in the future by directing surveys to acupuncture professionals and their patients.

Given that CAM-based acupuncture procedures are not covered by the publicly-funded Ontario Health Insurance Plan (OHIP) and are rarely paid by private employers, the vast majority of people in the province purchase these services 'out of pocket' (although some cost can be recouped through income tax deductions). In this regard, primary acupuncturists, chiropractors and naturopaths are on relatively 'equal footing' in terms of vying for new customers; making factors such as spatial accessibility and advertising in conjunction with effectiveness (and perhaps uniqueness) of treatment and professional reputation potentially very important determinants in market share distribution. If primary acupuncturists seek to secure a greater presence in the periphery of the Toronto CMA, then two, not mutually exclusive, approaches are logical. Either these practitioners must set up directly in these municipalities and/or they must advertise aggressively and perhaps highlight differences in their treatment effectiveness from others. There is some evidence that the latter may be occurring. As demonstrated in this study, while PA establishments are low in numbers in the 'outer band' of the CMA, roughly one-third of these offices employ a high visibility approach in terms of advertising (31.37% and 38.89% for high and low visibility areas respectively) and these proportions are higher than both dentists and chiropractors/naturopaths in these peripheral areas.

While greater attention to advertising by PA specialists, such as the presently under-utilized construction of informative websites, may encourage greater commuting to treatment, it will not completely offset spatial accessibility disparities. Not everyone is willing to absorb both treatment and significant transportation (monetary and time) costs; meaning that accessibility disadvantages to primary acupuncturists must also be countered through a wider distribution of these offices throughout metropolitan Toronto. The faster growing municipalities of the outer band such as Milton, Oakville, Bradford-West Gwillimbury, Aurora, Whitchurch-Stouffville, and Ajax might be areas of particular opportunity and perhaps strong candidates for 'greenfield' PA office development. Successfully widening the allocation of PA offices would also be dependent on counteracting apparent cultural influences as there are presently dense settlements of PA offices in pockets of Toronto with high proportions of people of Chinese ethnic origins [29].

Certainly, spatial accessibility to acupuncture treatment is enhanced by greater integration between the complementary and alternative and conventional medical sectors. While institutional and attitudinal divisions have historically been considerable, particularly in some western countries, integration is occurring even if the magnitude of medical assimilation does vary by jurisdiction. If more professionals in conventional medicine become receptive to non-allopathic approaches, spatial accessibility to acupuncture and other CAM approaches is improved in at least two ways. First, the number of locations from where acupuncture procedures and referrals are made expands considerably as more conventional health care offices, which are often in places of high visibility, are included in the mix. Second, medical procedures are far more likely to be listed under public health care insurance programs and/or given personal income tax advantages with allopathic doctor involvement. If greater integration encourages policymakers to extend full or partial coverage, acupuncture treatment accessibility would be improved as it becomes more affordable to a wider population.

## Author details

Stephen P. Meyer

Address all correspondence to: smeyer@laurentian.ca

Department of Geography, Laurentian University, Ramsey Lake Road, Greater Sudbury, Ontario, Canada

## References

[1] Rosted, P, Buudgaard, M, & Gordon, S. Pedersen AML. Acupuncture in the Management of Anxiety Related to Dental Treatment: A Case Series. Acupuncture in Medicine (2010). 1759-9873, 28(1), 3-5.

[2] Rosted, P, & Carrotte, P. An Audit to Assess the Outcome of a 1-Day Acupuncture Course for Dentists. European Journal of Dental Education (2007). 1600-0579, 11(1), 23-28.

[3] Eitner, S, Wichmann, M, & Holst, S. Hypnopuncture"- Dental-Emergency Treatment Concept for Patients with a Distinctive Gag Reflex. Journal of Clinical and Experimental Hypnosis (2005). 0020-7144, 53(1), 60-73.

[4] CAMlineCAM Therapies and Practitioners- Acupuncture. http://www.camline.ca/ accessed 13 April 13 (2012).

[5] Buchmueller, T. C, Jacobson, M, & Wold, C. How Far to the Hospital? The Effect of Hospital Closures on Access to Care. Journal of Health Economics (2006). 0167-6296, 25(4), 740-761.

[6] Langford, M, & Higgs, G. Measuring Potential Access to Primary Healthcare Services: The Influence of Alternative Spatial Representations of Population. The Professional Geographer (2006). 1467-9272, 58(3), 294-306.

[7] Meyer, S. P. A Geographic Assessment of 'Total' Health Care Supply in Ontario: Complementary and Alternative Medicine and Conventional Medicine. The Canadian Geographer (2010). 1541-0064, 54(1), 104-122.

[8] Meyer, S. P. Comparing Spatial Accessibility to Conventional Medicine and Complementary and Alternative Medicine in Ontario, Canada. Health & Place (2012). 1353-8292, 18(2), 305-314.

[9] Monnet, E, Collin-naudet, E, Bresson-hadni, S, & Minello, A. Di Martino V, Carel D, Jooste V, Cagnaire A, Evrard P, Obert-Clerc B, Miguet JP, Hillon P. Place of Residence and Distance to Medical Care Influence the Diagnosis of Hepatitis C: A Population-Based Study. Journal of Hepatology (2006). 1527-3350, 44(3), 499-506.

[10] Pong, R. W, & Pitblado, J. R. Geographic Distribution of Physicians in Canada: Beyond How Many and Where. Ottawa: Canadian Institute for Health Information; (2005).

[11] Pong, R. W. DesMeules M, Heng D, Lagacé C, Guernsey JR, Kazanjian A, Manuel D, Pitblado JR, Bollman R, Koren I, Dressler MP, Wang F, Luo W. Patterns of Health Services Utilization in Rural Canada. Chronic Diseases and Injuries in Canada (2011). 2204-7772, 31(1), 1-36.

[12] Rosenthal, M. B, Zaslavsky, A, & Newhouse, J. P. The Geographic Distribution of Physicians Revised. Health Services Research (2005). 1475-6773, 40(6), 1931-1952.

[13] Schuurman, N, Berube, M, & Crooks, V. A. Measuring Potential Spatial Access to Primary Health Care Physicians Using a Modified Gravity Model. The Canadian Geographer (2010). 1541-0064, 54(1), 29-45.

[14] Andrews, G. J, Wiles, J, & Miller, K. L. The Geography of Complementary Medicine: Perspectives and Prospects. Complementary Therapies in Nursing & Midwifery (2004). 1353-6117, 10(3), 175-185.

[15] Andrews, G. J, & Boon, H. CAM in Canada: Places, Practices, Research. Complementary Therapies in Clinical Practice (2005). 1744-3881, 11(1), 21-27.

[16] Hollenberg, D, & Bourgeault, I. New Health Geographies of Complementary, Alternative and Traditional Medicines in Primary Health Care. In: Crooks VA, Andrews GJ (eds.) Primary Health Care: People, Practice, Place. Surrey: Ashgate; (2009). 978-0-75467-247-0, 167-182.

[17] Meyer, S. P. The Spatial Pattern of Complementary and Alternative Medical Offices across Ontario and within Intermediate-Sized Metropolitan Areas. Urban Geography (2008). 0272-3638, 29(7), 662-682.

[18] Meyer, S. P. Place-Specific Explanations for the Geographic Patterns of Complementary and Alternative Practitioners: Contrasting Chiropractor, Massage, Holistic, Acupuncture, Naturopathic and Homeopathic Operations in Ontario. International Journal of Business and Social Science (2012). 2219-1933, 3(8), 24-39.

[19] Albert, D. P. New York and Colorado as Critical States in the Diffusion of State Licensing of Naturopathic Physicians. Complementary Health Practice Review (2009). 1533-2101, 14(2), 59-69.

[20] Albert, D. P, & Butar, F. B. Distribution, Concentration and Health Care Implications of Naturopathic Physicians in the United States. Complementary Health Practice Review (2004). 1076-1675, 9(2), 103-117.

[21] Albert, D. P, & Butar, F. B. Diffusion of Naturopathic State Licensing in the United States and Canada. Complementary Health Practice Review (2004). 1076-1675, 9(3), 193-207.

[22] Alcantara, J, Ohm, J, & Kunz, D. The Chiropractic Care of Children. The Journal of Alternative and Complementary Medicine (2010). 1075-5535, 16(6), 621-626.

[23] Brindle, M, & Goodrick, E. Revisiting Maverick Medical Sects: The Role of Identity in Comparing Homeopaths and Chiropractors. Journal of Social History (2001). 1527-1897, 34(3), 569-589.

[24] Smith, M, & Carber, L. Chiropractic Health Care in Health Professional Shortage Areas in the United States. American Journal of Public Health (2002). 0090-0036, 92(12), 2001-2009.

[25] Waalen, J. K, & Mior, S. A. Practice Patterns of 692 Ontario Chiropractors ((2001). Journal of Canadian Chiropractors Association 2005;0008-3194, 49(1), 21-31.

[26] Williams, A. M. The Diffusion of Alternative Health Care: A Canadian Case Study of Chiropractic and Naturopathic Practices. The Canadian Geographer (2000). 1541-0064, 44(2), 152-166.

[27] Li, H. Y, Cui, L, Cui, M, & Tong, Y. Y. Active Research Fields of Acupuncture Research: A Document Co-Citation Clustering Analysis of Acupuncture Literature. Alternative Therapies in Health and Medicine (2010). 5571-4960, 16(6), 38-45.

[28] Bishop, F, Massey, Y, Yardley, L, & Lewith, G. How Patients Choose Acupuncturists: A Mixed-Methods Project. Journal of Alternative & Complementary Medicine (2011). 1075-5535, 17(1), 19-25.

[29] Meyer, S. P. A Spatial Analysis of Acupuncture Practitioners in Ontario, Canada: Assessing Regional and Intra-Metropolitan Trends. In: Saad M. (ed.) Acupuncture Concepts and Physiology. Rijeka: InTech; (2011). 978-9-53307-410-8, 189-206.

[30] Thompson, J. B. The New Visibility. Theory, Culture & Society (2005). 0263-2764, 35.

[31] InfoCanadaCanadian Business Directory, April (2012). edition. Mississauga: InfoCanada; 2012.

[32] Statistics CanadaRoad Network File, (2011). Census. http://www12.statcan.gc.ca/census-recensement/2011/geo/RNF-FRR/index-eng.cfmaccessed 12 June 2012)

[33] DMTI Spatial IncLand Use (LUR). http://geo2.scholarsportal.info/accessed 15 May (2012).

[34] Ebdon, D. Statistics in Geography. New York: Basil Blackwell; (1987). 0-63113-688-6

[35] Statistics CanadaBoundary Files, (2011). Census. http://www12.statcan.gc.ca/census-recensement/2011/geo/bound-limit/bound-limit-eng.cfmaccessed 1 June 2012).

[36] Statistics CanadaPopulation and Dwelling Count Highlight Tables, (2011). Census. http://www12.statcan.gc.ca/census-recensement/2011/dp-pd/hlt-fst/pd-pl/Tables-Tableaux.cfm?LANG=Eng&T=300accessed 1 June 2012).